Wilkins' Clinical Skills, Techniques, and Equipment for the Canadian Dental Assistant

Fourteenth Edition

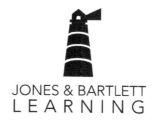

JONES & BARTLETT
LEARNING

World Headquarters
Jones & Bartlett Learning
25 Mall Road
Burlington, MA 01803
978-443-5000
info@jblearning.com
www.jblearning.com

Jones & Bartlett Learning books and products are available through most bookstores and online booksellers. To contact Jones & Bartlett Learning directly, call 800-832-0034, fax 978-443-8000, or visit our website, www.jblearning.com.

Disclaimer
This publication is sold with the understanding that the publisher is not engaged in rendering medical, legal, accounting, or other professional services. If medical, legal, accounting, or other professional service advice is required, the service of a competent professional should be sought. The authors, editor, and publisher have designed this publication to provide accurate information with regard to the subject matter covered. However, they are not responsible for errors, omissions, or for any outcomes related to the use of the contents of this publication and make no guarantee and assume no responsibility or liability for the use of the products and procedures described, or the correctness, sufficiency, or completeness of stated information, opinions, or recommendations. Treatments and side effects described in this publication are not applicable to all people; required dosages and experienced side effects will vary among individuals. Drugs and medical devices discussed herein are controlled by the Food and Drug Administration (FDA) and may have limited availability for use only in research studies or clinical trials. Research, clinical practice, and government regulations often change accepted standards. When consideration is being given to the use of any drug in the clinical setting, the health care provider or reader is responsible for determining FDA status of the drug, reading the package insert, and reviewing prescribing information for the most current recommendations on dose, precautions, and contraindications and for determining the appropriate usage for the product. This is especially important in the case of drugs that are new or seldom used. Any references in this publication to procedures to be employed when rendering emergency care to the sick and injured are provided solely as a general guide; other or additional safety measures might be required under particular circumstances. This publication is not intended as a statement of the standards of care required in any particular situation; circumstances and the physical conditions of patients can vary widely from one emergency to another. This publication is not intended in any way to advise emergency personnel concerning their legal authority to perform the activities or procedures discussed. Such local determination should be made only with the aid of legal counsel. Some images in this publication feature models; these models do not necessarily endorse, represent, or participate in the activities represented in the images.

Cover Image: © Photos.com

6048
Printed in the United States of America
27 26 25 24 23   10 9 8 7 6 5 4 3 2

Contents

Extraoral and Intraoral Examination

Lisa B. Johnson, RDH, MPH, DHS

CHAPTER OUTLINE

LEARNING OBJECTIVES

After studying this chapter, the student will be able to:

1. Explain the rationale for a comprehensive extra- and intraoral examination.
2. Explain the systematic sequence of the extra- and intraoral examination.
3. Identify normal hard and soft tissue anatomy of the head, neck, and oral cavity.
4. Describe and document physical characteristics (size, shape, color, texture, and consistency) and morphologic categories (elevated, flat, and depressed lesions) for notable findings.
5. Identify suspected conditions that require follow-up and referral for medical evaluation.

Rationale for the Extraoral and Intraoral Examination

- The extra- and intraoral examination is performed for early identification of abnormalities and pathologies, especially oral cancer.[1,2]
  - Although an essential goal of the examination is to detect cancer of the mouth at the earliest possible stage, a thorough examination may also reveal signs of thyroid disorders, eating disorders, nutritional deficiencies, sexually transmitted diseases, and a host of systemic conditions.
- Cancer prevention education for the patient is an essential component of the extra- and intraoral examination.

Components of Examination

- The standard of patient care is that the total patient is being treated, not only the oral cavity, and particularly not just the teeth and immediate surrounding tissues.
- The examination is all-inclusive to detect possible physical or psychological influences on the patient's oral health.
- Thorough examination is essential for each continuing care appointment so treatment for the control and prevention of oral diseases will be effective.
- Assessment of health-related risk factors, such as[3]:
  - History of previous cancer.
  - Family history of squamous cell carcinoma (SCC).
  - Tobacco use.
  - Alcohol use.
  - Cultural and genetic susceptibility.
  - Sun exposure and lack of use of sun protection.
  - Diet.
  - Certain surgeries such as organ or bone marrow transplant and subsequent long-term immunosuppressive medications.
  - Encounters involving orogenital contact may increase the risk of human papillomavirus (HPV) transmission.[4,5]
  - HPV vaccination status.[4,6]

I. Types of Examinations

- Comprehensive
  - A comprehensive examination includes a thorough summary of all the components of the assessment.
    - The extra- and intraoral examination is a component of a patient's complete assessment and is performed for all new patients and at each continuing care visit.
- Screening
  - Screening implies a brief, preliminary examination, usually for a particular purpose such as for initial patient assessment and triage to determine priorities for treatment.
- Limited examination
  - A type of brief examination made for an emergency situation. It may be used in the management of an acute condition.
- Follow-up
  - Brief follow-up examination to check healing following a treatment.
- Continuing care/reevaluation
  - After a specific period of time following the completion of the care plan and the anticipated restoration to health.
  - A continuing care examination is a complete reassessment from which a new dental hygiene diagnosis and care plan are derived.

II. Methods for Examination

The extra- and intraoral examination is accomplished by various visual and tactile, manual, and instrumental methods. Patient position, optimum lighting, and effective retraction for accessibility and visibility contribute to the accuracy and completeness of the examination.

- Visual examination
  - Direct observation: Visual observation is carried out in a systematic sequence to note surface appearance (color, contour, size) and to observe movement and other evidence of function.
  - Radiographic examination: The use of radiographs can reveal deviations from normal not observable by direct vision.
  - Transillumination: A strong light directed through a soft tissue or a tooth to enhance examination is useful for detecting irregularities of the teeth and locating calculus. Hold the mouth mirror to view from the lingual to see the translucency.
- Palpation
  - **Palpation** is examination using the sense of touch through tissue manipulation or pressure on an area with the gloved fingers of one hand or both.
  - Digital: The use of a single finger. Example: Index finger applied to the lingual side of

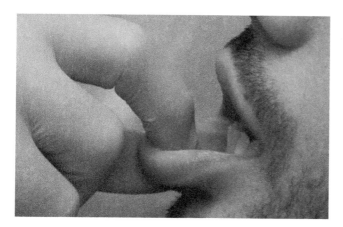

Figure 1 Palpation of the Lip to Illustrate the Use of a Finger and Thumb of the Same Hand

the mandible beneath the canine and premolar area to determine presence of a **torus** mandibularis.

- Bidigital: The use of finger and thumb of same hand. Example: Palpation of the lips (**Figure 1**).
- Bimanual: The use of finger or fingers and thumb from each hand applied simultaneously in coordination. Example: Index finger of one hand palpates on the floor of the mouth inside, while a finger or fingers from the other hand press on the same area from under the chin externally (**Figure 2A-B**).
- Bilateral: Two hands are used at the same time to examine corresponding structures on opposite sides of the body. Comparisons can be made. Example: Fingers placed beneath the chin to palpate the submandibular lymph nodes (**Figure 3**).

- Instrumentation
  - Examination instruments, such as a periodontal probe and an explorer, are used for specific examination of the teeth and periodontal tissues.
- Percussion
  - Percussion is the act of tapping a surface or tooth with an instrument.
  - Information about the status of health is determined either by the response of the patient or by the sound. When a tooth is known to be sensitive in any way, percussion needs to be avoided.
- Electrical test
  - An electric pulp tester may be used to detect the presence or absence of vital pulp tissue.
  - Methods for use of a pulp testing are described in Chapter 16.

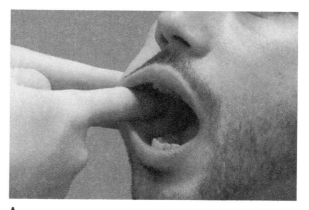

A

B

Figure 2 Bimanual Palpation. **A:** Examination of the buccal mucosa by simultaneous palpation extraorally and intraorally. **B:** Examination of the floor of the mouth by simultaneous palpation with fingers of each hand in apposition.

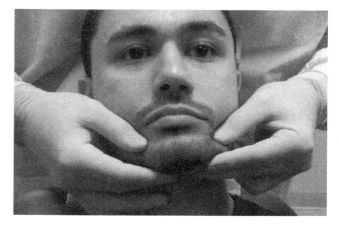

Figure 3 Bilateral Palpation. Bilateral palpation is used to examine corresponding structures on opposite sides of the body.

- Auscultation
  - Auscultation is the use of sound.
  - Example: The sound of clicking of the **temporomandibular joint** when the jaw is opened and closed. **Figure 4** shows examination of the temporomandibular joint.

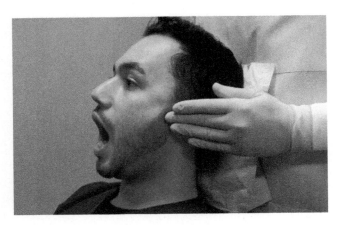

Figure 4 Assessment of the Temporomandibular Joint. The joint is palpated as the patient opens and closes the mouth.

III. Signs and Symptoms

- A specific objective for patient examination as a part of the complete assessment is the recognition of deviations from normal that may be signs or symptoms of disease.
- General signs and symptoms may occur in various disease conditions. Example: Fever, or increase in body temperature, accompanies most infections.
- A **pathognomonic sign or symptom** is unique to a disease and may be used to distinguish that condition from other diseases or conditions.

A. Signs

- A sign is any abnormality identified by a healthcare professional while examining a patient.
- A sign is objective information or data. Examples of signs include observable changes such as color, shape, and consistency, or abnormal findings revealed using a probe, explorer, radiograph, or other instrument for disease detection.

B. Symptoms

- A symptom is any departure from normal that may be indicative of disease.
- It is a subjective abnormality that can be observed by the patient.
- Examples are pain, tenderness, and bleeding when toothbrushing as described by the patient.

IV. Preparation for Examination

- Review the patient's health histories and dental/medical record, including risk factors,

radiographs, dental caries, and periodontal and oral cancer risk assessments.
- Examine dental radiographs.
- Explain the procedures to be performed and relevance of the procedures.
  - Example: "I am going to perform an extra-/intraoral examination to look for abnormalities that can affect your oral and overall health."
  - Patient understanding the rationale for an extra- and intraoral examination is critical to acceptance and education.
  - When a patient is wearing a scarf or other head/neck covering for cultural or religious reasons, the dental hygienist uses culturally sensitive communication skills. (See Chapter 3.)

Anatomic Landmarks of the Oral Cavity

Familiarization with structures (**Figure 5**, **Figure 6**, and **Figure 7**) and normal anatomy is a prerequisite to understanding abnormal presentations in the head and neck region.[1,3,5]

I. Oral Mucosa

The lining of the oral cavity, the oral mucosa, is a mucous membrane composed of connective tissue covered with stratified squamous epithelium. There are three divisions or categories of oral mucosa.

A. Masticatory Mucosa

- Covers the gingiva and hard palate, the areas most used during the mastication of food.

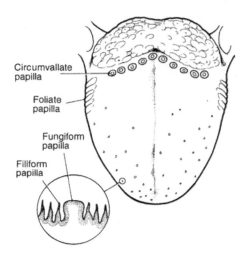

Circumvallate papilla

Foliate papilla

Fungiform papilla

Filiform papilla

Figure 5 Papillae of the Tongue

4

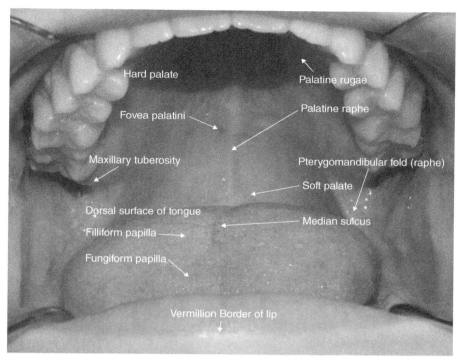

A

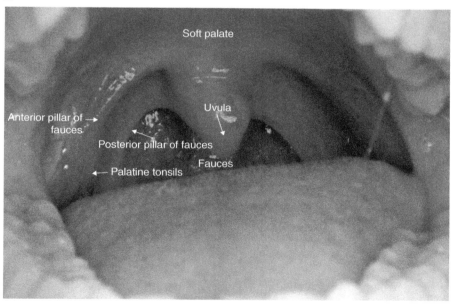

B

Figure 6 Anatomic Landmarks of the Oral Cavity—Dorsal Tongue View.
A: View of hard and soft palate. **B:** View of uvula and oropharynx.

- Except for the free margin of the gingiva, the masticatory mucosa is firmly attached to underlying tissues.
- The normal epithelial covering is keratinized.

B. Lining Mucosa

- Covers the inner surfaces of the lips and cheeks, floor of the mouth, underside of the tongue, soft palate, and alveolar mucosa.

- These tissues are not firmly attached to underlying tissue.
- The epithelial covering is not keratinized.

C. Specialized Mucosa

- Covers the dorsum (upper surface) of the tongue.
- Composed of many **papillae**; some contain taste buds.

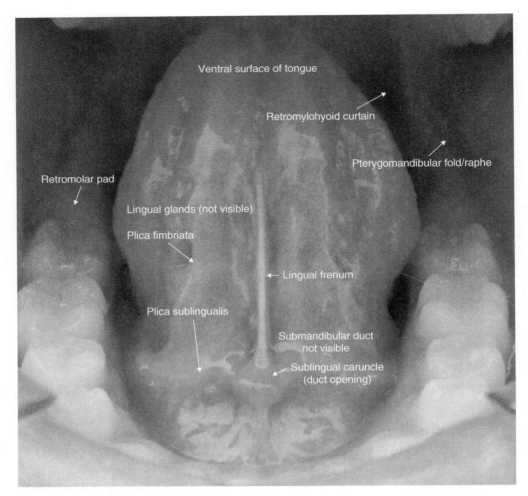

Figure 7 Anatomic Landmarks of the Oral Cavity—Ventral Tongue View

- The distribution of the four types of papillae is shown in Figure 5.
  - Filiform: Threadlike keratinized elevations that cover the **dorsal** surface of the tongue; they are the most numerous of the papillae.
  - Fungiform: Mushroom-shaped papillae interspersed among the filiform papillae on the tip and sides of the tongue; appear redder than the filiform papillae and contain variable numbers of taste buds. The inset enlargement in Figure 5 shows the comparative shape and size of the filiform and fungiform papillae.
  - Circumvallate (vallate): The 10–14 large round papillae arranged in a "V" between the body of the tongue and the base. Taste buds line the walls.
  - Foliate: Vertical grooves on the lateral posterior sides of the tongue; also contain taste buds.

Sequence of Examination

- Conducting an examination in a systematic sequence will minimize the possibility of excluding areas and overlooking details of importance. A systematic sequence improves efficiency, promotes professionalism, and inspires patient confidence.
- A recommended sequence for examination is outlined in **Box 1**, in which factors to consider during appointments are related to the actual observations made and recorded.
- This sequence is adapted from *Detecting Oral Cancer*, available from the National Institutes of Health and the National Cancer Institute.[1,2]
- In addition to proper sequence, familiarization of anatomic structures common to normal anatomy is critical to understanding abnormal findings (**Table 1**).

Box   1 Anatomic Landmarks of the Oral Cavity

- Lips
- Vermillion border
- Labial commissure
- Labial mucosa
- Buccal mucosa
- Philtrum
- Nasolabial groove
- Fauces
- Oral pharynx (includes soft palate, side and back wall of the throat, tonsils and posterior third or base of tongue)
- Vestibule
- Buccal vestibule
- Buccinator muscle
- Labial
- Buccal
- Mucobuccal fold
- Buccal frenum
- Labial frenum
- **Exostosis**
- Wharton's duct
- Lingual vein
- Sublingual fold
- Plica fimbriata
- Sublingual caruncle
- Median sulcus
- Lingual tonsils
- Lingual frenum
- Ankyloglossia
- Marginal gingiva
- Attached gingiva
- Free gingival groove
- Canine eminence
- Pterygomandibular raphe
- Parotid papilla
- Midpalatine raphe
- Palatine rugae
- Fovea palatine
- Torus palatinus
- Incisive papilla
- Uvula
- Palatine tonsils
- Pharyngeal adenoid tonsils
- Tonsillar pillars
- Tongue:
  - Dorsal
  - **Ventral**
  - Lateral border
- Filiform papilla
- Fungiform papilla
- Folate papillae
- Circumvallate papilla
- Lingual tonsils
- Stensen's duct
- Maxillary tuberosity
- Retromolar pad
- Ramus of mandible
- Zygomatic arch
- **Mandibular tori** (prevalence varies)
- Alveolar mucosa
- Mylohyoid muscle

Refer to Figures   6 and   7.

Table   1 Extraoral and Intraoral Examination

Sequence of Examination	Observe	Indication and Influences on Appointments
1. Overall appraisal of patient	Posture, gait General health status; size Hair; scalp Breathing; state of fatigue Voice, cough, hoarseness	Response, cooperation, attitude toward treatment Length of appointment
2. Face	Expression: Evidence of fear or apprehension Shape: Twitching; paralysis Jaw movements during speech Injuries; signs of abuse	Need for alleviation of fears Evidence of upper respiratory or other infections Enlarged masseter muscle (related to bruxism)
3. Skin	Color, texture, blemishes Traumatic lesions Eruptions, swellings Growths, **scars**, moles	Relation to possible systemic conditions Need for supplementary history Biopsy or other treatment to recommend Influences on instruction in diet

(continues)

Table 1 Extraoral and Intraoral Examination

Sequence of Examination	Observe	Indication and Influences on Appointments
4. Eyes	Size of pupils Color of sclera Eyeglasses (corrective) Protruding eyeballs	Dilated pupils or pinpoint may result from drugs, emergency state Eyeglasses essential during instruction Hyperthyroidism

5. Nodes (palpate) (**Figure 8**)
  a. Pre- and postauricular
  b. Occipital
  c. Submental; submandibular
  d. Cervical chain (Figure 8)
  e. Supraclavicular
	Adenopathy;
	lymphadenopathy
	Induration or pain
		Need for referral
		Medical consultation
		Ear infection
		Coordinate with intraoral examination

6. Glands (palpate)
  a. Thyroid (Figure 8B)
  b. Parotid
  c. Submental
  d. Submandibular
    (Figure 3)
	Enlargement or pain
	Induration longer than 2 wk
		Referral for medical consult

7. Temporomandibular joint (palpate) (Figure 4)	Limitations or deviations of movement **Trismus** Tenderness; sensitivity Noises: Clicking, popping, grating	Disorder of joint; limitation of opening Discomfort during appointment and during oral self-care

8. Lips
  a. Observe closed, then open
  b. Palpate (Figure 1)
	Color, texture, size
	Cracks, angular cheilosis
	Blisters, ulcers
	Traumatic lesions
	Irritation from lip-biting
	Limitation of opening; muscle elasticity; muscle tone
	Evidence of mouth breathing
	Induration
		Need for further examination: referral
		Immediate need for postponement of appointment when a lesion may be communicable or could interfere with procedures
		Care during retraction
		Accessibility during intraoral procedures
		Patient instruction: dietary, special biofilm control for mouth breather

9. Breath odor	Severity Relation to oral hygiene, gingival health	Possible relation to systemic condition Alcohol use history; special needs

10. Labial and buccal mucosa, left and right examined systematically
  a. Vestibule
  b. Mucobuccal folds
  c. Frena
  d. Opening of Stensen's duct
  e. Palpate cheeks
    (Figure 2A)
	Color, size, texture, contour
	Abrasions, traumatic lesions, cheek bite
	Effects of tobacco use
	Ulcers, growths
	Moistness of surfaces
	Relation of frena to free gingiva
	Induration
		Need for referral, biopsy, cytology
		Frena and other anatomic parts that need special adaptation for radiography or impression tray
		Avoid sensitive areas during retraction

11. Tongue
  a. Vestibule
  b. Dorsal (Figure 6A)
  c. Lateral borders
  d. Base of tongue
    (Figure 10)
  e. Deviation on extension
	Shape: normal asymmetric
	Color, size, texture, consistency
	Fissures; papillae
	Coating
	Lesions: elevated, depressed, flat
	Induration
		Need for referral, biopsy, cytology
		Need for instruction in tongue cleaning

Sequence of Examination	Observe	Indication and Influences on Appointments

12. Floor of mouth
  a. Ventral surface of tongue (Figure 7)
  b. Palpate (Figure 2B)
  c. Duct openings
  d. Mucosa, frena
  e. Tongue action
	Varicosities
	Lesions: Elevated, flat, depressed, traumatic
	Induration
	Limitation or freedom of movement of tongue
	Frena; tongue-tie
		Large muscular tongue influences retraction, gag reflex, accessibility for instrumentation
		Film placement problems

13. Saliva	Quantity; quality (thick, ropy) Evidence of dry mouth; lip wetting Tongue coating	Reduced in certain diseases, by certain drugs Special dental caries control program Influence on instrumentation Need for saliva substitute
14. Hard palate (Figure 6A)	Height, contour, color Appearance of rugae Tori, growths, ulcers	Need for referral, biopsy, cytology Signs of tongue thrust, deviate swallow Influence on radiographic film placement
15. Soft palate, uvula (Figure 6B)	Color, size, shape Petechiae Ulcers, growths	Referral, biopsy, cytology Large uvula influences gag reflex
16. Tonsillar region, throat (Figure 6B)	Tonsils: Size and shape Color, size, surface characteristics Lesions, trauma	Referral, biopsy, cytology Enlarged tonsils encourage gag reflex Throat infection, a sign for appointment postponement

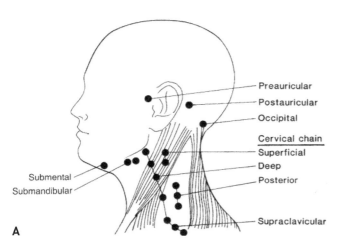
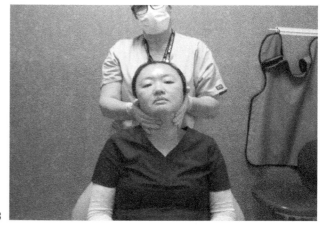

Figure 8 Lymph Node and Thyroid Gland Assessment. **A:** Lymph nodes. The locations of the major lymph nodes into which the vessels of the facial and oral regions drain. **B:** Examination of the thyroid gland. Identify the isthmus (center) of the thyroid gland. The butterfly-shaped gland sits below the bony protuberance or cricoid cartilage ring. Place two digits from each hand at the center of the gland and then slide digits laterally, approximately 1–2 cm from the center. Ask the patient to swallow slowly, several times and simultaneously palpate one lobe at a time while assessing for asymmetry. Observe the gland moving up and down as the patient swallows. Document any enlargement and asymmetry. Refer any aberration from normal to the patient's primary care provider for further evaluation. Note: The thyroid can be palpated from an anterior or posterior approach.[7]

I. Extraoral Examination

1. Observe patient during reception and seating to note physical characteristics and abnormalities and make an overall appraisal.

2. Observe head, face, eyes, and neck, and evaluate the skin of the face and neck.

3. Request the patient remove prosthesis prior to performing the intraoral examination. Explain how

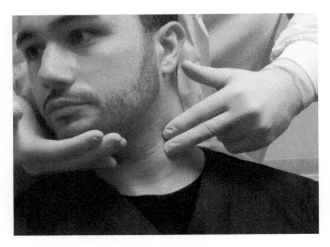

Figure 9 Cervical Node Palpation. Left anterior cervical lymph node chain is examined. Fingertips gently press and roll nodes along the length of the sternocleidomastoid muscle.

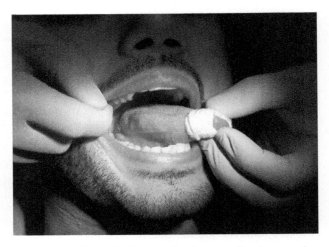

Figure 10 Examination of the Tongue. To observe the posterior third of the tongue and the attachment to the floor of the mouth, hold the tongue with a gauze sponge, retract the cheek, and move the tongue out, first to one side and then the other, as each section of the mucosa is carefully examined.

this will improve the ability to inspect all areas of the mouth adequately.

- If the patient is embarrassed to be seen without prosthesis, provide a tissue for them to cover their mouth when you are not examining the tissues.

4. Palpate the lymph nodes and the salivary and thyroid glands. Figure 8 shows the location of the major lymph nodes of the face, oral regions, and neck. Palpation is a significant component of the extra-/intraoral examination (**Figure 9**).

- Note any of the following symptoms or experiences:
  - ◦ Pain or discomfort upon palpation and/or upon swallowing.
  - ◦ Persistent difficulty swallowing in the absence of pain.
  - ◦ Any recent noticeable lumps the patient may have experienced without pain.
  - ◦ Persistent earache or hoarseness of voice.[5]

5. Observe mandibular movement and palpate the temporomandibular joint (Figure 4). Relate to items from questions in the medical/dental history.

II. Intraoral Examination

1. Make a preliminary examination of the lips and intraoral mucosa by using a mouth mirror or a tongue depressor.
2. View and palpate lips, labial and buccal mucosa, and mucobuccal folds (Figures 1 and 2A).
3. Examine and palpate the tongue, including the dorsal and ventral surfaces, lateral borders, and

base. Retract to observe posterior third, first to one side and then the other (**Figure 10**).

4. Observe mucosa of the floor of the mouth. Palpate the floor of the mouth (Figure 2B).
5. Examine the hard and soft palates, tonsillar areas, and pharynx (Figure 6A and B). Use a mirror to observe the oropharynx, nasopharynx, and if possible, the larynx.
6. Note amount and consistency of the saliva and evidence of dry mouth (xerostomia).

III. Documentation of Findings

A. History

Question the patient to gather necessary information about the history of an oral lesion. Take care not to alarm the patient as you are just fact finding to determine the best way to proceed.

- Whether the lesion is known or not known to the patient; previous evaluation.
- If known, when first noticed; if recurrence, previous date when lesion was first noticed.
- Duration, symptoms, changes in size and appearance.

B. Location and Extent

- When a lesion is first seen, its location is noted in relation to adjacent structures.
- Document a complete description of each finding, including the location, extent, size, color,

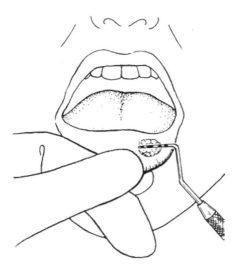

Figure 11 Use of a Probe to Measure a Lesion. In addition to the exact location, the width and length of a lesion are recorded. Using the probe provides a convenient method.

surface texture or configurations, consistency, **morphology**, and history.

- Intraoral photography can be of value to record images of anatomic deviations, location, and proportions.
- Descriptive words to define the location and extent include the following:
    - Localized: Lesion limited to a small focal area.
    - Generalized: Involves most of an area or segment.
    - Single lesion: One lesion of a particular type with a distinct margin.
    - Multiple lesions: More than one lesion of a particular type. Lesions may be:
        ○ Separate: discrete, not running together; may be arranged in clusters.
        ○ Coalescing: close to each other with margins that merge.

C. Physical Characteristics

- Size and shape
    - Record length and width in millimeters.
    - The height of an elevated lesion may be significant.
    - Use a probe to measure, as shown in **Figure 11**.
- Color
    - Red, pink, white, and red and white are the most commonly seen.
    - Other rarer lesions may be blue, purple, gray, yellow, black, or brown.
- Surface texture
    - A lesion may have a smooth or an irregular surface.
    - The texture may be papillary, verrucous or wart-like, fissured, corrugated, or crusted.
- Consistency
    - Lesions may be soft, spongy, resilient, hard, or indurated.

Morphologic Categories

- Most lesions can be classified as elevated, depressed, or flat as they relate to the normal level of the skin or mucosa.
- Flowcharts of elevated lesions (**Figure 12A**), depressed lesions (**Figure 12B**), and flat lesions (**Figure 12C**) break down the terms used for describing lesions in each category.

I. Elevated Lesions

An elevated lesion (Figure 12A) is above the plane of the skin or mucosa. Elevated lesions are considered blisterform or nonblisterform.

- Blisterform lesions contain fluid and are usually soft and translucent. They may be vesicles, pustules, or bullae.
    - Vesicle: A vesicle is a small (1 cm or less in diameter), circumscribed lesion with a thin surface covering. It may contain serum or mucin and appear white.
    - Pustule: A pustule may be more than or less than 5 mm in diameter and contain pus, giving it a yellowish color.
    - Bulla: A bulla is large (>1 cm). It is filled with fluid, usually mucin or serum, but may contain blood. The color depends on the fluid content.
- Nonblisterform lesions are solid and do not contain fluid. They may be papules, nodules, tumors, or plaques. Papules, nodules, and tumors are also characterized by the base or attachment. As shown in **Figure 13**, the **pedunculated** lesion is attached by a narrow stalk or pedicle, whereas the **sessile** lesion has a base as wide as the lesion itself.
    - Papule: A small (pinhead to 5 mm in diameter), solid lesion that may be pointed, rounded, or flat topped.
    - Nodule: Larger than a papule (>5 mm but <2 cm).
    - Tumor: 2 cm or greater in width. In this context, "tumor" means a general swelling or enlargement and does not refer to neoplasm, either benign or malignant.

- Plaque: Slightly raised lesion with a broad, flat top. It is usually larger than 5 mm in diameter, with a "pasted on" appearance.

II. Depressed Lesions

A depressed lesion (Figure 12B) is below the level of the skin or mucosa. The outline may be regular or irregular, and there may be a flat or raised border around the depression. The depth can be described as superficial or deep. A lesion greater than 3 mm is a deep lesion.

- Ulcer: Most depressed lesions are ulcers and represent a loss of continuity of the epithelium. The center is often gray to yellow, surrounded by a red border. An ulcer may result from the rupture of an elevated lesion (vesicle, pustule, or bulla).
- **Erosion**: An erosion is a shallow, depressed soft tissue lesion in which the epithelium above the basal layer is denuded. It does not extend through the epithelium to the underlying tissue.

III. Flat Lesions

A flat lesion (Figure 12C) is on the same level as the normal skin or oral mucosa. Flat lesions may occur as single or multiple lesions and have a regular or irregular form.

- A macule is a circumscribed area not elevated above the surrounding skin or mucosa.
  - It may be identified by its color, which contrasts with the surrounding normal tissues.

IV. Other Descriptive Terms

- **Crust**: An outer layer, covering, or scab that may have formed from coagulation or drying of blood, serum, or pus, or a combination. A crust may form after a vesicle breaks; for example, the

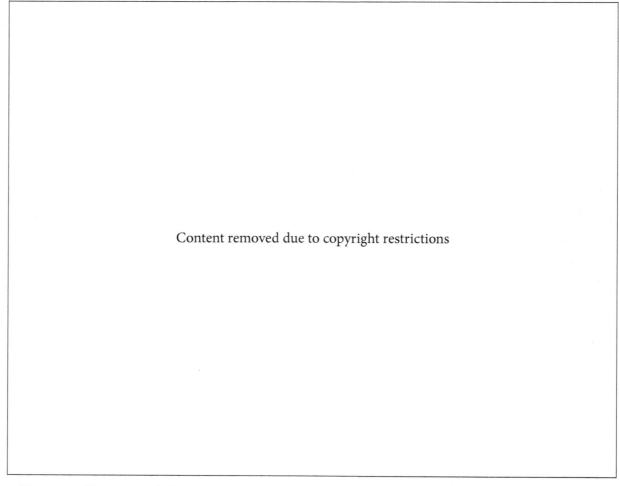

Content removed due to copyright restrictions

Figure 12 Flowcharts. **A:** Description of elevated soft tissue lesions. Elevated lesions are blisterform or nonblisterform.

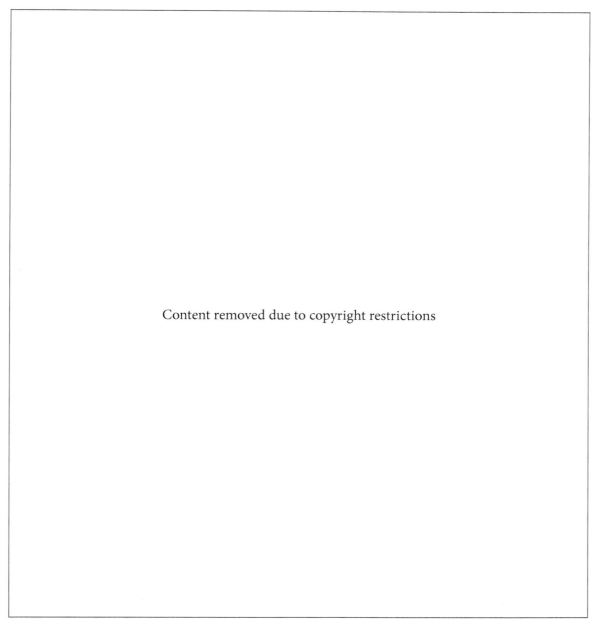

Content removed due to copyright restrictions

Figure 12 (*Continued*) **B:** Description of depressed soft tissue lesions. Depressed lesions are below the normal plane of the mucosa, usually an ulcer where there is a loss of continuity of epithelium. **C:** Description of flat soft tissue lesions. Flat lesions are level with the normal plane of the mucosa.

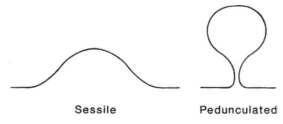

Sessile   Pedunculated

Figure 13 Attachment of Nonblisterform Lesions. The sessile lesion has a base as wide as the lesion itself; the pedunculated lesion is attached by a narrow stalk or pedicle.

skin lesion of chickenpox is first a macule, then a papule, then a vesicle, and then a crust.
- **Aphtha**: A small white or reddish ulcer.
- **Cyst**: A closed, epithelial-lined sac, normal or pathologic, that contains fluid or other material.
- **Erythema**: Red area of variable size and shape.
- **Exophytic**: Growing outward.
- **Idiopathic**: Of unknown etiology.
- **Indurated**: Hardened or abnormally hard.
- **Papillary**: Resembling a small, nipple-shaped projection or elevation.

- **Petechiae**: Minute hemorrhagic spots of pin-head to pinpoint size.
- **Pseudomembrane**: A loose membranous layer of exudate containing organisms, precipitated fibrin, necrotic cells, and inflammatory cells produced during an inflammatory reaction on the surface of a tissue.
- **Polyp**: Any mass of tissue that projects outward or upward from the normal surface level.
- **Punctate**: Marked with points or dots differentiated from the surrounding surface by color, elevation, or texture.
- **Purulent**: Containing, forming, or discharging pus.
- **Rubefacient**: Reddening of the skin.
- **Torus**: Bony elevation or prominence usually found on the midline of the hard palate (torus palatinus) and the lingual surface of the mandible (torus mandibularis) in the premolar area.
- **Verruca** (*verrucous* [verrucose]): A rough, wart-like growth.

Oral Cancer

- The oral cavity, oropharynx, larynx, paranasal sinuses and nasal cavity, and salivary glands are regions of the head and neck where cancer can begin.[2]
  - Cancers of the head and neck begin in the squamous cells that line moist, mucosal surfaces of the mouth, nose, and throat.[8,9]
  - Salivary glands contain different types of cells that can also become cancerous.[8,9]
- Because the early lesions are generally asymptomatic, they may go unnoticed and unreported by the patient. Observation by the dentist or dental hygienist is the principal method for the detection of oral cancer.
- The first step is to examine the entire face, neck, and oral mucous membrane of each patient at the initial examination and at each continuing care appointment (Table 1).
- It is necessary to know how to conduct the oral examination, most frequent sites where oral cancer occurs, characteristics of an early cancerous lesion, and procedure for referral and follow-up of when a lesion is found.
- In addition to the early lesions of oral cancers, the oral manifestations of neoplasms or abnormal growth of tissue elsewhere in the body, as well as the oral manifestations of chemotherapy, can be recognized.

- Most oral cancers are related to tobacco and/or excessive alcohol use.[5,10]
- Additional risk factors for cancer of the head and neck region include infection with HPV-16 and 18 types, multiple sex partners, weakened immune system, age 40 years and more, sun exposure to the lips, and history of cancer.[3,5,11]
- Increasing incidence of head and neck cancers in adults younger than 40 years suggests all patients, regardless of age or risk factors, must be screened for oral cancer.[10]

I. Location
- The most common sites for oral cancer are the lateral borders of the tongue, floor of the mouth, the lips, and the soft palate.

II. Appearance of Early Cancer
Early oral cancer takes many forms and may resemble a variety of common oral lesions. All types need to be examined with suspicion. Five basic forms are listed here[3,8,10]:

- White areas
  - White areas vary from a filmy, barely visible change in the mucosa to heavy, thick, heaped-up areas of dry white keratinized tissue.
  - Fissures, ulcers, or areas of induration or **sclerosis** in a white area are most indicative of malignancy.
  - Leukoplakia is a white **patch** or plaque that cannot be scraped off or characterized as any other disease. It may be associated with physical or chemical agents and the use of tobacco.
- Red areas
  - Erythroplakia is a term used to designate lesions of the oral mucosa that appear as bright red patches or plaques.
  - Lesions appear red, have a velvety consistency, and may coincide with small ulcers.
  - Erythroplakia is an oral lesion that cannot be characterized as any specific disease. It is less common than leukoplakia and more likely to manifest as dysplasia (precancerous) or malignancy.
- Ulcers
  - Ulcers may have flat or raised margins.
  - Palpation may reveal induration.
- Masses
  - Papillary masses, sometimes with ulcerated areas, occur as elevations above the surrounding tissues.

- Other masses may occur below the normal mucosa and may be found only by palpation.
- Pigmentation
  - Brown or black pigmented areas may be located on mucosa where pigmentation does not normally occur.

Clinical Recommendations for Evaluation of Oral Lesions

- Updated medical, social, and dental history along with the extra- and intraoral examination is recommended for all adult patients.[5]
- Adult patients with lesions considered to be innocuous or not suspicious for malignancy should be followed to confirm no further evaluation is needed.[5]
- Biopsy is indicated for adult patients with lesions considered to be suspicious of potential malignancy or malignant disorder or other symptoms.[5]
- Although not recommended for potential malignancy, cytologic adjuncts for minimally invasive detection of oral cancer can be performed when a patient refuses biopsy of the lesion or referral to a specialist. Cytologic adjuncts include brush cytology and toluidine blue, diffuse tissue reflectance, and laser-induced autofluorescence.[12] The rationale for performing adjunctive cytologic testing is to reinforce the need for biopsy or referral.[12]

I. Biopsy

- Biopsy is the removal and microscopic examination of a section of tissue or other material from the body for the purposes of diagnosis.
  - A biopsy is either excisional, when the entire lesion is removed, or incisional, when a representative section from the lesion is taken.
  - Considered the "gold standard" in oral cancer diagnosis.[3,8]
- Indications for biopsy
  - Any unusual oral lesion that cannot be identified with clinical certainty must be biopsied.
  - Any lesion that has not healed in 2 weeks is considered suspicious for malignancy until proven otherwise.
  - A persistent, thick, white, hyperkeratotic lesion and any mass (elevated or not) that does not break through the surface epithelium.

- Pathology report.
- Diagnostic criteria may vary, but one of the most recent guidelines for oral cytology includes the following[5]:
  - NILM (negative for intraepithelial lesion or malignancy): Normal, infection, inflammation, benign epithelial lesion, etc.
  - LSIL (low-grade squamous intraepithelial lesion): Mild to moderate dysplasia (cell changes).
  - HSIL (high-grade squamous intraepithelial lesion): Severe dysplasia.
  - SCC (squamous cell carcinoma).
  - Other malig (other malignancy).
  - IFN (indefinite for neoplasia or non-neoplasia).

Role of the Dental Hygienist in Thorough Intraoral/Extraoral Examination

- Identification of risk factors for oral cancer is an integral role in prevention of disease.
- In addition, dental hygienists play an important role educating patients about these risks, particularly as they pertain to tobacco cessation, alcohol reduction, and HPV vaccination.
- Professional continuing education and adherence to evidence-based practice guidelines can enhance the dental hygienist's confidence with current recommendations.[4,11]

Documentation

Documentation in the permanent record of a patient who had a biopsy (or smear) because of a questionable cancerous lesion is needed and must contain a minimum of the following:

- Details of the oral examination and follow-up procedures with reports from consultants, laboratories, medical follow-up, and outcomes.
- Recommendations for the frequency of a complete oral examination at future dental hygiene maintenance appointments.
- Review of lifestyle habits that may be a risk factor for an oral lesion with recommendations for specific preventive methods.
- A progress note at the patient's maintenance appointment following the biopsy with the results may be reviewed in **Box 2**.

Box 2 Example Documentation: Patient with an Oral Lesion

- **S**—50-year-old female presents for routine preventive maintenance with no current concerns at today's appointment. When questioned during intraoral examination, patient recalls accidentally biting her tongue recently.
- **O**—Patient smokes 1 pack cigarettes daily for the past 35 years and admits to drinking 1–2 beers nightly; left lateral border of tongue erythematous lesion 1 cm × 5 mm, flat.
- **A**—High risk for oral cancer, erythematous lesion requires further evaluation.
- **P**—Discuss concerns with patient regarding high-risk behaviors of tobacco use and alcohol. Recommend 2-week follow-up for reevaluation of lesion and further referral if no improvement. Recommended and offered tobacco cessation information.

Signed: _____, RDH

Date: _____

Factors to Teach the Patient

- Reasons for a careful extra- and intraoral examination at each maintenance appointment.
- Guidance and support on tobacco cessation and provide appropriate referral.
- How to conduct self-examination monthly to watch for changes in oral tissues and identify lesions that last longer than 2 weeks. Examination includes the face, neck, lips, gingiva, cheeks, tongue, palate, and throat. Any changes are reported to the dentist and the dental hygienist.
- General dietary and nutritional influences on the health of the oral tissues.
  - Benefits of diet rich in fruits and vegetables.
- How the oral cavity tends to reflect the general health.
- The warning signs of oral cancer from the American Cancer Society including the following[12]:
  - A swelling, lump, or growth anywhere, with or without pain.
  - White scaly patches or red velvety areas.
  - Any sore that does not heal promptly (within 2 weeks).
  - Numbness or tingling.
  - Excessive dryness or wetness.
  - Prolonged hoarseness, sore throats, persistent coughing, or the feeling of a "lump in the throat."
  - Difficulty with swallowing.
  - Difficulty in opening the mouth.

References

1. National Institute of Health, National Institute of Dental and Craniofacial Research. *Detecting Oral Cancer: A Guide for Health Care Professionals*. Published August 2020. https://www.nidcr.nih.gov/sites/default/files/2020-10/Detecting-Oral-Cancer-Healthcare-Professionals.pdf. Accessed September 6, 2021.

2. National Cancer Institute. Oral cavity and nasopharyngeal cancer screening (PDQ®)–health Professional Version. Published August 6, 2021. https://www.cancer.gov/types/head-and-neck/hp/oral-screening-pdq. Accessed September 17, 2021.

3. Rivera C. Essentials of oral cancer. *Int J Clin Exp Pathol*. 2015;8(9):11884-11894.

4. National HPV Vaccination Roundtable. *Cancer Prevention Through HPV Vaccination: An Action Guide for Dental Health Care Providers*. Published September 2019. http://hpvroundtable.org/wp-content/uploads/2018/04/DENTAL-Action-Guide-WEB.pdf. Accessed September 6, 2021.

5. Lingen MW, Abt E, Agrawal N, et al. Evidence-based clinical practice guideline for the evaluation of potentially malignant disorders in the oral cavity: a report of the American Dental Association. *J Am Dent Assoc*. 2017;148(10):712-727.e10.

6. Patton LL, Villa A, Bedran-Russo AK, et al. Human papillomavirus vaccine: an American Dental Association clinical evaluators panel survey. *J Am Dent Assoc*. 2020;151(4):303-304.e2.

7. University of Washington Department of Medicine. Technique: thyroid exam. *Advanced Physical Diagnosis Learning and Teaching at the Bedside*. https://depts.washington.edu/physdx/thyroid/tech.html. Accessed October 27, 2021.

8. Rethman MP, Carpenter W, Cohen EEW, et al. Evidence-based clinical recommendations regarding screening for oral squamous cell carcinomas. *J Am Dent Assoc*. 2010;141(5):509-520.

9. Warnakulasuriya S. Clinical features and presentation of oral potentially malignant disorders. *Oral Surg Oral Med Oral Pathol Oral Radiol*. 2018;125(6):582-590.

10. American Cancer Society. Oral cavity and oropharyngeal cancer key statistics 2021. Published March 23, 2021. https://www.cancer.org/cancer/oral-cavity-and-oropharyngeal-cancer/about/key-statistics.html. Accessed September 17, 2021.

11. Viens LJ, Henley SJ, Watson M, et al. Human papillomavirus-associated cancers, United States, 2008-2012. *MMWR Morb Mortal Wkly Rep*. 2016;65(26):661-666.

12. Lingen MW, Tampi MP, Urquhart O, et al. Adjuncts for the evaluation of potentially malignant disorders in the oral cavity. *J Am Dent Assoc*. 2017;148(11):797-813.e52.

Dental Soft Deposits, Biofilm, Calculus, and Stain

Catherine A. McConnell, RDH, BDSc, MEd, GCCT
Linda D. Boyd, RDH, RD, EdD

CHAPTER OUTLINE

LEARNING OBJECTIVES

After studying this chapter, the student will be able to:

1. Define acquired pellicle and discuss the significance and role of the pellicle in the maintenance of oral health.
2. Describe the different stages in biofilm formation and identify the changes in biofilm microorganisms as biofilm matures.
3. Differentiate between the types of soft and hard deposits.
4. Recognize the factors that influence the accumulation of biofilm, calculus, and stain.
5. Explain the location, composition, and properties of dental biofilm, calculus, and stain.
6. Identify the modes of attachment of supra- and subgingival calculus to dental structure.
7. Describe the clinical and radiographic characteristics of supra- and subgingival calculus and its detection.
8. Educate patients regarding the etiology and prevention of dental biofilm, calculus, and stain.
9. Differentiate between exogenous and endogenous stains and identify extrinsic and intrinsic dental stains and discolorations.
10. Determine the appropriate clinical approaches for stain removal and maintenance.
11. Design biofilm, calculus, and stain management strategies to meet each patient's individual needs.

Dental Biofilm and Other Soft Deposits

During clinical examination of the teeth and surrounding soft tissues, soft and hard deposits are assessed. The presence of **dental biofilm** is a primary risk factor for gingivitis, inflammatory periodontal diseases, and dental caries.[1]

- The soft deposits are referred to as acquired pellicle, dental biofilm, **materia alba**, and food debris.
- A comparison of the types of dental deposits with descriptions is found in **Table 1**.

Acquired Pellicle

- The acquired pellicle is a thin, **acellular** tenacious film formed of proteins, carbohydrates, and lipids.[2,3]
- Pellicle is uniquely positioned at the interface between the tooth surfaces and the oral environment. It forms over exposed enamel, dentin, mucosa, and restorative materials.

- The thickness of the enamel pellicle varies from 100 to 1,300 nm and thickness of the dentin pellicle varies from 300 to 1,200 nm.[2,4]
  - Thickness is dependent on its intra-oral location, time of formation, variations between individuals, and permanent versus primary dentition.[2]
  - The pellicle is thickest near the buccal gingival margin and thinner palatally where it is exposed to the forces of the tongue.[2]

I. Pellicle Formation

- Immediately upon exposure to saliva after eruption or after all soft and hard deposits have been removed from the tooth surfaces (such as by rubber cup or air polishing), the pellicle begins to form and is fully formed within 30 to 90 minutes.[3,4]
- Composition: Primarily glycoproteins, selectively **adsorbed** by the hydroxyapatite of the tooth surface.
  - Protein components are derived from the saliva, oral mucosal cells, gingival crevicular fluid (GCF), and **microorganisms**.[3]

Table 1 Tooth Deposits

Tooth Deposit	Description	Derivation	Removal Method
Acquired enamel pellicle	Translucent, homogeneous, thin, structured film covering and adherent to the surfaces of the teeth, restorations, calculus, and other surfaces	Supragingival: Saliva, oral mucosa, microorganism Subgingival: Gingival crevicular fluid	Toothbrush and appropriate interdental aid such as floss
Acquired dentin pellicle[2]	Translucent, two-layer structure, adheres to exposed dentin and restorative materials	Saliva, gingival crevicular fluid, and dentinal fluid	Toothbrush and appropriate interdental aid
Microbial (bacterial) biofilm Nonmineralized	Dense, organized bacterial communities embedded in EPS matrix adheres tenaciously to the teeth, calculus, prostheses, and other surfaces in the oral cavity	Colonization of oral microorganisms	Toothbrush and appropriate interdental aid such as floss
Materia alba Nonmineralized	Loosely adherent, unstructured, white or grayish-white mass of oral debris and bacteria that lies over dental biofilm	Incidental accumulation	Vigorous rinsing and water irrigation can remove materia alba
Food debris Nonmineralized	Unstructured, loosely attached particulate matter	Food retention following eating	Self-cleansing activity of tongue and saliva Rinsing vigorously removes debris Toothbrushing, flossing, and other aids
Calculus Mineralized	Calcified dental biofilm; Hard, tenacious mass that forms on the clinical crowns of the natural teeth and on dentures and other oral appliances	Biofilm **mineralization**	
a. Supragingival	Occurs coronal to the margin of the gingiva; is covered with dental biofilm	Source of minerals is saliva	Manual instrumentation Ultrasonic instrumentation
b. Subgingival	Occurs apical to the margin of the gingiva; is covered with dental biofilm	Source of minerals is gingival crevicular fluid	Manual instrumentation Ultrasonic instrumentation

- Initial attachment of bacteria to the pellicle is by selective adherence of microorganisms and occurs about 30 minutes after pellicle formation begins.[2,3]
  - Salivary proteins have a high affinity for the hydroxyapatite tooth surface and contribute to pellicle adherence and formation.[2]

II. Types of Acquired Pellicle

A. Acquired Enamel Pellicle

- Acquired enamel pellicle (AEP) is translucent and not readily visible until application of a disclosing agent.
  - Pellicle can take on extrinsic stain and become gradations of brown, gray, or other colors.
  - When stained with a disclosing agent, pellicle appears thin, with a pale staining that contrasts with the thicker, darker staining of dental biofilm.

B. Acquired Dentin Pellicle

- Acquired dentin pellicle (ADP) occurs on dentin exposed by recession.[2]

III. Functions of Pellicle

The pellicle plays an important role in the maintenance of oral health.[2,3] The various functions of the pellicle include[2,3]:

- Regulation of mineral homeostasis
  - Protects against acid-induced enamel demineralization (this role is more limited on dentin surfaces).
  - The pellicle structure may serve as a scaffold for remineralization.
  - May protect against erosion.
- Host defense and microbial colonization
  - About 8% of the proteins in the pellicle have antimicrobial functions.

- The bacterial colonization depends on specific protein binders in the pellicle. Some protein components inhibit binding and others promote adherence.
- Bacterial adherence and aggregation begin the process of biofilm formation.
- Lubrication
  - Pellicle keeps surfaces moist and prevents drying, which in turn enhances the efficiency of speech and mastication.
  - The AEP lubricating properties may also protect against abrasive damage.

IV. Removal of Pellicle

- Pellicle is not resilient enough to withstand oral self-care.
- Extrinsic factors that may interfere with pellicle formation and **maturation** include[5]:
  - Abrasive toothpastes.
  - Whitening products.
  - Intake of acidic foods and beverages.

Dental Biofilm

The **oral microbiome** is composed of microorganisms, their genetic makeup, and the environments found in the oral cavity.[6]

- The mouth has a number of environments, including the teeth, gingival sulcus, attached gingiva, tongue, oral mucosa, lips, and hard and soft palates, with their own microbial inhabitants.[6]
- The permanent teeth, as the only nonshedding surface in the body, serve as a unique environment for biofilm formation and maturation.[6]
- The microorganisms in the oral cavity perform both pro- and anti-inflammatory activities, which maintain homeostasis in health.[6]
- Dental biofilm is a dynamic, structured community of microorganisms, encapsulated in a self-produced **extracellular polymeric substance (EPS)** forming a **matrix** around microcolonies.
  - The matrix is composed of polysaccharides, proteins, and other compounds; it acts to protect the biofilm from the host's immune system and antimicrobial agents.
  - The microcolonies are separated by a network of open water channels that supply nutrients deep within the biofilm community.
- The three-dimensional structure of biofilms enhances their ability to communicate with each other, adapt, and respond to their environment.

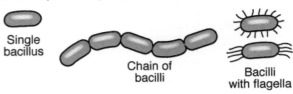

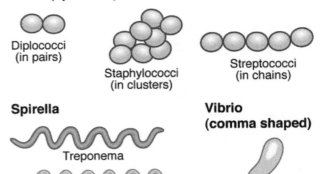

Figure 1 Bacilli, Cocci, Spirella, and Vibrio

Reproduced from Sakai J. *Practical Pharmacology for the Pharmacy Technician*. Baltimore, MD: Lippincott Williams & Wilkins; 2008.

- Adheres to the pellicle coating on all hard and soft oral structures, including teeth, existing calculus, and fixed and removable restorations.
- There are over 700 distinct microorganisms in the oral cavity, including bacteria, viruses, protozoa, and yeast.[6] Morphologic forms of bacteria found within biofilms are shown in **Figure 1**.

I. Steps in the Formation of Oral Biofilm

Biofilm formation involves a series of complex microbial interactions (**Figure 2**).

- The close proximity of microbial species allows for changes in gene expression, which impact the growth and capabilities of the biofilm community to cause disease.[1]

A. Step 1—Pellicle Formation

- The acquired pellicle provides the glycoproteins for microorganism adhesion.

B. Step 2—Initial Adhesion

- Biofilm formation begins with initial attachment of **planktonic** bacterial cells to the pellicle on the tooth surface.[7]

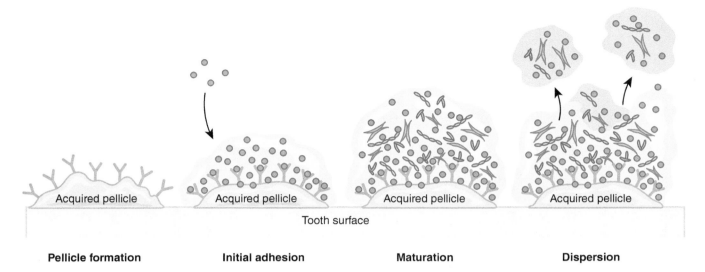

| Pellicle formation | Initial adhesion | Maturation | Dispersion |

Figure **2** Biofilm Microorganisms

Data from Huang R, Li M, Gregory RL. Bacterial interactions in dental biofilm. Virulence. 2011 Sep 1;2(5):435-44

- Microbes attach to the pellicle by means of fimbriae and pilli along with electrostatic interactions.[8]
- Initially, the adherent cells are not "committed" to this process and it is reversible. When cells are disrupted (with oral self-care activities), they may dislodged from the surface.[7]
- The early colonizers attached to the pellicle begin to excrete extracellular polymeric substance (EPS) to help bacteria bind together (co-adhesion) and to the pellicle.[7]

  Components of the EPS include:
  - Polysaccharides, glucans, and fructans, or levans produced by certain bacteria within the community and from dietary sucrose.
  - EPS provides a scaffold to anchor the bacteria together, increasing adherence to dental and other structures and providing protection as the bacterial community continues to grow.[6]
  - EPS contains components such as antimicrobial enzymes to protect the biofilm.[6]
- At this stage, the cocci adhere to filamentous bacteria, creating structural components of biofilm such as *corn cob* or *bristle brush* forms.[6,7]

C. Step 3—Maturation

- Later colonizing bacteria attach to the early colonizers to form microcolonies.[7] The metabolism of one species of bacteria may be a source of nutrients to another species, resulting in food chains or webs within the biofilm.[1,7]
- This stage is also characterized by further development of the biofilm architecture to enhance the

cell-to-cell communication process, also known as **quorum sensing**.[6]
- Quorum sensing controls the growth of the microbial community and signals microorganisms when to leave the biofilm to find new sites.[7]
- Maturation occurs by 72 hours.[6]

D. Step 4—Detachment and Dispersion

- Bacterial colonies mature and release planktonic cells to spread and colonize other areas within the oral cavity.
- Bacteria convert to motile forms in order to disperse.[7]
- Bacteria can disperse as single cells or in clumps.[7]

II. Changes in Biofilm Microorganisms

- Dental biofilm consists of a complex mixture of microorganisms in microcolonies. The microbial density is very high and increases as biofilm ages and matures.
- The potential for the development of dental caries and/or gingivitis increases with more microorganisms, especially as the numbers of **pathogenic** microorganisms outnumber the nonpathogenic microorganisms.[6,9]
- With undisrupted biofilm for approximately 7 days, gram-negative anaerobic bacteria growth is favored, which increases risk for dental caries and gingivitis, and eventually other inflammatory periodontal diseases increase.[6]

Time Frame	Microbiologic Findings
Day 1–2	Early biofilm consists primarily of gram-positive cocci with small accumulations of **leukocytes**
Day 2–4	The cocci still dominate while increasing numbers of gram-positive filamentous form and slender rods join the surface of the cocci colonies, along with more leukocytes
Day 5–10 (on average)	Filaments increase in numbers, and a mixed **flora** appears comprising rods, filamentous forms, and fusobacteria with heavy accumulations of leukocytes
Day 10–21	Gingivitis is clinically evident in 10 to 21 days

- Although there is significant variability between individuals in the pattern of dental biofilm development, the changes in **oral flora** follow a general pattern (Figure   2).
- The formation of dental biofilm may vary by days of accumulation (**Box   1**).

Supragingival and Subgingival Dental Biofilm

Recent technology innovations in DNA sequencing and fluorescent in situ hybridization (FISH) have allowed for a more in-depth understanding of the science of biofilms.[11,12]

I. Supragingival Biofilm

- Supragingival biofilm has greater variability in architecture than subgingival biofilm and typically consists of two layers of predominantly gram-positive **aerobic** bacteria[12]:
  - The first layer (basal layer) adheres to the tooth surface and is composed of streptococci, *Actinomyces*, filamentous bacteria, yeast, and *Lactobacillus*.
  - The second layer forms on top of the basal layer and includes streptococci and *Lactobacillus*.

II. Subgingival Biofilm

A. Subgingival Biofilm Architecture

- Subgingival biofilm is made up of four layers, which includes predominantly gram-negative **anaerobic** and motile organisms. The organisms present will vary in health and disease, but may contain the following[11]:
  - The first layer (basal layer) contains bacteria such as *Actinomyces*.
  - Intermediate layers contain bacteria such as *Tannerella forsythia* and *Fusobacterium nucleatum*.
  - Top layers contain spirochetes and this is typically where the periodontal pathogens such as *Porphyromonas gingivalis* and *P. endodontalis* may be located.

B. Subgingival Biofilm

The subgingival microbiome is very complex, and the bacteria present in health versus disease shift to a disease-associated community.[13] There are core species of bacteria that do not change from health to disease, such as Campylobacter gracilis and Fusobacterium nucleatum ss. Vincentii.[13]

- Subgingival microbiome in health[11]
  - Primarily gram-positive cocci and rods with a few gram-negative species.
  - *Corynebacterium* aid in forming the structure of early biofilm.
  - *Rothia* are involved with cell-cell aggregation in early biofilm formation.
- Subgingival microbiome associated with gingivitis[11,13]
  - There is a greater biofilm mass with more diversity and a higher number of bacterial species in gingivitis.
  - There is a shift from gram-positive species to gram-negative aerobic organisms in gingivitis.
  - Bacteria most associated with clinical signs of gingivitis and inflammation are *Prevotella* and *Selenomonas*.
- Periodontal-associated subgingival microbiome[11,13]
  - Significant shifts in the composition of the biofilm communities occur with more bacterial species in periodontitis as compared to health. Increased diversity in the microbiome is a unique feature of periodontitis.
  - Bacteria seen in health are still present, but **dysbiosis** results in shifts to periodontitis-associated species. Periodontal

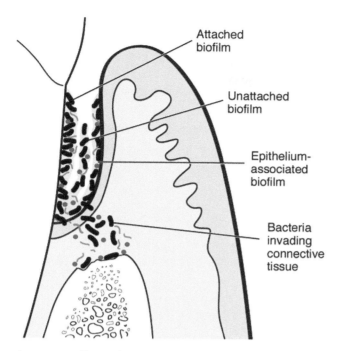

Figure 3 Bacterial Invasion. Diagram of a periodontal pocket shows attached and unattached biofilm (planktonic) bacteria within the pocket epithelium, in the connective tissue, and on the surface of the bone.

Labels on figure: Attached biofilm; Unattached biofilm; Epithelium-associated biofilm; Bacteria invading connective tissue

pathogens have been found to be present in the adjacent epithelial cells and underlying connective tissue (**Figure 3**).[14]

Composition of Dental Biofilm

- Microorganisms and EPS comprise 20% of the biofilm that are organic and inorganic solids. The other 80% is water.
- Composition differs among individuals and among tooth surfaces.

I. Inorganic Elements

A. Calcium and Phosphorus

- Calcium, phosphorus, and magnesium are more concentrated in biofilm than in saliva.[15]
- Saliva transports the minerals during the mineralization and demineralization processes.

B. Fluoride

- Fluoride concentration in biofilm is higher in the presence of fluoridated water, following professional topical fluoride applications, and with the use of fluoride-containing dentifrices and oral rinses for 3 to 6 hours before returning to baseline.[16]

II. Organic Elements

The organic EPS forms a scaffold for biofilm development and contains primarily polysaccharides and proteins, with small amounts of lipids.[17]

A. Polysaccharides (Carbohydrates)

- In addition to dietary sucrose and starch, polysaccharides are metabolized by bacteria such as *S. mutans* to produce glucans and fructans.[17]
- The glucans provide binding sites for microorganisms, especially *S. mutans*, which facilitates clustering and adherence of the bacteria to the tooth.[17]

B. Proteins

- The proteins of supragingival biofilm bind with glucans supporting further growth of biofilm.[17]

Clinical Aspects of Dental Biofilm

I. Distribution of Biofilm

A. Location

- *Supragingival biofilm*: Coronal to the gingival margin.
- *Gingival biofilm*: Forms on the external surfaces of the oral epithelium and attached gingiva.
- *Subgingival biofilm*: Located between the epithelial attachment and the gingival margin, within the sulcus or pocket.
- *Fissure biofilm*: Develops in pits and fissures of the teeth.

B. By Surfaces

- *During formation*
  - Supragingival biofilm formation begins at the gingival margin, particularly on proximal surfaces, and extends coronally when left undisturbed.
  - It spreads over the gingival third and on toward the middle third of the crown.
- *Tooth surfaces involved*
  - Biofilm is heaviest on lingual, posterior, and proximal surfaces.[18]
  - Anterior surfaces have the least biofilm.[18]

C. Factors Influencing Biofilm Accumulation

- Dental biofilm accumulates readily around crowded teeth as shown in **Figure 4**. With effective biofilm control, biofilm accumulation around crowded teeth is not greater than that around well aligned teeth.
  - Special accommodations such as using a toothbrush placed in a vertical position can remove thick biofilm on the lingual surface of the crowded mandibular anterior.
- Rough surfaces: Biofilm develops more rapidly on rough tooth surfaces, existing calculus, poorly contoured restorations, and removable appliances; thick, dense deposits can be difficult to remove.
- Occlusion: Deposits may extend over an entire crown of a tooth that is unopposed, out of occlusion, or not actively used during mastication.

D. Removal of Biofilm

- Toothbrushing and interdental cleaning are the most universal daily mechanical disruption methods.

II. Detection of Biofilm

A. Direct Vision

- *Thin biofilm:* May be translucent and therefore not visible without a disclosing agent.

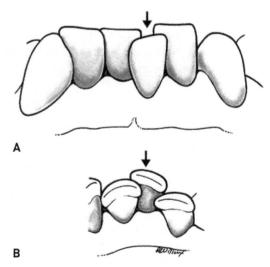

Figure 4 Biofilm Accumulation in Protected Areas. **A:** Crowded mandibular anterior teeth demonstrate dental biofilm after use of a disclosing agent. Thickest biofilm is on proximal surfaces and at cervical thirds of teeth. **B:** Note central incisors with thick extensive biofilm on the less accessible protected surfaces.

- *Stained biofilm:* Extrinsic stains may make biofilm more visible (e.g., yellow, green, tobacco stains).
- *Thick biofilm:* The tooth may appear dull and dingy, with a matted fur-like surface. Materia alba or food debris may collect over the biofilm.

B. Use of Explorer or Probe

- *Biofilm disruption:* Biofilm may be disturbed by passing the side of an explorer or probe over the tooth surface.

C. Use of Disclosing Agent

- When a disclosing agent is applied, biofilm takes on the color and becomes readily visible (Figure 4).

D. Clinical Record

- A Biofilm Control record should be used to document initial biofilm accumulation, followed by continuing changes over the treatment and follow-up appointments.
- Record biofilm by location and thickness (slight, moderate, or heavy). For objective evaluations, use of an index or a biofilm score is recommended. (See Chapter 21.)

Significance of Dental Biofilm

- Biofilm plays a major role in the initiation and progression of dental caries and periodontal diseases, caused by pathogenic microorganisms found in oral biofilms.[1]
- Biofilm is significant in the formation of **dental calculus**, which is essentially mineralized dental biofilm.

I. Dental Caries

- Dental caries is a disease of the dental calcified structures (enamel, dentin, and cementum) characterized by demineralization of the mineral components and dissolution of the organic matrix. (See Chapter 16.)
- The sequence of events leading to demineralization and dental caries is shown in **Figure 5**.

A. The Caries Microbiome

- Dysbiosis of the microbiome results in changes in the microbiome communities with reduced

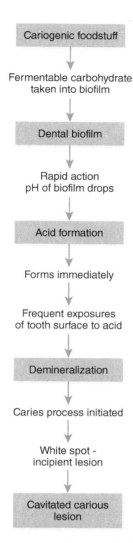

Figure 5 Development of Dental Caries. Flowchart shows the step-by-step action within the microbial biofilm on the tooth surface.

Cariogenic foodstuff

↓ Fermentable carbohydrate taken into biofilm

Dental biofilm

↓ Rapid action pH of biofilm drops

Acid formation

↓ Forms immediately

↓ Frequent exposures of tooth surface to acid

Demineralization

↓ Caries process initiated

↓ White spot - incipient lesion

Cavitated carious lesion

diversity to favor caries initiation. This dysbiosis may occur due to decreased salivary flow resulting in a reduced buffering capacity and/or frequent fermentable carbohydrate exposure.[19,20]

- Acid tolerant *S. mutans* and *S. sobrinus*, predominantly, and lactobacilli are thought to be the major bacteria associated with caries, particularly in those with poor biofilm removal without access to regular dental care.[19,21]
- For populations with lower caries rates, *S. mutans* may be lower and other acidogenic bacteria such as *Actinomyces* may be predominant.[19,21]

B. The pH of Biofilm

- Acid formation begins *immediately* once a **cariogenic** substance is taken into the biofilm, resulting in a rapid drop in the pH of the biofilm.[22]

- Critical pH for enamel demineralization averages 5.5, although other factors impact decalcification.[23]
- The critical pH for root surface demineralization may be higher because of the lower mineral content of dentin and cementum.[23]
    - The critical pH for demineralization of dentin is approximately 6.7, which is particularly relevant for patients with multiple areas of recession and xerostomia.[24]
- The extent of demineralization depends on the length of time and frequency the pH is below critical level; biofilm composition, pH-lowering ability of the microorganisms, and action of saliva are additional factors that affect the caries process.[22]

C. Effect of Diet on Biofilm

- Cariogenic foods
    - In a diet high in fermentable carbohydrates, biofilm communities shift to bacteria with higher pH-lowering ability.[22]

Materia Alba

I. Clinical Appearance and Content

- Materia alba is a soft, whitish tooth deposit that is clinically visible without application of a disclosing agent. It may have a cottage cheese–like texture and appearance.
- Materia alba is an unorganized accumulation of living and dead bacteria, desquamated epithelial cells, disintegrating **leukocytes**, salivary proteins, and food debris. This differentiates it from organized oral biofilms.

II. Prevention

- Materia alba can be removed with the basic mechanical oral self-care procedures. (See Chapters 26 and 27.)

Food Debris

- After food consumption, food remnants may collect in areas of the cervical third and proximal embrasures of the teeth.
- Vertical **food impaction** results during mastication as food is forced into open contact areas (loss of proximal contact), dental diastemas, poorly contoured restorations, or occlusal irregularities such as plunger cusps.[25]

- Left unattended, the accumulation of food debris adds to a general unsanitary condition of the mouth and may contribute to the initiation of dental caries and oral malodor.[26]

Calculus

Dental calculus is dental biofilm mineralized by crystals of calcium phosphate mineral salts between previously living microorganisms.[27]

- The calculus is covered with a layer of nonmineralized dental biofilm containing live bacteria.[27]
- The hard, tenacious mass forms on the clinical crowns of natural teeth, dental implants, dentures, and other dental prostheses.
- Dental calculus is classified by its location on a tooth surface as related to the adjacent free gingival margin, that is, *supragingival* and *subgingival* calculus as shown in **Figure 6**.

I. Supragingival Calculus

A. Location

- Forms on clinical crowns coronal to the margin of the gingiva.
- Forms on implants, complete and partial dentures.

B. Distribution: Most Frequent Sites

- On the lingual surfaces of mandibular anterior teeth and the facial surfaces of maxillary first and second molars, opposite the openings of the ducts of the submandibular and parotid salivary glands.
  - **Figure 7** shows heavy supragingival calculus forming a continuous "bridge" across several teeth.

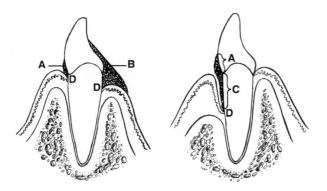

Figure 6 Dental Calculus. **A:** Supragingival calculus on the cervical third of a mandibular anterior tooth extends slightly subgingivally. **B:** Supragingival calculus over crown, exposed root surface, and the margin of the gingiva. **C:** Subgingival calculus along root to the base of a periodontal pocket. **D:** Base of pocket.

- On the crowns of teeth out of occlusion, nonfunctioning teeth, or teeth that are neglected during daily biofilm removal (toothbrushing or interdental care).
- On surfaces of dentures, dental prostheses, and oral piercings.

II. Subgingival Calculus

A. Location

- Forms apical to the margin of the gingiva and extending toward the clinical attachment on the root surface.
- Forms on dental implants.

B. Distribution

- May be generalized or localized on single teeth or a group of teeth.
- Heaviest deposits are related to areas most difficult for the patient to access during personal oral biofilm removal procedures.
- **Figure 8** illustrates subgingival calculus on an extracted molar and premolar. In **Figure 9A** and **B**, ledges of interproximal calculus can be seen radiographically.
  - The calculus typically will form at the cementoenamel junction as recession and pocket formation continue.
  - The color of subgingival calculus comes from exposure to the products of blood and blood breakdown products.

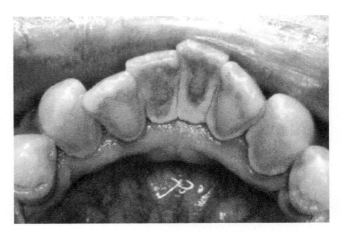

Figure 7 Supragingival Calculus. Heavy calculus deposits on the lingual surfaces of the mandibular anterior teeth. These deposits are so large that they interfere with the patient's oral self-care efforts. In addition, calculus deposits harbor living bacteria that are in constant contact with the gingival tissue.

Reproduced from Nield-Gehrig J, Willmann D. *Foundations of Periodontics for the Dental Hygienist.* 3rd ed. Philadelphia, PA: Lippincott Williams & Wilkins; 2011.

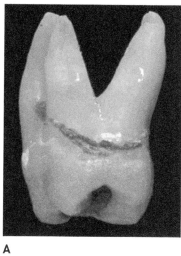

A

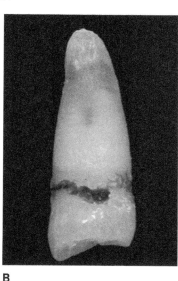

B

Figure 8 Subgingival Calculus on Extracted Teeth. **A:** On a maxillary first molar, calculus that formed in the subgingival environment is dark brown because elements of blood were incorporated during calcification. Additionally, some of the bacteria that are formed in calculus produce pigment. It can be seen here on surfaces where it most commonly forms and is often missed during periodontal instrumentation: near the cementoenamel junction (CEJ), at line angles, in grooves (the concavity just coronal to the buccal furcation), and furcations. **B:** Calculus at and apical to the CEJ on a premolar.

Reproduced from Weiss G, Scheid R. *Woelfel's Dental Anatomy.* 8th ed. Philadelphia, PA: Lippincott Williams & Wilkins; 2012.

Calculus Composition

- Calculus is composed of inorganic and organic components and water.
- The percentages vary depending on the age, hardness of a deposit, and location of the calculus (supragingival calculus in maxillary molar areas tends to be higher in calcium, phosphorus, and

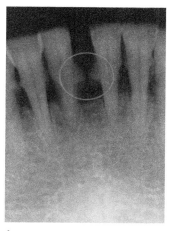

A

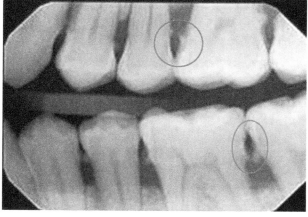

B

Figure 9 Subgingival Calculus in Radiographs. **A:** Heavy supra- and subgingival proximal calculus is shown on the mandibular anterior teeth (#24–25). **B:** The bitewing radiographs show heavy ledges or spines of subgingival calculus in the proximal areas of premolar and molar areas.

ash content than on the lingual of mandibular anterior teeth).[24]

- Mature calculus usually contains inorganic components; the rest is organic components and water.

I. Inorganic Content

A. Major Inorganic Components

- The main components are calcium (Ca), phosphorus (P), carbonate (CO_3), sodium (Na), and magnesium (Mg).[28]

B. Trace Elements

- Trace elements include copper (Cu), zinc (Zn), strontium (Sr), manganese (Mn), silicon (Si), fluorine (F), iron (Fe), and potassium (K).[28]

C. Fluoride in Calculus

- Fluoride is present primarily as part of hydroxyapatite in supragingival dental calculus.[28]
- The concentration of fluoride in calculus varies depending on the patient's exposure to fluoridated drinking water, topical applications, dentifrices, or any form in contact with the external surface of the calculus.

D. Crystals

- Dental calculus contains four types of calcium phosphate crystals:
  - Brushite
  - Octocalcium phosphate
  - Hydroxyapatitie
  - Whitlockite[27]

E. Composition of Calculus

- Dental enamel is the most highly mineralized tissue in the body and contains 95% to 97% inorganic salts; dentin contains 65% and cementum and bone contain 45% to 70%.[28]
- Supragingival calculus has an average mineral content of 37% with amounts as high as 80%.[27]
  - The predominant inorganic component in exterior layers of supragingival calculus is octacalcium phosphate, with hydroxyapatite being more dominant in older calculus.[27]
- Subgingival calculus has an average mineral content of 58% with maximum content of 60–80%.[27]
  - The predominant inorganic component of subgingival calculus is whitlockite.[27]

II. Organic Content

- The organic proportion of calculus consists of various types of microorganisms, desquamated epithelial cells, leukocytes, and mucin from the saliva.
- Substances identified in the organic matrix include lipids such as free fatty acids and phospholipids and a protein portion.[29]

Calculus Formation

- Calculus results from the deposition of minerals into a biofilm organic matrix.
- Mineralization of supragingival and subgingival calculus is essentially the same, although the source of the elements for mineralization is not the same.

I. Factors in Rate of Calculus Formation

- Genetic and individual variation in saliva composition and flow.[27]
  - In heavy calculus formers, saliva contains higher levels of calcium and three times greater levels for phosphorus than light calculus formers.[27]
- Diet, especially alkaline food, foods high in silicon like rice, and refined carbohydrates.[27,29]
- Individual variations in bacterial load.[27]
- Age, race, and gender.[27]
- More severe periodontal disease.[30]
- Malposition and crowding of teeth.[30]
- Lower levels of S. mutans.[30]
- Inhibitors of calculus formation (i.e., urea, zinc, and pyrophosphates).[28,29]

II. Precursor to Calculus Mineralization

- Nonmineralized biofilm is necessary for initiation of calculus formation.
- In supragingival biofilm, filamentous microorganisms are oriented at a right angle to the tooth and provide the matrix for the deposition of minerals.[27]
- In subgingival biofilm, cocci, rods, and filamentous bacteria do not form a distinct pattern in relation to the tooth.[27]

III. Mechanism of Calculus Mineralization

- **Supersaturation** of saliva is the driving force for mineralization.[29,31]
- Dead microorganisms degrade and mineral deposition begins using the cell walls of the bacteria.[29]
- The initial calcium phosphate crystals form by binding with phospholipids in the cell membranes of the bacteria.[29]
- These early crystals are typically brushite, which progress through transformation stages of maturation as mineralization continues to octacalcium phosphate, whitlockite, and finally to a stable hydroxyapatite phase.[28]
- The final stable phase occurs around 8 months.[28]
- Calculus forms in layers.
  - In supragingival calculus, the layers are heterogeneous and each may have a different mineral content.[27]

- In subgingival calculus, the layers are more similar or homogeneous with equal mineral density.[27]
- The layers of calculus are called *incremental lines*.[29] The lines are evidence calculus grows or increases by apposition of new layers.

IV. Types of Calculus Deposits

The surface of the calculus is typically rough and can be detected with an explorer. The exception is veneer-type calculus, which is smooth and difficult to detect with an explorer.

- Crusty, spiny, or nodular deposits.
- Ledge or ring formation.
- Thin, smooth veneers.
- Finger- and fern-like formations.
- Individual calculus islands or spots.

V. Formation Time

- The average time required for the primary soft deposit to change to the mature mineralized stage is about 12 days.[27]
  - Half of mineralization can begin in the first two days when a patient's daily oral self-care is inadequate.[27]
- Formation time depends on individual factors previously mentioned.

Attachment of Calculus

- The ease or difficulty of calculus removal is related to the manner of attachment of the calculus to the tooth surface.

I. Attachment by Means of an Acquired Pellicle

- In early calculus formation, the attachment is superficial because no interlocking with the tooth surface occurs and calculus can be easily removed.

II. Attachment to Minute Irregularities in the Tooth Surface

- Dentin irregularities include cracks, resorption, and carious defects.[32]
  - Cemental irregularities include tiny spaces left at previous locations of **Sharpey's fibers**, resorption lacunae, root gouging from improper scaling, and cemental tears.

- Calculus is difficult to remove when it is attached by this method because it becomes locked into the irregularities.

III. Attachment by Direct Contact with the Tooth Surface

- Interlocking of inorganic apatite crystals of the enamel and cementum with the calcium phosphate crystals of the calculus.[33]
- Research suggests this mode of attachment results in a portion of the calculus that is prone to fracture during removal, but it may leave calculus crystals attached to the tooth surface.[33]

Clinical Implications of Dental Calculus

- There has been a long-standing debate over whether subgingival calculus has a role in periodontal disease.[27]
- Given calculus is always covered by a layer of unmineralized viable biofilm, it is likely the biofilm is responsible for the initiation of the immune response in gingivitis and periodontitis.[27]
  - Calculus is a *secondary* etiologic factor in periodontitis because it acts as a reservoir for bacteria and endotoxins.[27]
  - The progression of calculus apically is responsible for the deepening of the pocket and loss of attachment due to the layer of biofilm covering it.
  - Research has shown that removal of the biofilm on subgingival calculus results in healing of periodontal tissues.[27]
- The cornerstone of nonsurgical periodontal therapy is the daily control of biofilm by the patient, supplemented by definitive professional supra- and subgingival instrumentation to reduce or eliminate gingival inflammation and bleeding on probing and regular periodontal maintenance or supportive care.[27,34]
  - However, understanding the mode of attachment is important to recognize that calculus is prone to fracture during removal and may leave calculus crystals attached to the tooth surface.[33]
  - These remaining calcium phosphate crystals may then serve as a nidus for continued biofilm formation.[33]
  - It is important to meticulously debride subgingival biofilm given complete removal of calculus is not feasible.[27]

Clinical Characteristics

- Identification of calculus prior to removal depends on knowledge of its appearance, consistency, and distribution.
- Appointment planning, selection of instruments, and techniques depend on understanding the texture, morphology, and mode of attachment of calculus. **Table** 2 lists a summary of clinical characteristics.

I. Supragingival Examination
A. Direct Examination

- Supragingival deposits may be seen directly or indirectly, using a mouth mirror.

Table 2 Clinical Characteristics of Dental Calculus[27,29,30,33]

Characteristic	Supragingival Calculus	Subgingival Calculus
Color	White, creamy yellow, or gray May be stained by tobacco, food, tea, or coffee Slight deposits may be invisible until dried with compressed air	Light to dark brown, dark green, or black due to gingival crevicular fluid, blood and blood breakdown products
Shape	**Amorphous**, bulky Gross deposits may: ■ Form interproximal bridge between adjacent teeth (Figure 7) ■ Extend over the margin of the gingiva ■ Form based on the anatomy of the teeth; contour of gingival margin; and pressure of the tongue, lips, cheeks	Conforms to the root surface due to constraints of the pocket wall Calculus formations occur in the following forms: ■ Crusty, spiny, or nodular ■ Ledge or ringlike ■ Thin, smooth veneers ■ Finger- and fern-like ■ Individual calculus islands
Consistency and texture	Moderately hard Newer deposits less mineralized (37%) Porous surface covered with nonmineralized biofilm	Harder and more mineralized (58%) than supragingival calculus Surface covered with dental biofilm
Size and quantity	Quantity has direct relationship to: ■ Personal oral self-care ■ Diet ■ Individual characteristics, such as diet and salivary flow ■ Position of the teeth ■ Use of tobacco products	Quantity is related to: ■ Personal oral self-care ■ Individual characteristics, such as age ■ Bacterial load ■ Disease severity
Distribution on individual tooth	Coronal to margin of gingiva	Apical to margin of gingiva Extends to bottom of the pocket and follows contour of soft-tissue attachment
Distribution on teeth	Symmetrical arrangement on teeth, except when influenced by: ■ Malpositioned teeth ■ Unilateral hypofunction ■ Inconsistent personal oral self-care Location related to openings of the salivary gland ducts: ■ Facial surface of maxillary molars ■ Lingual surface of mandibular anterior teeth	Heaviest on proximal surfaces, lightest on facial surfaces Occurs with or without associated supragingival deposits

Data from Akcalı A, Lang NP. Dental calculus: the calcified biofilm and its role in disease development. *Periodontol 2000*. 2018;76(1):109-115. doi:10.1111/prd.12151; Jin Y, Yip H-K. Supragingival calculus: formation and control. *Crit Rev Oral Biol Med*. Published online 2002:16; Fons-Badal C, Fons-Font A, Labaig-Rueda C, Fernanda Solá-Ruiz M, Selva-Otaolaurruchi E, Agustín-Panadero R. Analysis of predisposing factors for rapid dental calculus formation. *J Clin Med*. 2020;9(3):E858. doi:10.3390/jcm9030858; Rohanizadeh R, LeGeros RZ. Ultrastructural study of calculus–enamel and calculus–root interfaces. *Arch Oral Biol*. 2005;50(1):89-96. doi:10.1016/j.archoralbio.2004.07.001

B. Use of Compressed Air

- Small amounts of calculus may be invisible when they are wet with saliva.
- With adequate light and drying with air, small deposits usually become visible.

II. Subgingival Examination

A. Visual Examination

- Dark edges of calculus may be seen at or just beneath the gingival margin.
- Gentle air blast can deflect the gingival margin from the tooth to gain some visibility into the coronal portion of the pocket.

B. Gingival Tissue Color Change

- Dark calculus may be visible as a dark shadow along the gingiva and suggest the presence of subgingival calculus.

C. Tactile Examination

- *Probe*: While probing for sulcus/pocket characteristics, a rough subgingival tooth surface may be felt when calculus is present.
- *Explorer*: With a subgingival explorer like an ODU 11/12, each tooth is explored carefully to the base of the pocket to detect any calculus deposits.

D. Radiographic Examination

- Radiographic examination may detect large calculus deposits on proximal surfaces (see Figure 9A and B).

E. Dental Endoscopy

- The use of the dental endoscope in deep pockets and furcations can detect otherwise undetectable calculus, especially burnished or veneer-type calculus.[35]

Prevention of Calculus

- Risk factors related to calculus formation are similar to those for dental biofilm formation and relate to the patient's daily biofilm removal regime.

I. Personal Dental Biofilm Control

A. Objective

- Regular removal of dental biofilm by appropriately selected brushing, interdental care, and supplementary methods is a major factor in the control of dental calculus reformation.

B. Oral Self-Care Education

- Patient education includes[34]:
  - Identification and hands-on demonstration of the oral hygiene aids appropriate for the patient's needs.
  - Follow-up at continuing care appointments to commend the patient's successes and review and refine techniques as necessary to overcome barriers.
  - Identification of dietary behaviors that may be enhancing biofilm growth, such as sugar-sweetened beverages and sugary snacks between meals.

II. Regular Professional Continuing Care

- Professional maintenance or supportive periodontal care appointments on a regular basis supplement daily oral self-care.[34]
- With emphasis on good oral hygiene and routine professional removal, low levels of supragingival and subgingival calculus can be maintained.[27]

III. Anticalculus Dentifrice

A. Objective

- Calculus-control dentifrices aim to inhibit calculus crystal growth, which may lessen the amount of calculus formation.[29] (See Chapter 28.)
- Dentifrices do not have an effect on existing calculus deposits; however, they may prevent formation of new supragingival calculus.
- For a patient who cannot control supragingival calculus, and hence cannot achieve optimum gingival tissue health, an anticalculus dentifrice may provide motivation, as well as be a supplement to mechanical biofilm removal efforts.

B. Chemotherapeutic Anticalculus Agents

- Agents used in "tartar-control" mouth rinses or dentifrices are mineralization inhibitors.
  - Examples include pyrophosphates and zinc citrate.[29]

Dental Stains and Discolorations

- Discolorations of the teeth and restorations occur in three general ways[36]:
  - Adhered directly to the tooth surfaces.
  - Contained within calculus or pellicle.
  - Incorporated within the tooth structure or the restorative material.

Significance of Dental Stains

- The significance of stain is primarily the appearance or cosmetic (esthetic) effect.[37]
- In general, any detrimental effect on the teeth or gingival tissues is related to the dental calculus in which the stain occurs.
- Certain stains provide a means of evaluating adequate oral self-care for management of dental biofilm.

I. Classification of Stains

A. Classified by Location

- **Extrinsic** stain: Occurs on the external surface of the tooth and may be removed by procedures of toothbrushing, scaling, and/or polishing.
  - Origins are metallic and nonmetallic.[36]
- **Intrinsic** stain: Occurs due to changes in structural composition or thickness of the enamel.
  - Internalized discoloration: Extrinsic stain is internalized into the tooth structure following development.[36]
  - Occurs in development defects and acquired defects like restorative materials.

B. Classified by Source

- **Exogenous** stain: Develops or originates from sources outside the tooth.
  - Exogenous stains may be extrinsic and stay on the outer surface of the tooth or intrinsic and become incorporated within the tooth structure.
- **Endogenous** stain: Develops or originates from within the tooth.
  - Endogenous stains are always intrinsic and usually are discolorations of the dentin reflected through the enamel.

II. Recognition and Identification

More than one type of stain may occur and more than one etiologic factor may cause the stains and discolorations of an individual's dentition. A differential diagnosis may be needed in order to plan whether an appropriate intervention is indicated.

A. Medical and Dental History

- Developmental delays; medications; use of tobacco, marijuana, or betel or areca nut; and fluoride histories all contribute necessary information.
- Thorough medical, dental, and social histories and cultural practices can provide information to supplement clinical observations.

B. Food Diary

- Assessment of a patient's food diary may aid in identifying certain contributing factors.
  - Examples of staining from beverages include tea, coffee, dark-colored juices, and wine.

C. Oral Hygiene Habits

- The history of oral self-care routines may help explain the presence of certain stains.

III. Application of Procedures for Stain Removal

A. Stains Occurring Directly on the Tooth Surface

- Stains directly associated with the pellicle on the surface of the enamel or exposed cementum are removed as much as possible during toothbrushing or interdental cleaning.
- Certain stains can be removed with debridement and/or polishing. (See Chapter 42.)
- When stains are tenacious, avoid excessive polishing. Use the most conservative approach with the least abrasive polishing agent to prevent the following:
  - Excess tooth structure or abrasion of the gingival margin.
  - Removal of a layer of fluoride-rich tooth surface.
  - Overheating of the dental structure with a power-driven polisher.

B. Stains Incorporated within Acquired Pellicle

- When stain is included within the acquired pellicle, it can be removed with a toothbrush and interdental aid(s).

C. Stains Incorporated within the Tooth

- When stain is intrinsic, whether exogenous or endogenous, it cannot be removed by scaling or polishing. Evaluation for possible whitening procedures may be considered. (See Chapter 43.)
- If stain removal is inadequate, microabrasion is another noninvasive approach that can be used.[37]
- For more extensive deep staining, porcelain veneers or crowns may be necessary to restore esthetics.[37]

Extrinsic Stains

There are two broad categories for extrinsic stains[36]:

- Directed extrinsic stains caused by compounds, organic chromogens, attached to the pellicle producing a stain.
- Indirect extrinsic stains result from chemical interaction with the tooth surface that creates a colored stain.

The most frequently observed stains—yellow, green, black line, and tobacco—are described first; descriptions of the less common orange, red, and metallic stains follow.

I. Yellow Stain

A. Clinical Features

- Dull, yellowish discoloration of dental biofilm is illustrated in **Figure 10**.

B. Distribution on Tooth Surfaces

- Yellow stain can be generalized or localized.

C. Occurrence

- More common in older adults.
- More evident when oral self-care is inadequate.

D. Etiology

- Dietary sources.
- Tobacco use.

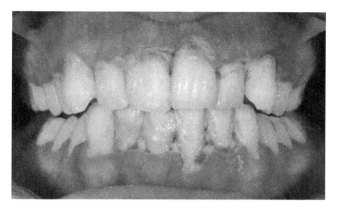

Figure 10 Yellow Stain. Generalized, dull, yellowish discoloration of dental biofilm.
© Danielzgombic/E+/Getty Images.

II. Green Stain

A. Clinical Features

- Light or yellowish green to very dark green.[38]
- Occurs in three general forms:
  - Small curved line following contour of facial gingival margin.
  - Irregular coverage of flat tooth surfaces.
  - Streaked, following grooves or lines in enamel.

B. Distribution on Tooth Surfaces

- Most frequently facial gingival third of maxillary anterior teeth.[38]

C. Composition

- **Chromogenic** bacteria.
- Decomposed hemoglobin.
- Inorganic elements include copper, nickel, and other elements in small amounts.[38]

D. Occurrence

- May occur at any age; primarily found in childhood.
- Collects on both permanent and primary teeth.

E. Recurrence

- Recurrence depends on thoroughness of oral self-care.

F. Etiology

- Green stain results from poor oral hygiene, dental biofilm retention, chromogenic bacteria, and gingival hemorrhage.[38]

- Chromogenic bacteria are nourished in dental biofilm where the green stain is produced.[38]
- Blood pigments from hemoglobin are decomposed by bacteria.[38]

G. Clinical Approach

- The patient may be able to remove the soft deposits with a toothbrush during oral self-care education.
- Choose the least abrasive polishing agent for stain removal.

H. Other Green Stains

- In addition to the clinical entity known as "green stain" that was just described, dental biofilm and acquired pellicle may become stained a green color by a variety of substances.
- Differential distinction may be determined by questioning the patient or from items in the medical or dental histories. Green discoloration may result from the following:
  - **Chlorophyll** preparations.
  - Metallic dust produced by some industries.
  - Green tea.
  - Certain drugs, such as smoking marijuana.

III. Black-Line Stain

- Black-line stain is a highly retentive black or dark-brown calculus-like stain that forms along the gingival third near the gingival margin. It may occur on primary or permanent teeth.

A. Other Names

- Pigmented dental biofilm, brown stain, black stain.

B. Clinical Features

- Continuous or interrupted fine line formed by pigmented spots, 1-mm wide (average), no appreciable thickness.
  - May be a wider band or even occupy entire gingival third in severe cases (rare).
- Appears black at bases of pits and fissures.
- Lower numbers of cariogenic microorganisms compared to dental biofilm that is not discolored.[39]
  - Although more research is needed, some studies have found a lower prevalence of caries in children with black-line stain.[39,40]

C. Distribution on Tooth Surfaces

- Facial and lingual surfaces; follows contour of gingival margin onto proximal surfaces.

- Rarely on facial surfaces of maxillary anterior teeth.
- Most frequently: Lingual and proximal surfaces of maxillary posterior teeth and occlusal pits.

D. Composition and Formation

- Black-line stain is composed of chromogenic microorganisms embedded in a ferric matrix with a higher phosphorus–calcium content.[39]
- Attachment of black-line stain to the tooth is by a pellicle-like structure.

E. Occurrence

- Occurrence increases with age, although most research has been done with children.[39]

F. Recurrence

- Black-line stain tends to form again despite regular personal care.
- Quantity may be less when biofilm control procedures are meticulous.

G. Predisposing Factors

- No definitive etiology, but several have been proposed, including[39]:
  - *Actinomyces* may be involved in growth of the black pigmentation.
  - Dietary habits.
  - Conflicting data exist about a connection between black-line stain and poor oral hygiene.
  - Iron supplements may promote development.

IV. Tobacco Stain

A. Clinical Features

- Light brown to dark leathery brown or black (**Figure 11**).
- Incorporated in calculus deposit.
- Heavy deposits (particularly from smokeless tobacco) may penetrate irregularities in the enamel and become exogenous intrinsic.

B. Distribution on Tooth Surface

- Diffuse staining of dental biofilm.
- Narrow band that follows contour of gingival crest, slightly above the crest.
- Wide, firm, tar-like band may cover the cervical third and extend to the central third of the crown, primarily on lingual surfaces.

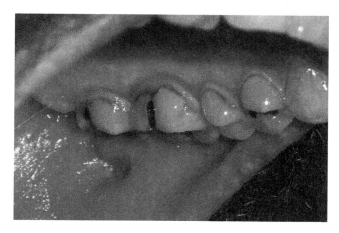

Figure 11 Tobacco Stain. Dark brown band following contour of gingival crest.

Photograph used by permission of Dr. Julius Manz, San Juan College, NM.

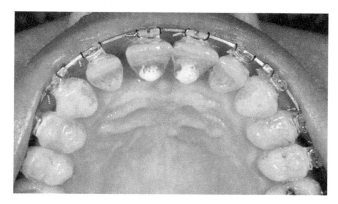

Figure 12 Brown Stain. Most likely caused by pigmented foods or drinks.

© Danielzgombic/E+/Getty Images.

C. Composition

- Tar and products of combustion.[38]
- Brown pigment from smokeless tobacco.

D. Predisposing Factors

- Smoking or chewing tobacco or use of hookah to inhale tobacco. The quantity of stain is not necessarily proportional to the amount of tobacco used.
- Inadequate oral self-care.
- Extent of dental biofilm and calculus available for adherence.

V. Brown Stains

A. Clinical Features

- The pellicle can take on stains of various colors that result from chemical alterations.
- Found primarily on buccal of maxillary molars and lingual of mandibular anterior surfaces.

B. Predisposing Factors

- Poor oral hygiene may be associated with it.
- Tannins in tea, coffee, soy sauce, and other foods may also deposit in the pellicle, resulting in brown stain (**Figure 12**).

C. Stannous Fluoride

- Light brown, sometimes yellowish, stain forms on the teeth in the pellicle.
  - Studies suggest minimal stain accumulation after 6 months with twice daily use, so it is important to weigh the risk of stain with the benefits of use in reducing gingivitis and as an antiplaque agent.[41]

- The brown stain results from the formation of stannous sulfide or brown tin oxide from the reaction of the tin ion in the fluoride compound.[41]

D. Antimicrobial Agents

- Chlorhexidine and essential oil/phenol are used in mouth rinses and are effective against biofilm formation.[42]
- Chromogenic polyphenols in the diet such as coffee, tea, and wine may interact with chlorhexidine and worsen the staining.[36]
- A brownish stain on the tongue and tooth surfaces may result, usually more pronounced on proximal and other surfaces less accessible to routine biofilm control procedures.[36]
- The stain also tends to form more rapidly on exposed roots than on enamel. Tooth staining is considered a significant side effect.
- Clinical implications
  - Stain may not be removable from enamel defects, anterior composite, and crown- or veneer-type restorations.
  - Careful consideration of risk versus benefit of use as an antimicrobial agent is needed by the patient and clinician.

E. Betel/Areca

- The betel nut is a seed of the *Areca catechu*, a type of palm tree.
  - The nut is ground and other ingredients such as flavoring and tobacco may be added to create a "chew" or "**quid**." Betel chewing is common among people of all ages in Micronesian islands, such as Guam, and Asian countries, particularly China.[43] In the Polynesian islands,

the use has cultural connections and is used in religious ceremonies.

- The discoloration imparted to the teeth is a dark mahogany brown, sometimes almost black. It may become thick and hard, with partly smooth and partly rough surfaces.
- Microscopically, the black deposit consists of microorganisms and mineralized material with a laminated pattern characteristic of subgingival calculus.[44]

F. Swimmer Stain

- Frequent exposure to pools disinfected with chlorine or bromine can cause yellowish or dark brown stains on the facial surfaces of maxillary and mandibular incisor teeth.[45]

VI. Orange and Red Stains

A. Clinical Appearance

- Orange or red stains appear at the cervical third.

B. Distribution on Tooth Surfaces

- More frequently on anterior than on posterior teeth.

C. Occurrence

- Rare (red rarer than orange).

D. Etiology

- Possibly chromogenic bacteria.
- Poor oral hygiene.[36]

VII. Metallic Stains

A. Metals or Metallic Salts from Metal-Containing Dust of Industry

- Clinical appearance/examples of colors on teeth[36]:
  - Copper or brass: Green or bluish-green.
  - Iron: Brown to greenish-brown.
  - Nickel: Green.
  - Cadmium: Yellow or golden brown.
- Distribution on tooth surfaces
  - Primarily anterior; may occur on any teeth.
  - Cervical third more commonly affected.
- Manner of formation
  - Industrial workers inhale dust through the mouth, bringing aerosolized metallic particles in contact with teeth.
  - Metal imparts color to pellicle.
  - Occasionally, stain may penetrate tooth surface and become exogenous intrinsic stain.

- Prevention
  - Workers need to be advised to wear a mask while working.

Endogenous Intrinsic Stains

I. Pulpless or Traumatized Teeth

Not all pulpless teeth discolor. However, traumatized teeth that have not been treated endodontically often discolor.

A. Clinical Appearance

- A wide range of colors exists; stains may be light yellow-brown, slate gray, reddish-brown, dark brown, bluish-black, or black. Others have an orange or greenish tinge.

B. Etiology

- Blood and other pulp tissue elements may be available for breakdown as a result of hemorrhages in the pulp chamber, root canal treatment, or necrosis and decomposition of the pulp tissue.[36]
- Pigments from the decomposed hemoglobin and pulp tissue penetrate and discolor the dentinal tubules.

II. Disturbances in Tooth Development

- Stains incorporated within the tooth structure may be related to the period of tooth development.[36,46]
- Defective tooth development may result from factors of genetic abnormality or environmental influences during tooth development.

A. Hereditary: Genetic

- **Amelogenesis imperfecta**: The enamel is partially or completely missing due to a generalized disturbance of the ameloblasts. Teeth are yellow to yellowish-brown.
- **Dentinogenesis imperfecta** (*opalescent dentin*): The dentin is abnormal as a result of disturbances in the odontoblastic layer during development. The teeth appear translucent or opalescent and vary in color from yellow-brown to blue-gray.[46]

B. Developmental Enamel Defects

- Development enamel defects (DDE) include enamel hypoplasia, enamel opacity, and molar-incisor hypomineralization (MIH) and result from damage to the tooth germ during development; the location of the defect(s) is typically related to the timing of the injury during development.[47]

- *Generalized* **hypoplasia** (**chronologic** hypoplasia resulting from ameloblastic disturbance of short duration) may extend across multiple teeth and color may vary from chalky white to yellow or brown.[48]
- *Local hypoplasia* affects a single tooth (e.g., individual white spots, caused by trauma to a primary tooth).

- Clinical appearance[48]:
  - Teeth erupt with white spots, pits, or grooves depending on the severity of the injury to the tooth germ.
  - Over time, the enamel hypoplasia defects are prone to extrinsic stain.
- Etiology[47,48]
  - Trauma or **infection** of an individual tooth.
  - Rubella infection or disease causing a high fever.
  - Drug intake during pregnancy.
  - Preterm birth.
  - Hypocalcemia (low calcium) levels such as in premature infants.

C. Dental Fluorosis

- Dental fluorosis was originally called "brown stain." Later, Dr. Frederick S. McKay studied the condition and described it in the dental literature as "mottled enamel."
- Etiology
  - Enamel hypomineralization results from ingestion of excessive fluoride ion from any source during the period of mineralization. The enamel alterations are a result of toxic damage to the ameloblasts.
  - Severity is related to the age and dose of fluoride exposure.[49,50]
- Fluorosis classification
  - There are several indices for classifying fluorosis.[50] (See Chapter 34.)
- Clinical appearance
  - When the teeth erupt, the color of the enamel ranges from chalky white spots to brown. Depending on the severity of the enamel defect(s), discoloration may occur over time.[49]
  - Severe effects of excess fluoride during development may produce cracks or pitting. This condition and appearance led to the name *mottled enamel*.

III. Drug-Induced Stains and Discolorations

A. Tetracycline

- Tetracycline antibiotics have an affinity for calcium and form complexes with hydroxyapatite crystals in mineralized tissues (**Figure 13**).[51]
- Discoloration of a child's teeth may result when the drug is administered to the mother during the fourth month of pregnancy or to the child in infancy and early childhood.[51]
- Etiology
  - The discoloration depends on the dosage, length of time used, and type of tetracycline prescribed.[51]
- Clinical appearance[51]
  - Discoloration may be generalized or localized to individual teeth that were developing at the time of administration of the antibiotic.
  - Color of teeth may be light green to dark yellow, or a gray-brown, with or without banding and approximate age when the antibiotic was taken.
  - The patient's medical history may reveal the illness for which the antibiotic was prescribed.

B. Minocycline

- Unlike tetracycline, minocycline has been reported to cause generalized intrinsic staining posteruption.[52]
- Clinical appearance
  - Use of minocycline can result in a generalized intrinsic blue-gray to gray staining of the permanent teeth.[52]

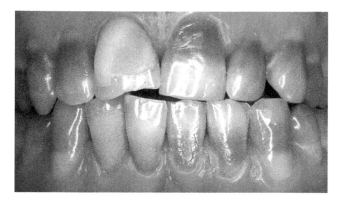

Figure 13 Tetracycline Stain. Tetracycline staining in this permanent dentition resulted from the administration of tetracycline antibiotic during the time that crowns formed. Teeth have the appearance of yellow to gray-brown horizontal bands across the crowns. (The staining on tooth no. 8 has been covered with a tooth-colored restorative material such as composite resin.)

Courtesy of Carl Allen, DDS, MSD.

- Etiology
  - Several theories exist about the mechanism related to intrinsic and extrinsic mechanisms for the stain.[52]

Exogenous Intrinsic Stains

- When intrinsic stains come from an outside source, not from within the tooth, the stain is called exogenous intrinsic.
- Extrinsic stains result from stain in the tooth following development and may occur when the stain penetrates enamel defects and exposed dentin to become intrinsic (**Figure 14**). These may also be called internalized discoloration.[36]
- The sources of these stains may include:[36]
  - Developmental defects.
  - Acquired defects such as tooth wear and gingival recession.
  - Dental caries.
  - Restorative materials.

I. Restorative Materials

A. Silver Amalgam

- Silver amalgam can impart a gray to black discoloration to the tooth structure around a restoration.
- Tin migrates from the amalgam restoration into the enamel and dentin.[36]

B. Endodontic Therapy

- Discoloration tends to be most evident on the cervical third of the crown and root surface.[53]
- Materials used during endodontic therapy can cause intrinsic staining.[53]

- Endodontic sealers may cause stain ranging in color from orange-red to gray.
- Endodontic medicaments, which may include tetracycline, may cause a dark brown intrinsic stain.
- Portland cement–based materials may cause a gray intrinsic stain.
- Antibiotic pastes used in regenerative endodontic procedures may also contain tetracycline, but also ciprofloxacin, metronidazole, or minocycline, and result in a green-brown staining.

II. Stain in Dentin

- Discoloration resulting from a carious lesion is an example.
- Arrested decay or secondary dentin can present as black stain on severely decayed teeth. The surface is hard and glossy, and stain cannot be removed.

III. Other Local Causes

- Enamel erosion is the loss of hard tissue by chemical means such as acidic foods (including carbonated drinks), eating disorders (bulimia), and gastroesophageal reflux disease.[54,55]
  - Resulting thinner enamel allows the yellow color of the underlying dentin to show through and cause the teeth to appear duller gray or yellow (**Figure 15**).
- Attrition of occlusal surfaces can result in loss of enamel, allowing a yellow or brown outline of dentin to show through (**Figure 16**).

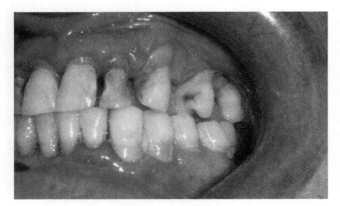

Figure 14 Exogenous Intrinsic Stain. Most likely from an outside source such as tobacco or food and becomes intrinsic over time. Areas of attrition allow yellow color of underlying dentin to be exposed and become further stained.

Photograph used by permission of Dr. Julius Manz, San Juan College, NM.

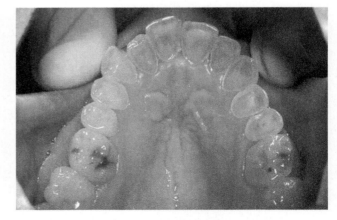

Figure 15 Enamel Erosion. The extensive enamel erosion reveals the yellow color of the dentin on the lingual surfaces of anterior teeth and premolars. This individual had chronic severe gastroesophageal reflux disease (GERD) of more than 10 years' duration.

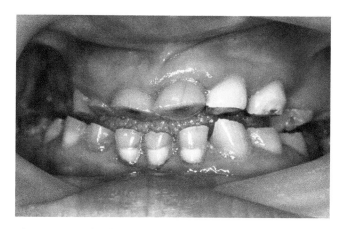

Figure 16 Attrition. Attrition of the maxillary teeth exposing the yellow dentin and brown of the pulp chamber.

Courtesy of Dr. Richard Foster, Guilford Technical Community College, Jamestown, NC.

Documentation

The permanent records for each patient should include information relating to the soft deposits, calculus, and stain, including:

- Clinical description of appearance of the teeth relative to the biofilm, materia alba, or food debris as indications of the personal oral care on a daily basis.
- The extent of supragingival and subgingival deposits (slight, moderate, or heavy) should be described in the initial examination record and charted to show location for reference during the clinical removal and during teaching personal care for prevention.
- Record color, type, extent, and location of stains with the patient's examination and assessment.
- Personal patient care procedures demonstrated, preventive measures discussed, and frequency of continuing care appointments recommended.
  See **Box 2** for a sample documentation note.

Factors to Teach the Patient

- Location, composition, and properties of dental biofilm and calculus with emphasis on its role in dental caries and periodontal infections.
- Effects of personal oral care procedures in the prevention of dental biofilm, calculus, and stain.
- Biofilm control procedures with special adaptations for individual needs.
- Sources of cariogenic foodstuff in the diet and frequency of consumption in relation to dental caries formation.
- What calculus is and how it forms from dental biofilm.
- Etiology of individual's dental stains and discolorations with suggestions for modification of sources of extrinsic stain.
- Advantages of a smoking cessation program.
- Effect of tetracyclines on developing teeth. Need to avoid use during pregnancy and by children to age 12 years.
- Select products with an American Dental Association or Canadian Dental Association Seal of Acceptance.

References

1. Marsh PD, Zaura E. Dental biofilm: ecological interactions in health and disease. *J Clin Periodontol*. 2017;44(S18):S12-S22.

2. Rasputnis W, Schestakow A, Hannig M. The dentin pellicle: a neglected topic in dental research. *Arch Oral Biol*. 2021;129:105212.

3. Siqueira WL, Custodio W, McDonald EE. New insights into the composition and functions of the acquired enamel pellicle. *J Dent Res*. 2012;91(12):1110-1118.

4. Hannig M. Ultrastructural investigation of pellicle morphogenesis at two different intraoral sites during a 24-h period. *Clin Oral Investig*. 1999;3(2):88-95.

5. Hara AT, Zero DT. The caries environment: saliva, pellicle, diet, and hard tissue ultrastructure. *Dent Clin North Am*. 2010;54(3):455-467.

6. Seneviratne C, Zhang C, Samaranayake L. Bacterial biofilm and associated infections. Chin J Dent Res. 2011;14(2):87-94.

7. Huang R, Li M, Gregory RL. Bacterial interactions in dental biofilm. *Virulence*. 2011;2(5):435-444.

8. Jamal M, Ahmad W, Andleeb S, et al. Bacterial biofilm and associated infections. J Chin Med Assoc. 2018;81(1):7-11.

9. Kilian M, Chapple ILC, Hannig M, et al. The oral microbiome - an update for oral healthcare professionals. *Br Dent J*. 2016;221(10):657-666.

10. Loe H, Theilade E, Jensen SB. Experimental gingivitis in man. *J Periodontol*. 1965;36:177-187.

11. Abusleme L, Hoare A, Hong B-Y, Diaz PI. Microbial signatures of health, gingivitis, and periodontitis. *Periodontol 2000*. 2021;86(1):57-78.

12. Zijnge V, van Leeuwen MBM, Degener JE, et al. Oral biofilm architecture on natural teeth. *PLoS One*. 2010;5(2):e9321.

13. Curtis MA, Diaz PI, Van Dyke TE. The role of the microbiota in periodontal disease. *Periodontol 2000*. 2020;83(1):14-25.

14. Tribble GD, Lamont RJ. Bacterial invasion of epithelial cells and spreading in periodontal tissue. *Periodontol 2000*. 2010;52(1):68-83.

15. Tanaka M, Matsunaga K, Kadoma Y. Correlation in inorganic ion concentration between saliva and plaque fluid. *J Med Dent Sci*. 2000;47(1):55-59.

16. Naumova EA, Kuehnl P, Hertenstein P, et al. Fluoride bioavailability in saliva and plaque. *BMC Oral Health*. 2012;12:3.

17. Koo H, Allan RN, Howlin RP, Stoodley P, Hall-Stoodley L. Targeting microbial biofilms: current and prospective therapeutic strategies. *Nat Rev Microbiol*. 2017;15(12):740-755.

18. Sreenivasan PK, Prasad KVV. Distribution of dental plaque and gingivitis within the dental arches. *J Int Med Res*. 2017;45(5):1585-1596.

19. Tanner ACR, Kressirer CA, Rothmiller S, Johansson I, Chalmers NI. The caries microbiome: implications for reversing dysbiosis. *Adv Dent Res*. 2018;29(1):78-85.

20. Ribeiro AA, Azcarate-Peril MA, Cadenas MB, et al. The oral bacterial microbiome of occlusal surfaces in children and its association with diet and caries. *PLoS One*. 2017;12(7):e0180621.

21. Johansson I, Witkowska E, Kaveh B, Lif Holgerson P, Tanner ACR. The microbiome in populations with a low and high prevalence of caries. *J Dent Res*. 2016;95(1):80-86.

22. Lingström P, van Ruyven FO, van Houte J, Kent R. The pH of dental plaque in its relation to early enamel caries and dental plaque flora in humans. *J Dent Res*. 2000;79(2):770-777.

23. Bowen WH. The Stephan Curve revisited. *Odontology*. 2013;101(1):2-8.

24. Hoppenbrouwers PM, Driessens FC, Borggreven JM. The mineral solubility of human tooth roots. *Arch Oral Biol*. 1987;32(5):319-322.

25. Khairnar M. Classification of food impaction - revisited and its management. *Indian J Dent Res*. 5(1):1113-1119.

26. Aylıkcı BU, Çolak H. Halitosis: from diagnosis to management. *J Nat Sci Biol Med*. 2013;4(1):14-23.

27. Akcalı A, Lang NP. Dental calculus: the calcified biofilm and its role in disease development. *Periodontol 2000*. 2018;76(1):109-115.

28. Abraham J, Grenón M, Sánchez HJ, Pérez C, Barrea R. A case study of elemental and structural composition of dental calculus during several stages of maturation using SRXRF. *J Biomed Mater Res Part A*. 2005;75A(3):623-628.

29. Jin Y, Yip H-K. Supragingival calculus: formation and control. *Crit Rev Oral Biol Med*. 2002;13(5):426-441.

30. Fons-Badal C, Fons-Font A, Labaig-Rueda C, Fernanda Solá-Ruiz M, Selva-Otaolaurruchi E, Agustín-Panadero R. Analysis of predisposing factors for rapid dental calculus formation. *J Clin Med*. 2020;9(3):E858.

31. Carino A, Ludwig C, Cervellino A, Müller E, Testino A. Formation and transformation of calcium phosphate phases under biologically relevant conditions: experiments and modelling. *Acta Biomater*. 2018;74:478-488.

32. Selvig KA. Attachment of plaque and calculus to tooth surfaces. *J Periodontal Res*. 1970;5(1):8-18.

33. Rohanizadeh R, LeGeros RZ. Ultrastructural study of calculus–enamel and calculus–root interfaces. *Arch Oral Biol*. 2005;50(1):89-96.

34. Sanz M, Herrera D, Kebschull M, et al. Treatment of stage I-III periodontitis-the EFP S3 level clinical practice guideline. *J Clin Periodontol*. 2020;47(Suppl 22):4-60.

35. Osborn JB, Lenton PA, Lunos SA, Blue CM. Endoscopic vs. tactile evaluation of subgingival calculus. *J Dent Hyg*. 2014;88(4):229-236.

36. Watts A, Addy M. Tooth discolouration and staining: a review of the literature. *Br Dent J*. 2001;190(6):309-316.

37. Kapadia Y, Jain V. Tooth staining: a review of etiology and treatment modalities. *Acta Sci Dent Sci*. 2018;2(6):67-70.

38. Prathap S, Rajesh H, Boloor VA, Rao AS. Extrinsic stains and management: a new insight. *J Acad Indus Res*. 2013;1(8):435-442.

39. Elelmi Y, Mabrouk R, Masmoudi F, Baaziz A, Maatouk F, Ghedira H. Black stain and dental caries in primary teeth of Tunisian preschool children. *Eur Arch Paediatr Dent*. 2021;22(2):235-240.

40. Asokan S, Varshini KR, Geetha Priya PR, Vijayasankari V. Association between black stains and early childhood caries: a systematic review. *Indian J Dent Res*. 2020;31(6):957-962.

41. Milleman KR, Patil A, Ling MR, Mason S, Milleman JL. An exploratory study to investigate stain build-up with long term use of a stannous fluoride dentifrice. *Am J Dent*. 2018;31(2):71-75.

42. Figuero E, Herrera D, Tobías A, et al. Efficacy of adjunctive anti-plaque chemical agents in managing gingivitis: a systematic review and network meta-analyses. *J Clin Periodontol*. 2019;46(7):723-739.

43. Saraswat N, Pillay R, Everett B, George A. Knowledge, attitudes and practices of South Asian immigrants in developed countries regarding oral cancer: an integrative review. *BMC Cancer*. 2020;20(1):477.

44. Reichart PA, Lenz H, König H, Becker J, Mohr U. The black layer on the teeth of betel chewers: a light microscopic, microradiographic and electronmicroscopic study. *J Oral Pathol*. 1985;14(6):466-475.

45. Escartin JL, Arnedo A, Pinto V, Vela MJ. A study of dental staining among competitive swimmers. *Community Dent Oral Epidemiol*. 2000;28(1):10-17.

46. American Academy of Pediatric Dentistry, Council on Clinical Affairs. Guideline on dental management of heritable dental developmental anomalies. *Pediatr Dent*. 2016;38(6):302-307.

47. Bensi C, Costacurta M, Belli S, Paradiso D, Docimo R. Relationship between preterm birth and developmental defects of enamel: a systematic review and meta-analysis. *Int J Paediatr Dent*. 2020;30(6):676-686.

48. Rodd HD, Graham A, Tajmehr N, Timms L, Hasmun N. Molar incisor hypomineralisation: current knowledge and practice. *Int Dent J*. 2021;71(4):285-291.

49. Fejerskov O, Manji F, Baelum V. The nature and mechanisms of dental fluorosis in man. *J Dent Res*. 1990;69 Spec No:692-700; discussion 721.

50. Rozier RG. Epidemiologic indices for measuring the clinical manifestations of dental fluorosis: overview and critique. *Adv Dent Res*. 1994;8(1):39-55.

51. Thomas MS, Denny C. Medication-related tooth discoloration: a review. *Dent Update*. 2014;41(5):440-447.

52. Good M, Hussey D. Minocycline: stain devil?: your access options. *Br J Dermatol*. 2003;149(2):237-239.

53. Krastl G, Allgayer N, Lenherr P, Filippi A, Taneja P, Weiger R. Tooth discoloration induced by endodontic materials: a literature review. *Dent Traumatol*. 2013;29(1):2-7.

54. Ortiz ADC, Fideles SOM, Pomini KT, Buchaim RL. Updates in association of gastroesophageal reflux disease and dental erosion: systematic review. *Expert Rev Gastroenterol Hepatol*. 2021;15(9):1037-1046.

55. Chan AS, Tran TTK, Hsu YH, Liu SYS, Kroon J. A systematic review of dietary acids and habits on dental erosion in adolescents. *Int J Paediatr Dent*. 2020;30(6):713-733.

Indices and Scoring Methods

Lisa F. Mallonee, RDH, RD, LD, MPH
Charlotte J. Wyche, RDH, MS

CHAPTER OUTLINE

After studying this chapter, the student will be able to:

1. Identify and define key terms and concepts related to dental indices and scoring methods.
2. Identify the purpose, criteria for measurement, scoring methods, range of scores, and reference or interpretation scales for a variety of dental indices.
3. Select and calculate dental indices for a use in a specific patient or community situation.

This chapter provides an introduction to scoring methods used by clinicians, researchers, and community practitioners to evaluate **indicators** of oral health **status**. It is not possible to explain all of the many dental indices that have been used in a variety of settings, but the most notable, current, and widely used indices and scoring methods are described in this chapter.

Types of Scoring Methods

Indices and scoring methods are used in clinical practice and by community programs to determine and record the oral health status of individuals and groups.

I. Individual Assessment Score

A. Purpose

In clinical practice, an **index**, or a scoring system, for an individual patient can be used to measure the amount or condition of oral disease or related condition in individuals or a population for purposes of evaluation, education or motivation.[1]

- An index is based on a graduated scale with defined upper and lower limits.
- Used for data collection and comparisons of individuals or population groups using established criteria.
- Frequently used in clinical trials.

B. Uses

- To provide individual assessment to help a patient recognize an oral problem.
- To reveal the degree of effectiveness of oral hygiene practices.
- To motivate the patient during preventive and professional care for the elimination and control of oral disease.
- To evaluate the success of individual oral self-care, professional treatment, and status of oral disease over a period of time by comparing index scores.

II. Clinical Trial

A. Purpose

A clinical trial is planned to determine the effect of an agent or a procedure on the prevention, progression, or control of a disease.

- The trial is conducted by comparing an experimental group with a control group that is similar to the experimental group in every way, except for the variable being studied.
- Examiners who collect dental index data for research are **calibrated** or trained to measure the index in exactly the same way each time.
- Examples of indices used for clinical trials are the biofilm index (BI)[2,3] and the patient hygiene performance (PHP).[4]

B. Uses

- To determine baseline **data** before experimental factors are introduced.
- To measure the effectiveness of specific agents for the prevention, control, or treatment of oral conditions.
- To measure the effectiveness of mechanical devices for personal care, such as toothbrushes, interdental cleaning devices, or irrigators.

III. Epidemiologic Survey

A. Purpose

The word **epidemiology** denotes the study of disease characteristics of populations rather than individuals. Epidemiologic surveys provide information on the trends and patterns of oral health and disease in populations.

B. Uses

- To determine the **prevalence** and **incidence** of a particular condition occurring within a given population.
- To provide baseline data on indicators that show existing dental health status in populations.

- The *Surgeon General's Report(s) on Oral Health in America* used epidemiologic data to identify oral health disparities in certain populations.[5,6]
- To provide data to support recommendations for public health interventions to improve the health status of populations, such as those provided in the U.S. *Healthy People 2030* document.[7]

IV. Community Surveillance

A. Purpose

Community oral health assessment is a multifaceted process of identifying factors that affect the oral health status of a selected population. Community **surveillance** of oral health indicators and **determinants** can be accomplished at many levels.

- Government agencies, local community-based service-providing agencies, and professional associations are examples of groups that collect data to determine oral health status by conducting oral health **screenings**.
- Information from community-wide oral screenings can be used when planning local community-based oral health services or education.
- An example of a system designed to be used by a community-based group is the Association of State and Territorial Dental Directors' (ASTDD) Basic Screening Survey.[8]

B. Uses

- To assess the needs of a community.
- To help plan community-based health promotion/disease prevention programs.
- To compare the effects or evaluate the results of community-based programs.

Indices

An index is a way of expressing clinical observations by using numbers. The use of numbers can provide standardized information to make observations of a health condition consistent and less subjective than a word description of that condition.

I. Descriptive Categories of Indices

A. General Categories

- Simple index: Measures the presence or absence of a condition. An example is the biofilm index

that measures the presence of dental biofilm without evaluating its effect on the gingiva.
- Cumulative index: Measures all the evidence of a condition, past and present. An example is the DMFT index for dental caries.

B. Types of Simple and Cumulative Indices

- Irreversible index: Measures conditions that will not change. An example is an index that measures dental caries experience.
- Reversible index: Measures conditions that can be changed. Examples are indices that measure dental biofilm.

II. Selection Criteria

A useful and effective index:
- Is simple to use and calculate.
- Requires minimal equipment, expense, and time to complete.
- Is acceptable to the individuals being measured; does not cause discomfort.
- Has clear-cut criteria that are readily understandable.
- Is objective—free from subjective interpretation.
- Has **validity**—measures what it is intended to measure
- Has **reliability**—is reproducible by the same examiner or different examiners.
- Is quantifiable—statistics can be applied to data collected.

Oral Hygiene Status (Biofilm, Debris, and Calculus)

Indices that measure oral hygiene status can be used in a clinical setting to educate and motivate an individual patient. When data are collected in a community setting, such as a nursing home, the findings can help determine how daily oral care is being provided and monitor the results of oral hygiene education programs.

I. Biofilm Index (BI)

This index was historically known as plaque index (PI).[2,3]

A. Purpose

- To assess the thickness of biofilm at the gingival area.

B. Selection of Teeth

- The entire dentition or selected teeth can be evaluated.
- *Areas examined:* Examine four gingival areas (distal, facial, mesial, and lingual) systematically for each tooth.
- *Modified procedures:* Examine only the facial, mesial, and lingual areas. Assign double score to the mesial reading and divide the total by 4.

C. Procedure

- Dry the teeth and examine visually using adequate light, mouth mirror, and probe or explorer.
- Evaluate dental biofilm on the cervical third; pay no attention to biofilm that has extended to the middle or incisal thirds of the tooth.
- Use probe to test the surface when no biofilm is visible. Pass the probe or explorer across the tooth surface in the cervical third and near the entrance to the sulcus. When no biofilm adheres to the probe tip, the area is scored 0. When biofilm adheres, a score of 1 is assigned.
- Use a disclosing agent, if necessary, to assist evaluation for the 0–1 scores. When the Pl I is used in conjunction with the gingival index (GI), the GI is completed first because the disclosing agent masks the gingival characteristics.
- Include biofilm on the surface of calculus and on dental restorations in the cervical third in the evaluation.
- Criteria

Biofilm Index

Score	Criteria
0	No biofilm.
1	A film of biofilm adhering to the free gingival margin and adjacent area of the tooth. The biofilm may be recognized only after application of disclosing agent or by running the explorer across the tooth surface.
2	Moderate accumulation of soft deposits within the gingival pocket that can be seen with the naked eye or on the tooth and gingival margin.
3	Abundance of soft matter within the gingival pocket and/or on the tooth and gingival margin.

D. Scoring

- BI for area
  - Each area of a tooth (distal, facial, mesial, lingual, or palatal) is assigned a score from 0 to 3.
- BI for a tooth
  - Scores for each area are totaled and divided by 4.
- BI for groups of teeth
  - Scores for individual teeth may be grouped and totaled and divided by the number of teeth. For instance, a BI may be determined for specific teeth or groups of teeth. The right side of the dentition may be compared with the left.
- BI for the individual
  - Add the scores for each tooth and divide by the number of teeth examined. The BI score ranges from 0 to 3.
- Suggested range of scores for patient reference

Rating	Scores
Excellent	0
Good	0.1–0.9
Fair	1.0–1.9
Poor	2.0–3.0

- BI for a group
  - Add the scores for each member of a group and divide by the number of individuals.

II. Biofilm Control Record (BCR)

This index was previously known as the plaque control record.[9]

A. Purpose

- To record the presence of dental biofilm on individual tooth surfaces to permit the patient to visualize progress while learning biofilm control.

B. Selection of Teeth and Surfaces

- All teeth are included. Missing teeth are identified on the record form by a single, thick horizontal line.
- Four surfaces are recorded: Facial, lingual, mesial, and distal.
- Six areas may be recorded. The mesial and distal segments of the diagram may be divided to

provide space to record proximal surfaces from the facial separately from the lingual or palatal surfaces (**Figure 1**).[10]

C. Procedure

- Apply disclosing agent or give a chewable tablet. Instruct patient to swish and rub the solution over the tooth surfaces with the tongue before rinsing.
- Examine each tooth surface for dental biofilm at the gingival margin. No attempt is made to differentiate the quantity of biofilm.
- Record by making a dash or color in the appropriate spaces on the diagram (Figure 1) to indicate biofilm on facial, lingual, palatal, mesial, and/or distal surfaces.

D. Scoring

- Total the number of teeth present and multiply by 4 to obtain the number of available surfaces. Count the number of surfaces with biofilm.
- Multiply the number of biofilm-stained surfaces by 100 and divide by the total number of available surfaces to derive the percentage of surfaces with biofilm.
- Compare scores over subsequent appointments as the patient learns and practices biofilm control. Ten percent or less biofilm-stained surfaces can be considered a good goal, but if the biofilm is regularly left in the same areas, special instruction is indicated.

- Calculation: Example for biofilm control record
  - Individual findings: 26 teeth scored; 8 surfaces with biofilm.
  - Multiply the number of teeth by 4: $26 \times 4 = 104$ surfaces.
  - Percentage with biofilm =

$$\frac{Number\ of\ surfaces\ with\ biofilm \times 100}{Number\ of\ available\ tooth\ surfaces} = \frac{8 \times 100}{104}$$

$$= \frac{800}{104}$$

$$= 7.7\%$$

- Interpretation
  - Although 0% is ideal, less than 10% biofilm-stained surfaces has been suggested as a guideline in periodontal therapy. After initial therapy and when the patient has reached a 10% level of biofilm control or better, necessary additional periodontal and restorative procedures may be initiated.[9] In comparison, a similar evaluation using a biofilm-free score would mean that a goal of 90% or better biofilm-free surfaces would have to be reached before the surgical phase of treatment could be undertaken.

III. Biofilm-Free Score (BFS)

This index was historically called the plaque-free score.[11]

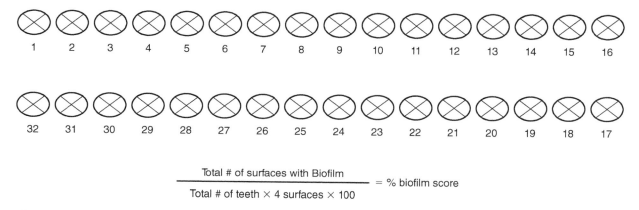

$$\frac{Total\ \#\ of\ surfaces\ with\ Biofilm}{Total\ \#\ of\ teeth \times 4\ surfaces \times 100} = \%\ biofilm\ score$$

Figure 1 Biofilm Control Record. Diagrammatic representation of the teeth includes spaces to record biofilm on six areas of each tooth. The facial surfaces are on the outer portion and the lingual and palatal surfaces are on the inner portion of the arches. Teeth are numbered by the American Dental Association system on the inside and by the Fédération Dentaire Internationale system on the outside.

A. Purpose

- To determine the location, number, and percentage of biofilm-free surfaces for individual motivation and instruction. Interdental bleeding can also be documented.

B. Selection of Teeth and Surfaces

- All erupted teeth are included. Missing teeth are identified on the record form by a single, thick horizontal line through the box in the chart form.
- Four surfaces are recorded for each tooth: Facial, lingual or palatal, mesial, and distal.

C. Procedure

- Biofilm-free score
  - Apply disclosing agent or give chewable tablet. Instruct patient to swish and rub the solution over the tooth surfaces with the tongue before rinsing.
  - Examine each tooth surface for evidence of biofilm using adequate light and a mouth mirror.
  - The patient needs a hand mirror to see the location of the biofilm missed during personal hygiene procedures.
  - Use an appropriate tooth chart form or a diagrammatic form, such as that shown in **Figure** 2. Red ink for recording the biofilm is suggested when a red disclosing agent is used to help the patient associate the location of the biofilm in the mouth with the recording.
- Papillary bleeding on probing
  - The small circles between the diagrammatic tooth blocks in Figure 2 are used to record proximal bleeding on probing.
  - Improvement in the gingival tissue health will be demonstrated over a period of time as fewer bleeding areas are noted.

Content removed due to copyright restrictions

Figure 2 Biofilm-Free Score. **A:** Diagrammatic representation of the teeth used to record biofilm and papillary bleeding. **B:** Enlargement of one section of the diagram shows tooth surfaces. Teeth are numbered by the American Dental Association system inside each block and by the Fédération Dentaire Internationale system outside each block.

D. Scoring: Biofilm-Free Score

- Total the number of teeth present.
- Total the number of surfaces with biofilm that appear in red on the tooth diagram.
- To calculate the biofilm-free score:
  - Multiply the number of teeth by 4 to determine the number of available surfaces.
  - Subtract the number of surfaces with biofilm from the total available surfaces to find the number of biofilm-free surfaces.
  - Biofilm-free score

$$\frac{Number\ of\ Biofilm\text{-}free\ surface \times 100}{Number\ of\ available\ surfaces}$$

$$= Percentage\ of\ biofilm\text{-}free\ surfaces$$

- Evaluate biofilm-free score: Ideally, 100% is the goal. When a patient maintains a percentage under 85%, check individual surfaces to determine whether biofilm is usually left in the same areas. To prevent the development of specific areas of periodontal infection, remedial instruction in the areas usually missed is indicated.
- Calculation: Example for biofilm-free score
  - Individual findings: 24 teeth scored and 37 surfaces with biofilm.
  - Multiply the number of teeth by 4: $24 \times 4 = 96$ available surfaces.
  - Subtract the number of surfaces with biofilm from total available surfaces: $96 - 37 = 59$ biofilm-free surfaces.
  - Percentage of biofilm-free surfaces

$$\frac{59 \times 100}{96} = 61.5\%$$

- Interpretation
  - On the basis of the ideal 100%, 61.5% is poor. More personal daily oral care instruction is indicated.

E. Scoring: Papillary Bleeding on Probing

- Total the number of small circles marked for bleeding. A patient with 32 teeth has 30 interdental areas. The mesial or distal surface of a tooth adjacent to an edentulous area is probed and counted.
- Evaluate total interdental bleeding. In health, bleeding on probing does not occur.

IV. Patient Hygiene Performance (PHP)[4]

A. Purpose

- To assess the extent of biofilm and debris over a tooth surface. Debris is defined for the PHP as a soft foreign material consisting of dental biofilm, materia alba, and food debris loosely attached to tooth surfaces.

B. Selection of Teeth and Surfaces

- Teeth examined:

Maxillary	Mandibular
No. 3 (16)[a]	No. 19 (36)
Right first molar	Left first molar
No. 8 (11)	No. 24 (31)
Right central incisor	Left central incisor
No. 14 (26)	No. 30 (46)
Left first molar	Right first molar

[a]Fédération Dentaire Internationale system tooth numbers are in parentheses.

- Substitutions
  - When a first molar is missing, is less than three-fourths erupted, has a full crown, or is broken down, the second molar is used.
  - The third molar is used when the second is missing.
  - The adjacent central incisor is used for a missing incisor.
- Surfaces
  - The facial surfaces of incisors and maxillary molars and the lingual surfaces of mandibular molars are examined.

C. Procedure

- Apply disclosing agent. Instruct the patient to swish for 30 seconds and expectorate, but not rinse.
- Examination is made using a mouth mirror.

- Each tooth surface to be evaluated is subdivided (mentally) into five sections (**Figure 3A**) as follows:
  - Vertically: Three divisions—mesial, middle, and distal.
  - Horizontally: The middle third is subdivided into gingival, middle, and occlusal or incisal thirds.
- Each of the five subdivisions is scored for the presence of stained debris as follows:

Patient Hygiene Performance

Score	Criteria
0	No debris (or questionable).
1	Debris definitely present.
M	When all three molars or both incisors are missing.
S	When a substitute tooth is used.

D. Scoring

- Debris score for individual tooth
  - Add the scores for each of the five subdivisions. The scores range from 0 to 5. Examples are shown in **Figure 3B** and **Figure 3C**.
- PHP for the individual
  - Total the scores for the individual teeth and divide by the number of teeth examined. The PHP ranges from 0 to 5.
- Suggested range of scores for evaluation

Rating	Scores
Excellent	0 (no debris)
Good	0.1–1.7
Fair	1.8–3.4
Poor	3.5–5.0

- Calculation: Example for an individual

Tooth	Debris Score
No. 3 (16)	5
No. 8 (11)	3
No. 14 (26)	4
No. 19 (36)	5
No. 24 (31)	2
No. 30 (46)	3
Total	22

$$\frac{Total\ debris\ score}{Number\ of\ teeth\ scored} = \frac{22}{6} = 3.67$$

- Interpretation
  - According to the suggested range of scores, this patient with a PHP of 3.67 would be classified as exhibiting poor hygiene performance.
- PHP for a group
  - To obtain the average PHP score for a group or population, total the individual scores and divide by the number of people examined.

V. Simplified Oral Hygiene Index (OHI-S)[12,13]

A. Purpose

- To assess oral cleanliness by estimating the tooth surfaces covered with debris and/or calculus.

B. Components

- The simplified oral hygiene index (OHI-S) has two components: the simplified debris index (DI-S) and the simplified calculus index (CI-S). The two scores may be used separately or may be combined for the OHI-S.

C. Selection of Teeth and Surfaces

- Identify the six specific teeth (see **Figure 4**)
  - Posterior: The facial surfaces of the maxillary molars and the lingual surfaces of the

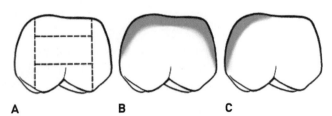

A   **B**   **C**

Figure 3 Patient Hygiene Performance. **A:** Oral debris is assessed by dividing a tooth into five subdivisions, each of which is scored 1 when debris is shown to be present after use of a disclosing agent. **B:** Example of debris score of 3. Shaded portion represents debris stained by disclosing agent. **C:** Example of debris score of 1.

Data from Podshadley AG, Haley JV. A method for evaluating oral hygiene performance. *Public Health Rep.* 1968;83(3):259-264.

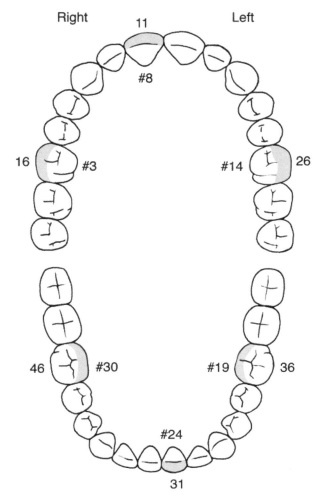

Right 11 Left

#8

16 #3 #14 26

46 #30 #19 36

#24

31

Figure 4 Simplified Oral Hygiene Index. Six tooth surfaces are scored as follows: facial surfaces of maxillary molars and of the maxillary right and mandibular left central incisors, and the lingual surfaces of mandibular molars. Teeth are numbered by the American Dental Association system on the lingual surface and by the Fédération Dentaire Internationale system on the facial surface.

mandibular molars are scored. Although usually the first molars are examined, the first fully erupted molar distal to each second premolar is used if the first molar is missing.

- Anterior: The facial surfaces of the maxillary right and the mandibular left central incisors are scored. When either is missing, the adjacent central incisor is scored.
- Extent
  - Either the facial or lingual surfaces of the selected teeth are scored, including the proximal surfaces to the contact areas.

D. Procedure

- Qualification: At least two of the six possible surfaces are examined to calculate an individual score.

- Record six debris scores
  - Definition of oral debris: Oral debris is a soft foreign matter, such as dental biofilm, material alba, and food debris on the surfaces of the teeth.
- Examination: Move the side of the tip of a probe or an explorer across the tooth surface to estimate the surface area covered by debris.
- Criteria (see **Figure 5** and the Debris Index table next).

Simplified Debris Index (DI-S)

Score	Criteria
0	No debris or stain present.
1	Soft debris covering not more than one-third of the tooth surface being examined, or presence of extrinsic stains without debris, regardless of surface area covered.
2	Soft debris covering more than one-third but not more than two-thirds of the exposed tooth surface.
3	Soft debris covering more than two-thirds of the exposed tooth surface.

- Record six calculus scores
- Examination: Use an explorer to estimate surface area covered by supragingival calculus deposits. Identify subgingival deposits by exploring and/or probing. Record only definite deposits of hard calculus.
  - Criteria: Location and tooth surface areas scored are illustrated in **Figure 6**.

Simplified Calculus Index (CI-S)

Score	Criteria
0	No calculus present.
1	Supragingival calculus covering not more than one-third of the exposed tooth surface being examined.
2	Supragingival calculus covering more than one-third but not more than two-thirds of the exposed tooth surface, or the presence of individual flecks of subgingival calculus around the cervical portion of the tooth.
3	Supragingival calculus covering more than two-thirds of the exposed tooth surface or a continuous heavy band of subgingival calculus around the cervical portion of the tooth.

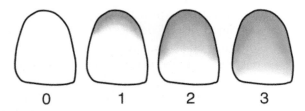

Figure 5 Simplified Oral Hygiene Index. For the debris index, six teeth (Figure 3) are scored. Scoring of 0–3 is based on tooth surfaces covered by debris as shown.

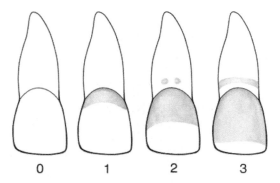

Figure 6 Simplified Oral Hygiene Index. For the calculus index, six teeth (Figure 3) are scored. Scoring of 0–3 is based on location and tooth surface area with calculus as shown. Note slight subgingival calculus recorded as 2 and more extensive subgingival calculus as 3.

E. Scoring

- *OHI-S individual score.*
- Determine separate DI-S and CI-S.
  - Divide each total score by the number of teeth scored (6).
  - DI-S and CI-S values range from 0 to 3.
- Calculate the OHI-S.
  - Combine the DI-S and CI-S.
  - OHI-S value ranges from 0 to 6.
- Suggested range of scores for evaluation[13]

Rating	Scores
Individual simplified debris index (DI-S) and the simplified calculus index (CI-S)	
Excellent	0
Good	0.1–0.6
Fair	0.7–1.8
Poor	1.9–3.0
OHI-S (combined DI-S and CI-S)	
Excellent	0
Good	0.1–1.2
Fair	1.3–3.0
Poor	3.1–6.0

- Calculation: Example for an individual

Tooth	Simplified Debris Index Score	Simplified Calculus Index Score
No. 3 (16)	2	2
No. 8 (11)	1	0
No. 14 (26)	3	2
No. 19 (36)	3	2
No. 24 (31)	2	1
No. 30 (46)	2	2
Total	13	9

$$DI\text{-}S = \frac{Total\ debris\ score}{Number\ of\ teeth\ scored} = \frac{13}{6} = 2.17$$

$$CI\text{-}S = \frac{Total\ calculus\ scores}{Number\ of\ teeth\ scored} = \frac{9}{6} = 1.50$$

$$OHI\text{-}S = DI\text{-}S + CI\text{-}S = 2.17 + 1.50 = 3.67$$

- Interpretation
  - According to the suggested range of scores, the score for this individual (3.67) indicates a poor oral hygiene status.
- OHI-S group score
  - Compute the average of the individual scores by totaling the scores and dividing by the number of individuals.

Gingival and Periodontal Health

Measurements for gingival and periodontal indices have varied over the years. Two indices, not completely described here, are of historic interest.

- The papillary-marginal-attached index, attributed to Schour and Massler[14] and later revised by Massler,[15] was used to assess the extent of gingival changes in large groups for epidemiologic studies.
- The periodontal index of Russell,[16] another acclaimed contribution to the study of disease incidence, was a complex index that accounted for both gingival and periodontal changes. Its aim was to survey large populations.
- For patient instruction and motivation, several bleeding indices and scoring methods have been developed.
- Bleeding on gentle probing or flossing is an early sign of gingival inflammation and precedes color changes and enlargement of gingival tissues.[17,18]

- Bleeding on probing is an indicator of the progression of periodontal disease, so testing for bleeding has become a significant procedure for assessment prior to treatment planning, after therapy to show the effects of treatment, and at maintenance appointments to determine continued control of gingival inflammation.

I. Periodontal Screening and Recording (PSR)[19,20,21]

A. Purpose

To assess the state of periodontal health of an individual patient.

- A modified form of the original community periodontal index of treatment needs (CPITN) index.[22]
- Designed to indicate periodontal status in a rapid and effective manner and motivate the patient to seek necessary complete periodontal assessment and treatment.
- Used as a screening procedure to determine the need for comprehensive periodontal evaluation.

B. Selection of Teeth

- The dentition is divided into sextants. Each tooth is examined. Posterior sextants begin distal to the canines.

C. Procedure

- Instrument: Probe originally designed for World Health Organization (WHO) surveys (**Figure 7**), with markings at intervals from tip: 3.5, 5.5, 8.5, and 11.5 mm.
- Color coded between 3.5 and 5.5 mm.
- Working tip: A ball 0.5 mm in diameter. The functions of the ball are to aid in the detection of calculus, rough overhanging margins of restorations, and other tooth surface irregularities, and also to facilitate assessment at the probing depth and reduce risk of overmeasurement.
- Probe application
  - Insert probe gently into a sulcus until resistance is felt.
  - Apply a circumferential walking step to probe systematically about each tooth through each sextant.
  - Observe color-coded area of the probe for prompt identification of probing depths.
  - Each sextant receives one code number corresponding to the deepest position of the color-coded portion of the probe.

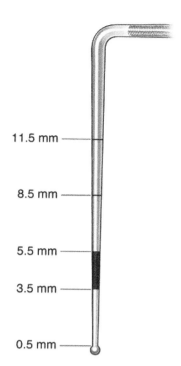

11.5 mm

8.5 mm

5.5 mm

3.5 mm

0.5 mm

Figure 7 World Health Organization (WHO) Periodontal Probe. The specially designed WHO probe measures 3.5-, 5.5-, 8.5-, and 11.5-mm intervals. This probe is used to make determinations for the periodontal screening and recording and the community periodontal index.

Data from Fédération Dentaire Internationale. A simplified periodontal examination for dental practices. Based on the Community Periodontal Index of Treatment Needs—CPITN. *Aust Dent J.* 1985;30(5):368-370.

- Criteria
  - Five codes and an asterisk are used. **Figure 8** shows the clinical findings, code significance, and patient management guidelines.
  - Each code may include conditions identified with the preceding codes; for example, Code 3 with probing depth from 3.5 to 5.5 mm may also include calculus, an overhanging restoration, and bleeding on probing.
  - One need not probe the remaining teeth in a sextant when a Code 4 is found. For Codes 0, 1, 2, and 3, the sextant is completely probed.
- Recording
  - Use a simple six-box form to provide a space for each sextant. The form can be made into peel-off stickers or a rubber stamp to facilitate recording in the patient's permanent record.
  - One score is marked for each sextant; the highest code observed is recorded. When indicated, an asterisk is added to the score in the individual space with the sextant code number.

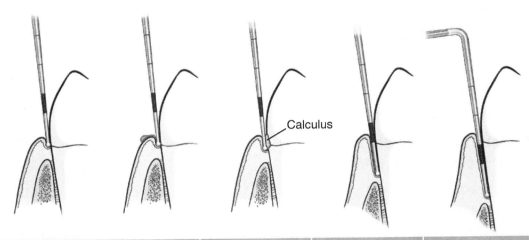

Calculus

PSR and CPI sextant scores	Code 0	Code 1	Code 2	Code 3	Code 4
CPI description	• Entire black band of the probe is visible.	• Entire black band of the probe is visible, but bleeding is present after gentle probing.	• Entire black band is visible, but calculus is present. • Bleeding may or may not be present.	• 4 to 5 mm pocket depth. • Black band on probe partially hidden by gingival margin.	• 6 mm or greater pocket depth. • Black band of probe completely hidden by gingival margin.
PSR sextant code description	• Colored area of probe completely visible. • No calculus, defective restoration margins, or bleeding.	• Colored area of probe completely visible. • No calculus or defective restoration margins. • Bleeding after gentle probing.	• Colored area of probe completely visible. • Supra- or subgingival rough surface or calculus. • Defective restoration margins.	• Colored area of probe only partially visible. • Calculus, defective restorations, and bleeding may or may not be present.	• Colored area of probe completely disappears (probing depth of 5.5 mm or greater).
PSR management guidelines	• Biofilm control instruction. • Preventive care.	• Biofilm control instruction. • Preventive care.	• Biofilm control instruction. • Complete preventive care. • Calculus removal. • Correction of defective restoration margins.	• Comprehensive periodontal assessment and treatment plan is indicated.	• Comprehensive periodontal assessment and treatment plan is indicated.

Figure 8 Community Periodontal Index (CPI) and Periodontal Screening and Recording (PSR) Codes

Data from Petersen PE, Baez RJ. *Oral Health Surveys: Basic Methods*. 5th ed. Geneva: World Health Organization; 2013. https://apps.who.int/iris/bitstream/handle/10665/97035/9789241548649_eng.pdf. Accessed April 25, 2022; American Academy of Periodontology. Parameter on comprehensive periodontal examination. *J Periodontol*. 2000;71(5 suppl):847-848.

D. Scoring

- Follow-up patient management
  - Patients are classified into assessment and treatment planning needs by the highest coded score of their periodontal screening and recording (PSR).
- Calculation: Example 1: PSR Sextant Score

4*	2	3
3	2*	4*

- Interpretation
  - With Codes 3 and 4, a comprehensive periodontal examination is indicated. The asterisks indicate furcation involvement in two sextants and a mucogingival involvement in the mandibular anterior sextant. When the patient is not aware of the periodontal involvement, counseling is important if cooperation and compliance are to be obtained.
- Calculation: Example 2: PSR Sextant Score

2	1	2
2	1*	2*

- Interpretation
  - An overall Code 2 can indicate calculus and overhanging restorations that can be removed. All restorations are checked for recurrent dental caries. Appointments for instruction in dental biofilm control are of primary concern.
    - In this example, the asterisks in two sextants indicate a notable clinical feature such as minimal attached gingiva.

II. Community Periodontal Index (CPI)[1,22]

A. Purpose

To screen and monitor the periodontal status of populations.

- Originally developed as the CPITN index that included a code to indicate an individual and group-summary recording of treatment needs. However, because of changes in management of periodontal disease, the treatment needs portion of the index has been eliminated.
- One component of a complete oral health survey[1] designed by the WHO that includes the assessment of many oral health indicators, including mucosal lesions, dental caries, fluorosis, prosthetic status, and dentofacial anomalies.
- Later modified to form the PSR index for scoring individual patients.

B. Selection of Teeth

- The dentition is divided into sextants for recording on the assessment form.
- Posterior sextants begin distal to canines.

Adults (20 Years and Older)

- A sextant is examined only if there are two or more teeth present that are not indicated for extraction.
- Ten index teeth are examined.
- The first and second molars in each posterior sextant. If one is missing, no replacement is selected and the score for the remaining molar is recorded.
- The maxillary right central incisor and mandibular left central incisor.
- If no index teeth or tooth is present in the sextant, then all remaining teeth in the sextant are examined and the highest score is recorded.

Children and Adolescents (7-19 Years of Age)

- Six index teeth are examined; the first molar in each posterior quadrant and the maxillary right and the mandibular left incisors.
- For children younger than age 15 years, periodontal pocket depth is not recorded to avoid the deepened sulci associated with erupting teeth. Only bleeding and calculus are considered.

C. Procedure

- Instrument: A specially designed probe is used to record both the community periodontal index (CPI) and PSR. The probe is described in Figure 7.
- Criteria: CPI score.
- Five codes are used to record bleeding, calculus, and periodontal pocket depth. Criteria for the CPI codes are similar to the criteria for the PSR, as illustrated in Figure 8 and the Community Periodontal Index table next.

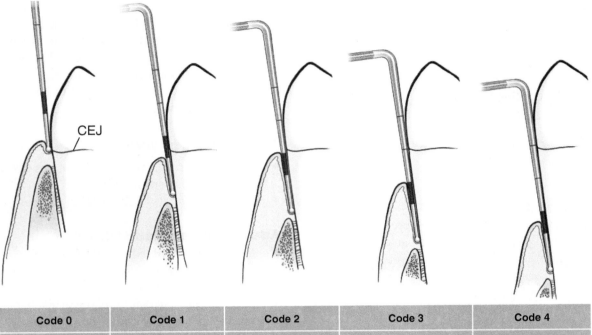

Code 0	Code 1	Code 2	Code 3	Code 4
• 0 to 3 mm loss of attachment. • Cementoenamel junction (CEJ) is covered by gingival margin and CPI score is 0 to 3. If CEJ is visible, or if CPI score is 4, LOA codes 1 to 4 are used.	• 3.5 to 5.5 mm loss of attachment. • CEJ is within the black band on the probe.	• 6 to 8 mm loss of attachment. • CEJ is between the top of the black band and the 8.5 mm mark on the probe.	• 9 to 11 mm loss of attachment. • CEJ is between the 8.5 mm and 11.5 mm marks on the probe.	• 12 mm or greater loss of attachment. • CEJ is beyond the highest (11.5 mm) marks on the probe.

Figure 9 Loss of Attachment (LOA) Codes

Data from Petersen PE, Baez RJ. *Oral Health Surveys: Basic Methods.* 5th ed. Geneva: World Health Organization; 2013. https://apps.who.int/iris/bitstream/handle/10665/97035/9789241548649_eng.pdf. Accessed April 25, 2022; American Academy of Periodontology. Parameter on comprehensive periodontal examination. *J Periodontol.* 2000;71(5 suppl):847-848.

Community Periodontal Index

Code	Criteria
0	Healthy periodontal tissues.
1	Bleeding after gentle probing; entire colored band of probe is visible.
2	Supragingival or subgingival calculus present; entire colored band of probe is visible.
3	4- to 5-mm pocket; colored band of probe is partially obscured.
4	6 mm or deeper; colored band on the probe is not visible.

- Criteria: Loss of attachment (LOA) code.
  - In conjunction with the CPI, the WHO probe is also used to record LOA. The five LOA codes used are illustrated in **Figure 9**. LOA is not recorded for individuals younger than 15 years of age.

Loss of Attachment (LOA) Code	Criteria
0	0–3 mm LOA
1	4–5 mm LOA
2	6–8 mm LOA
3	9–11 mm LOA
4	12 mm or greater LOA

III. Sulcus Bleeding Index (SBI)[17]

A. Purpose

- To locate areas of gingival sulcus bleeding and color changes in order to recognize and record the presence of early (initial) inflammatory gingival disease.

B. Areas Examined

- Four gingival units are scored systematically for each tooth: the labial and lingual marginal gingiva (M units) and the mesial and distal papillary gingiva (P units).

C. Procedure

- Use standardized lighting while probing each of the four areas.
- Walk the probe to the base of the sulcus, holding it parallel with the long axis of the tooth for M units, and directed toward the col area for P units.
- Wait 30 seconds after probing before scoring apparently healthy gingival units.
- Dry the gingiva gently if necessary to observe color changes clearly.
- Criteria

Sulcular Bleeding Index

Code	Criteria
0	Healthy appearance of P and M, no bleeding on sulcus probing.
1	Apparently healthy P and M showing no change in color and no swelling, but bleeding from sulcus on probing.
2	Bleeding on probing and change of color caused by inflammation. No swelling or macroscopic edema.
3	Bleeding on probing and change in color and slight edematous swelling.
4	Bleeding on probing and change in color and obvious swelling or bleeding on probing and obvious swelling.
5	Bleeding on probing and spontaneous bleeding and change in color, marked swelling with or without ulceration.

D. Scoring

- Sulcus bleeding index (SBI) for area
  - Score each of the four gingival units (M and P) from 0 to 5.
- SBI for tooth
  - Total scores for the four units and divide by 4.

- SBI for individual
  - Total the scores for individual teeth and divide by the number of teeth. SBI scores range from 0 to 5.

IV. Gingival Bleeding Index (GBI)[23]

A. Purpose

- To record the presence or absence of gingival inflammation as determined by bleeding from interproximal gingival sulci.

B. Areas Examined

Each interproximal area has two sulci, which can be scored as one interdental unit or scored separately.

- Certain areas may be excluded from scoring because of accessibility, tooth position, diastemata, or other factors, and if exclusions are made, a consistent procedure is followed for an individual and for a group if a study is to be conducted.
- A full complement of teeth has 30 proximal areas. In the original studies, third molars were excluded, and 26 interdental units were recorded.[23]

C. Procedure

- Instrument
  - Unwaxed dental floss is used.
- Steps
  - Pass the floss interproximally first on one side of the papilla and then on the other.
  - Curve the floss around the adjacent tooth and bring the floss below the gingival margin.
  - Move the floss up and down for one stroke, with care not to lacerate the gingiva. Adapt finger rests to provide controlled, consistent pressure.
  - Use a new length of clean floss for each area.
  - Retract for visibility of bleeding from both facial and lingual aspects.
  - Allow 30 seconds for reinspection of an area that does not show blood immediately either in the area or on the floss.
- Criteria
  - Bleeding indicates the presence of disease. No attempt is made to quantify the severity of bleeding.

D. Scoring

- The numbers of bleeding areas and scorable units are recorded. Patient participation in observing and recording over a series of appointments can increase motivation.

V. Eastman Interdental Bleeding Index (EIBI)[24,25]

A. Purpose

- To assess the presence of inflammation in the interdental area as indicated by the presence or absence of bleeding.

B. Areas Examined

- Each interdental area around the entire dentition.

C. Procedure

- Instrument
  - Triangular wooden interdental cleaner.
- Steps
  4. Gently insert a wooden cleaner into each interdental area in such a way as to depress the papilla 1–2 mm (**Figure 10**), then immediately remove.
  5. Make the path of insertion horizontal (parallel to the occlusal surface), taking care not to angle the point in an apical direction.
  6. Insert and remove four times; move to next interproximal area.
  7. Record the presence or absence of bleeding within 15 seconds for each area.

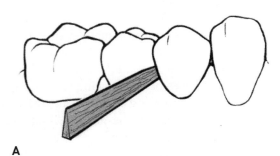

A

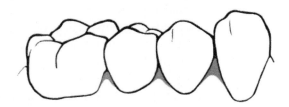

B

Figure 10 Eastman Interdental Bleeding Index. The test for interdental bleeding is made by inserting a wooden interdental cleaner into each interdental space. **A:** Wooden interdental cleaner inserted in a horizontal path, parallel with the occlusal surfaces. **B:** The presence or absence of bleeding is noted within a quadrant 15 seconds after final insertion. Bleeding indicates the presence of inflammation.

D. Scoring

- Number of bleeding sites
  - The number may be totaled for an individual score for comparison with scores over a series of appointments.
- Percentage scores
  - Index is expressed as a percentage of the total number of sites evaluated. Calculations can be made for total mouth, quadrants, or maxillary versus mandibular arches.
- Calculation example
  - An adult with a complete dentition has 15 maxillary and 15 mandibular interproximal areas. The Eastman interdental bleeding index revealed 13 areas of bleeding. To calculate percentage:

$$\frac{Number\ of\ bleeding\ areas}{Total\ number\ of\ areas} \times 100 = Percent\ bleeding\ area$$

$$\frac{13}{30} \times 100 = 43\%$$

VI. Gingival Index (GI)[3]

A. Purpose

- To assess the severity of gingivitis based on color, consistency, and bleeding on probing.

B. Selection of Teeth and Gingival Areas

A GI may be determined for selected teeth or for the entire dentition.

- Areas examined
  - Four gingival areas (distal, facial, mesial, and lingual) are examined systematically for each tooth.
- Modified procedure
  - The distal examination for each tooth can be omitted. The score for the mesial area is doubled and the total score for each tooth is divided by 4.

C. Procedure

- Dry the teeth and gingiva; under adequate light, use a mouth mirror and probe.
- Use the probe to press on the gingiva to determine the degree of firmness.
- Slide the probe along the soft-tissue wall near the entrance to the gingival sulcus to evaluate bleeding (**Figure 11**).
- Criteria

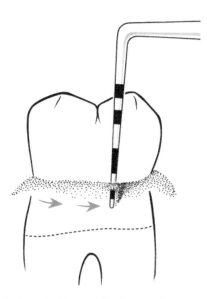

Figure 11 Gingival Index. Probe stroke for bleeding evaluation. The broken line represents the level of attachment of the periodontal tissues. The probe is inserted a few millimeters and moved along the soft-tissue pocket wall with light pressure in a circumferential direction. The stroke shown here is in contrast with the walking stroke used for probing depth evaluation and measurement.

Gingival Index Code	Criteria
0	Normal gingiva.
1	Mild inflammation—slight change in color, slight edema. *No bleeding* on probing.
2	Moderate inflammation—redness, edema, and glazing. *Bleeding* on probing.
3	Severe inflammation—marked redness and edema. Ulceration. Tendency to *spontaneous bleeding*.

D. Scoring

- GI for area
  - Each of the four gingival surfaces (distal, facial, mesial, and lingual) is given a score of 0–3.
- GI for a tooth
  - Scores for each area are totaled and divided by 4.
- GI for groups of teeth
  - Scores for individual teeth may be grouped and totaled and divided by the number of teeth. A GI may be determined for specific teeth, group of teeth, quadrant, or side of mouth.

- GI for the individual
  - Scores for each tooth are added up and divided by the number of teeth examined. Scores range from 0 to 3.
- Suggested range of scores for patient reference

Rating	Scores
Excellent (healthy tissue)	0
Good	0.1–1.0
Fair	1.1–2.0
Poor	2.1–3.0

- Calculation: Example for an Individual
  - Using six teeth for an example of screening; teeth selected are known as the **Ramfjord index teeth**.[26]

Tooth No.	M	F	D	L	
3 (16)	3	1	3	1	
9 (21)	1	0	1	1	
12 (24)	2	1	2	0	
19 (36)	3	1	3	3	
25 (41)	1	1	1	1	
28 (44)	2	1	2	0	
Total	12	5	12	6	= 35

$$Gingival\ index = \frac{Total\ score}{Number\ of\ surfaces} = \frac{35}{24} = 1.46$$

- Interpretation
  - According to the suggested range of scores, the score for this individual (1.46) indicates only fair gingival health (moderate inflammation).
  - The ratings for each gingival area or surface can be used to help the patient compare gingival changes and improve oral hygiene procedures.
- GI for a group
  - Add the individual GI scores and divide by the number of individuals examined.

VII. Modified Gingival Index (MGI)[27,28]

A. Purpose

- Adaptation of the original GI that eliminates probing in the sulcus; less sensitive measure of gingivitis since it relies only on visual observation.
- Probing requirement was removed to reduce disruption of plaque biofilm disruption, avoid potential gingival trauma, and eliminate need for multiple probing assessments to increase reliability.

B. Areas Examined

- Assesses full mouth or gingiva of selected teeth.
- Gingiva is divided into marginal and papillary units.

C. Scoring

- Scores the extent and severity of gingival inflammation using five ordinal numbers.
- Scoring of mild and moderate inflammation differs from original GI.
- Calculates mean scores for individuals and population groups.
- Criteria:

Modified Gingival Index Code	Criteria
0	Normal, healthy tissue.
1	Mild inflammation; involves any part of the gingiva *not entire* marginal or papillary gingival unit.
2	Mild inflammation involved the *entire* marginal or papillary gingival unit.
3	Moderate inflammation.
4	Severe inflammation.

Dental Caries Experience

Dental caries experience data are most useful when measuring the prevalence of dental disease in groups rather than individuals. The population scores can document such information as the number of persons in any age group who are affected by dental caries, the number of teeth that need treatment, or the proportion of teeth that have been treated.

I. Permanent Dentition: Decayed, Missing, and Filled Teeth or Surfaces (DMF, DMFT, or DMS)[29]

A. Purpose

- To determine total dental caries experience, past and present, by recording either the number of affected teeth or tooth surfaces.

B. Selection of Teeth and Surfaces

- The DMFT is based on 28 teeth.
- The decayed, missing, and filled surfaces (DMFS) is based on surfaces of 28 teeth; 128 surfaces.
  - 16 posterior teeth × 5 surfaces (facial, lingual, mesial, distal, and occlusal) = 80 surfaces.
  - 12 anterior teeth × 4 surfaces (facial, lingual, mesial, and distal) = 48 surfaces.
  - Teeth missing due to dental caries are recorded using five surfaces for posterior and four surfaces for anterior teeth.
- Teeth not counted.
  - Third molars.
  - Unerupted teeth. A tooth is considered erupted when any part projects through the gingiva. Certain types of research may require differentiation between clinical emergence, partial eruption, and full eruption.
  - Congenitally missing and supernumerary teeth.
  - Teeth removed for reasons other than dental caries, such as an impaction or during orthodontic treatment.
  - Teeth restored for reasons other than dental caries, such as trauma (fracture), cosmetic purposes, or use as a bridge abutment.
  - Primary tooth retained with the permanent successor erupted. The permanent tooth is evaluated because a primary tooth is never included in this index.

C. Procedures

- Examination
  - Examine each tooth in a systematic sequence.
  - Observe teeth by visual means as much as possible.
  - Use adequate light.
  - Review the stages of dental caries in Chapter 25.
- Criteria for recording[29]
  - Each tooth is recorded once when using the DMFT index.

- Five surfaces for posterior teeth and four surfaces for anterior teeth are recorded when using the DMFS index.
- DMF indices use a dichotomous scale (present or absent) to record decay.

DMF Rating	Criteria
Decayed (D)	Visible dental caries is present or both dental caries and a restoration are present.
Missing (M)	A tooth extracted because of dental caries or when it is carious, nonrestorable, and indicated for extraction.
Filled (F)	Any permanent or temporary restoration is present or a defective restoration without evidence of dental caries is present.

D. Scoring

- Individual DMF
  - Total each component separately.
    - *Total D + M + F = DMF*
  - *Example:* An individual presents with dental caries on the mesial and occlusal surfaces of a posterior tooth and caries on the mesial surface of an anterior tooth. A molar tooth and an anterior tooth are missing because of dental caries and there is an amalgam restoration on the mesial–distal–occlusal surfaces of a posterior tooth.
    - *DMFT = 2 + 2 + 1 = 5*
    - *DMFS = 3 + 9 + 3 = 15*
- A DMF score may have different interpretations. For example, an individual with a DMF score of 15 who has experienced regular dental care may have a distribution such as D = 0, M = 0, F = 15.
- Group DMF
  - Total the DMFs for each individual examined.
  - Divide the total DMFs by the number of individuals in the group.
- Calculation:
  - *Example:* A population of 20 individuals with individual DMF scores of 0, 0, 0, 0, 2, 2, 3, 3, 3, 4, 9, 9, 9, 10, 10, 10, 11, 11, 12, and 16 equals a group total DMF of 124.

$$\frac{124}{20} = 6.2 = the\ average\ DMF\ for\ the\ group$$

  - This DMF average represents accumulated dental caries experience for the group.

- The differences in caries experience between two groups of individuals within this population are notable and influence interpretation of the results. For the first 10 individuals, the group average is 17/10 = 1.7 and for the second 10 individuals the average DMF is 107/10 = 10.7.
- Scores for these two groups can be presented separately because of the wide difference.
- Average DMF scores can also be presented by age group.
- Specific treatment needs of a group
  - To calculate the percentage of DMF teeth that need to be restored, divide the total D component by the total DMF.
- Calculation:
  - *Example 1:* To calculate the *percentage of DMF teeth* that need to be restored, divide the total D component by the total number of DMF teeth.
    - *D = 175, M = 55, F = 18*
    - *Total DMFT = 248*

$$\frac{D}{DMF} = \frac{175}{248} = 0.71\ or$$

    71% of the teeth need restorations

  - *Example 2:* The same type of calculations can be used to determine the *percentage of all teeth missing* in a group of individuals.
    - *20 individuals have 28 × 20 = 560 permanent teeth.*
    - *D = 175, M = 55, F = 18 or nearly 10% of all their teeth lost because of dental caries.*

$$\frac{M}{Total\ \#\ of\ teeth} = \frac{55}{560} = 0.098$$

II. Primary Dentition: Decayed, Indicated for Extraction, and Filled (df and def)[30,31]

A. Purpose

- To determine the dental caries experience for the primary teeth present in the oral cavity by evaluating teeth or surfaces.

B. Selection of Teeth or Surfaces

- deft or dft: 20 teeth evaluated.
- defs or dfs: 88 surfaces evaluated.
  - Posterior teeth: Each has five surfaces: facial, lingual or palatal, mesial, distal, and occlusal. (8 teeth × 5 surfaces = 40 surfaces.)
  - Anterior teeth: Each has four surfaces: facial, lingual or palatal, mesial, and distal (12 teeth × 4 surfaces = 48 surfaces).

- Teeth not counted
  - Missing teeth, including unerupted and congenitally missing.
  - Supernumerary teeth.
  - Teeth restored for reasons other than dental caries are not counted as f.

C. Procedure

- Instruments and examination
  - Same as for DMF.
- Criteria

Decayed, Indicated for Extraction, Filled (df and def)

Rating	Criteria
d	Primary teeth (or surfaces) with dental caries but not restored.
e	Primary teeth (or number of surfaces) that are *indicated for extraction* because of dental caries.
f	Primary teeth (or surfaces) restored with an amalgam, composite, or temporary filling. Each tooth (or surface) is scored only once. A tooth with recurrent caries around a restoration receives a "d" score.

- Difference between deft/defs and dft/dfs
  - In the deft and defs, both "d" and "e" are used to describe teeth with dental caries. Thus, d and e are sometimes combined, and the index becomes the dft or dfs.

D. Scoring

- Calculation:
  - *Example 1:* Individual def: A 2½-year-old child has 18 teeth. Teeth A (55) and J (65) are unerupted. There is no sign of dental caries in teeth M (73), N (72), O (71), P (81), Q (82), and R (83). All other teeth have two carious surfaces each, except tooth B (54), which is broken down to the gum line.
    Summary:
    Total number of teeth = 18
    Number of "d" teeth = 11
    Number of "e" teeth = 1
    Number of "f" teeth = 0
    def = d + e + f = 11 + 1 + 0 = 12
- Interpretation
  - Twelve of 18 teeth (67%) with carious lesions indicates a serious need for dental treatment and a caries management program for the child.

- Calculation: Example 2: Individual dfs
  - Using the same 2½-year-old child to calculate dfs: Eleven teeth each have two carious surfaces: $11 \times 2 = 22$ carious surfaces
  Tooth B has $1 \times 5 = 5$ carious surfaces
    Total dfs: $d + f = 27 + 0 = 27$
- Interpretation
  - The child has 48 total anterior surfaces (12 teeth $\times$ 4 surfaces) and 30 total posterior surfaces (6 teeth $\times$ 5 surfaces) to total 78 surfaces.

$$\frac{dfs}{Number\ of\ surfaces} = \frac{27}{78}$$

= 0.35 or 35% of the surfaces in need of dental treatment

E. Mixed Dentition

- A DMFT or DMFS and a deft or defs are never combined or added together.

III. Primary Dentition: Decayed, Missing, and Filled (dmf)[30,31]

A. Purpose

- To determine dental caries experience for children. Only primary teeth are evaluated.

B. Selection of Teeth or Surfaces

- dmft: 12 teeth evaluated (8 primary molars; 4 primary canines).
- dmfs: 56 surfaces evaluated.
  - Primary molars: 8×5 surfaces each = 40
  - Primary canines: 4×4 surfaces each = 16
- Each tooth is counted only once. When both dental caries and a restoration are present, the tooth or surface is scored as "d."

C. Procedure

- Instruments and examination are the same as for DMF.
- Criteria for dmft or dmfs:

dmf Rating	Criteria
d	Primary molars and canines (or surfaces) that are carious.
m	Primary molars and canines (or surfaces) that are missing. A primary molar or canine is presumed missing because of dental caries when it has been lost before normal exfoliation.
f	Primary molars and canines (or surfaces) that have a restoration but are without caries.

Table 1 ECC and S-ECC Case Definition

Age	Birth to 3 Years (0–35 Months)	3–4 Years (36–47 Months)	4–5 Years (48–59 Months)	5–6 Years (60–71 Months)
ECC	One or more teeth with decayed (either cavitated or noncavitated), missing, or filled surfaces			
S-ECC	▪ Any sign of smooth surface caries	▪ One or more cavitated or filled smooth surfaces in primary maxillary anterior teeth ▪ One or more missing teeth due to caries OR dmfs score ≥4	▪ One or more cavitated or filled smooth surfaces in primary maxillary anterior teeth ▪ One or more missing teeth due to caries OR dmfs score ≥5	▪ One or more cavitated or filled smooth surfaces in primary maxillary anterior teeth ▪ One or more missing teeth due to caries OR dmfs score ≥6

Data from: Drury TF, Horowitz AM, Ismail AI, et al. Diagnosing and reporting early childhood caries for research purposes. *J Public Health Dent.* 1999;59(3):192-197.

D. Scoring

- Calculation: Example 1: Individual dmf
  - A 7-year-old boy has all primary molars and canines present. Examination reveals two carious surfaces on one molar tooth, one missing canine tooth, and one two-surface amalgam filling on a molar tooth:
    - $dmft = 1 + 1 + 1 = 3$
    - $dmfs = 2 + 4 + 2 = 8$

E. Mixed Dentition

- Permanent and primary teeth are evaluated separately. A DMFT or DMFS and a dmft or dmfs are never added together.

IV. Early Childhood Caries (ECC)[32]

A. Purpose

- To provide case definitions that determine dental caries experience and severity in children 5–6 years of age or younger.

B. Selection of Teeth or Surfaces

- Each surface (mesial, distal, facial, lingual, and occlusal) of each tooth visible in the child's mouth is evaluated. Only primary teeth are scored.

C. Procedure

- Visual examination of all surfaces of each erupted tooth.
- Categorized according to age and severity.
  - Early childhood caries (ECC) applies to children 6 years of age and younger.
  - Severe early childhood caries (S-ECC) applies to children 5 years of age and younger.
- Criteria for case definitions are included in **Table 1**.

D. Scoring

- A designation of early childhood caries (ECC) or severe early childhood caries (S-ECC) for a particular individual relates the age of the child with the status of DMFT surfaces observed.
- Community-based surveys identify the percentage of a population with ECC and/or S-ECC.

V. Root Caries Index (RCI)[33]

A. Purpose

- To determine total root caries experience for individuals and groups and provide a direct, simple method for recording and making comparisons.

B. Selection of Teeth

- Up to four surfaces (mesial, distal, facial, and lingual/palatal) are counted for each tooth.
- Only surfaces with visible gingival recession are counted.
- Teeth with multiple roots and extreme recession, though rare, could present with two or three lesions on the same surface. In this case, the most severe lesion is selected for recording and each surface is counted only once.

C. Procedure

- Examination
  - Use adequate retraction and light to examine each tooth.
  - Apply current knowledge of the stages of dental caries to prevent damage to remineralizing areas during examination. Only cavitated lesions are recorded.
- Record a rating for each root surface.

Root Caries Index Rating	Criteria
NoR	Root surface with a covered cementoenamel junction and no visible recession (R = recession).
R-D	Root surface with recession present and root caries present (D = decay).
R-F	Root surface with recession present and the surface is restored (F = filled).
R-N	Root surface with recession, but no caries or restoration is present.
M	The tooth is missing.

D. Scoring

- Calculation: Formula

$$\frac{[R-D]+[R-F]}{[R-D]+[R-F]+[R-N]} \times 100 = RCI$$

- Calculation: Example individual root caries index (RCI)
  - A man, aged 70, presents with 23 natural teeth (23 × 4 = 92 surfaces). Clinical examination reveals:

    $R - D = 26$

    $R - F = 8$

    $R - N = 58$

$$RCI = \frac{26+8}{26+8+58} = \frac{34}{92} \times 100 = 36.9\%$$

- Interpretation
  - A score of 36.9% means that of all tooth surfaces with visible gingival recession, 36.9% have a history of root caries (cavitated or restored) carious lesions.
- Group or community RCI
  - The R − D, R − F, and R − N scores for all individuals in the group are added together and the RCI formula is calculated using the total scores.

Dental Fluorosis

Dental indices such as the Thylstrup–Fejerskov index,[34] the fluorosis risk index,[35] and the developmental defects of dental enamel index[36,37] have been used to investigate the effects of fluoride concentration on dental enamel. The two indices described here are the most commonly used for community-based assessment.

I. Dean's Fluorosis Index[38]

A. Purpose

- To measure the prevalence and severity of dental fluorosis.
- Originally developed in the 1930s and refined in 1942 to relate the severity of hypomineralization of dental enamel to concentration of fluoride in the water supply.
- Considered less sensitive than some other measures of fluorosis, but still recommended for use in community studies.

B. Selection of Teeth

- The smooth surface enamel of all teeth is examined.

C. Procedure

- Each tooth is visually examined for signs of fluorosis and assigned a numerical score using the descriptive categories listed in **Table 2**.

D. Scoring

- An individual fluorosis score is assigned using the highest numerical score recorded for two or more teeth.
- Community levels of fluorosis are indicated by the percentage of individuals in the **sample** or population that receives scores in each category.

II. Tooth Surface Index of Fluorosis (TSIF)[39]

A. Purpose

- To measure the prevalence and severity of dental fluorosis.
- More sensitive than Dean's index in identifying the mildest signs of fluorosis.

B. Selection of Teeth

- The smooth surface enamel, cusp tips, and incisal edges of all teeth are examined.

C. Procedure

- Each tooth is examined visually and assigned a numerical score using the criteria in **Table 3**.

Table 2 Scoring System for Dean's Fluorosis Index

Category	Description	Numerical Score
Normal	Smooth, creamy white tooth surface	0
Questionable	Slight changes from normal transparency	1
Very mild	Small, scattered opaque areas; less than 25% of tooth surface	2
Mild	Opaque areas; less than 50% of tooth surface	3
Moderate	Significant opaque and/or worn areas; may have brown stains	4
Severe	Widespread, significant hypoplasia, pitting, brown staining, worn areas, and/or a corroded appearance	5

Data from Dean HT. The investigation of physiological effect by the epidemiological method. In: Moulton FR, ed. *Fluorine and Dental Health*. Washington, DC: American Association for the Advancement of Science; 1942:23-71.

D. Scoring

- Tooth surface index of fluorosis (TSIF) data are presented as a distribution citing the percentage of the population with each numerical score, rather than as mean scores for the entire group.

Community-Based Oral Health Surveillance

Community oral health screenings can be performed at every level: local, national, and worldwide. Data collected by such screenings are useful for monitoring health status and determining population access to or need for oral health services.

I. WHO Basic Screening Survey

The WHO screening survey includes the CPI and the LOA indices described earlier.[1]

A. Purpose

- To collect comprehensive data on oral health status and dental treatment needs of a population.

Table 3 Scoring System for Tooth Surface Index of Fluorosis

Content removed due to copyright restrictions

This system is suitable for surveying both adults and children.

B. Tissues/Areas Examined

Survey categories include the following:
- Orofacial (intraoral and extraoral) lesions and anomalies.
- Temporomandibular joint status.
- Periodontal status.
- Dentition status and treatment needs.
- Prosthetic status and need.
- Need for immediate care/referral.

C. Procedures

- Standardized assessment form with boxes for data entry identifies the codes and descriptive criteria for each **data collection** category.

- Standardized codes facilitate computerized data entry and analysis.
- Photographs in the training manual provide examples of criteria for each code.

D. Scoring

- Data can be analyzed by survey team or arrangements can be made for data entry forms to be analyzed by the WHO.

II. Association of State and Territorial Dental Directors' (ASTDD) Basic Screening Survey[8]

A. Purpose

- Developed by the ASTDD to provide oral screening for adult, school age, and/or preschool populations.
  - Data levels are consistent with monitoring the U.S. Public Health Service national health objectives.
  - Data collected can easily be compared with data collected by other communities and states using the data collection techniques.
- The system was designed to be used by screeners with or without dental background because:

- Sometimes nondental personnel have better access to some population groups.
- Some communities have little access to dental public health professionals.

B. Selection of Teeth

- All teeth are examined, but each individual patient receives one score for each category.

C. Procedure

- Oral screening can be combined with an optional questionnaire that collects additional data on demographics and access to dental care.
- Screeners are trained and calibrated. They record oral findings using photographs and detailed descriptions of associated criteria.

D. Scoring

- **Table 4** outlines the scoring criteria and categories recorded for preschool and school children.
- **Table 5** lists the scoring criteria and categories recorded for older adults.
- Data from each indicator can be compiled and expressed in frequency graphs or tables as a percentage of the population that exhibits a specific category trait.

Table 4 Association of State and Territorial Dental Directors' Basic Screening Survey Scoring Criteria: Preschool and School Children

Criteria	Score	Preschoolers	School Children
Untreated caries (≥0.5 mm discontinuity in tooth surface)	0 = No untreated caries 1 = Untreated caries	✓	✓
Treated decay (amalgam, composite, or temporary filling)	0 = No treated decay 1 = Treated decay	✓	✓
Sealants on permanent molars	0 = No sealants 1 = Sealants		✓
Treatment urgency	0 = No obvious problem (routine dental care indicated) 1 = Early dental care (within 2 wk) 2 = Urgent care (as soon as possible—presents with pain, swelling, etc.)	✓	✓

A ✓ mark indicates that the oral condition category is scored in that particular age group. Some categories (i.e., sealants) are not scored in all age groups.

Data from ASTDD Basic Screening Surveys. Association of State and Territorial Dental Director website. http://www.astdd.org/basic-screening-survey-tool. Updated January 2022. Accessed April 25, 2022.

Table 5 Association of State and Territorial Dental Directors' Basic Screening Survey Scoring Criteria: Older Adults

Criteria	Score
Removable upper denture	0 = No 1 = Yes
If yes: Do you wear upper denture when eating?	0 = No 1 = Yes
Removable lower denture	0 = No 1 = Yes
If yes: Do you wear lower denture when eating?	0 = No 1 = Yes
Number of upper natural teeth (include root fragments)	Range 0–16
Number of lower natural teeth (include root fragments)	Range 0–16
Root fragments	0 = No 1 = Yes 9 = Edentulous
Untreated decay	0 = No 1 = Yes 9 = Edentulous
Need for periodontal care	0 = No 1 = Yes 9 = Edentulous
Suspicious soft-tissue lesions	0 = No 1 = Yes 9 = Edentulous
Treatment urgency	0 = No obvious problem—next scheduled visit 1 = Early care—within next several weeks 2 = Urgent care—within next week—pain or infection
Obvious tooth mobility (optional indicator)	0 = No 1 = Yes 0 = Edentulous
Severe dry mouth (optional indicator)	0 = No 1 = Yes

Data from ASTDD Basic Screening Surveys. Association of State and Territorial Dental Director website. http://www.astdd.org/basic-screening-survey-tool. Updated January 2022. Accessed April 29, 2022.

Documentation

Factors related to dental indices to document in the patient records include:

- Name of the index or indices used.
- Score calculated for the index.
- Objective statement that provides an interpretation of the index score.
- Follow-up instructions provided to the patient.
- An example of documentation for use of a dental index appears in **Box 1**.

Factors to Teach Patient or Members of the Community

- How an index is used and calculated, and what the scores mean.
- Purpose for the selection of the particular index being used.
- Correlation of index scores with current oral health practices and procedures.
- Procedures to follow to improve index scores and bring the oral tissues to health.

References

NOTE: Many of the citations below may seem not to be current or even seem completely out-of-date; however, the reader will note that most are "classic" references, which refer to the development and first use of the index.

1. Petersen PE, Baez, RJ. *Oral Health Surveys: Basic Methods.* 5th ed. Geneva, Switzerland: World Health Organization; 2013. https://apps.who.int/iris/bitstream/handle/10665/97035/9789241548649_eng.pdf. Accessed April 25, 2022.

2. Silness J, Loe H. Periodontal disease in pregnancy. II. correlation between oral hygiene and periodontal condition. *Acta Odontol Scand.* 1964;22:121-135.

3. Löe H. The gingival index, the plaque index and the retention index systems. *J Periodontol.* 1967;38(6 suppl):610-616.

4. Podshadley AG, Haley JV. A method for evaluating oral hygiene performance. *Public Health Rep.* 1968;83(3):259-264.

5. U.S. Department of Health and Human Services. *Oral Health in America: A Report of the Surgeon General.* Rockville, MD: U.S. Department of Health and Human Services, National Institute of Dental and Craniofacial Research, National Institutes of Health; 2000:63-89.

6. National Institutes of Health. *Oral Health in America: Advances and Challenges.* Bethesda, MD: US Department of Health and Human Services, National Institutes of Health, National Institute of Dental and Craniofacial Research; 2021. https://www.nidcr.nih.gov/sites/default/files/2021-12/Oral-Health-in-America-Advances-and-Challenges.pdf. Accessed April 28, 2022.

7. Healthy People 2030. Objectives and data: oral conditions. https://health.gov/healthypeople/objectives-and-data/browse-objectives/oral-conditions. Accessed April 25, 2022.

8. Association of State and Territorial Dental Directors. *Basic Screening Surveys.* Reno, NV: ASTDD; 2022. http://www.astdd.org/basic-screening-survey-tool/. Accessed April 25, 2022.

9. O'Leary TJ, Drake RB, Naylor JE. The plaque control record. *J Periodontol.* 1972;43(1):38.

10. Ramfjord SP, Ash MM. *Periodontology and Periodontics.* Philadelphia, PA: WB Saunders Co; 1979:273.

11. Grant DA, Stern IB, Everett FG. *Periodontics.* 5th ed. St. Louis, MO: Mosby; 1979:529-531.

12. Greene JC, Vermillion JR. The simplified oral hygiene index. *J Am Dent Assoc.* 1964;68:7-13.

13. Greene JC. The Oral Hygiene Index—development and uses. *J Periodontol.* 1967;38(6 suppl):625-637.

14. Schour I, Massler M. Prevalence of gingivitis in young adults. *J Dent Res.* 1948;27(6):733.

15. Massler M. The P-M-A index for the assessment of gingivitis. *J Periodontol.* 1967;38(6 suppl):592-601.

16. Russell AL. A system of classification and scoring for prevalence surveys of periodontal disease. *J Dent Res.* 1956;35(3):350-359.

17. Mühlemann HR, Son S. Gingival sulcus bleeding—a leading symptom in initial gingivitis. *Helv Odontol Acta.* 1971;15(2):107-113.

18. Meitner SW, Zander HA, Iker HP, et al. Identification of inflamed gingival surfaces. *J Clin Periodontol.* 1979;6(2):93-97.

19. American Academy of Periodontology. Parameter on comprehensive periodontal examination. *J Periodontol.* 2000;71(5 suppl):847-848.

20. Khocht A, Zohn H, Deasy M, et al. Assessment of periodontal status with PSR and traditional clinical periodontal examination. *J Am Dent Assoc.* 1995;126(12):1658-1665.

21. Periodontal screening and recording training program kit. Chicago, IL: American Dental Association and American Academy of Periodontics; 1992.

22. Ainamo J, Barmes D, Beagrie G, et al. Development of the World Health Organization (WHO) community periodontal index of treatment needs (CPITN). *Int Dent J.* 1982;32(3):281-291.

23. Carter HG, Barnes GP. The gingival bleeding index. *J Periodontol.* 1974;45(11):801-805.

24. Abrams K, Caton J, Polson A. Histologic comparisons of interproximal gingival tissues related to the presence or absence of bleeding. *J Periodontol.* 1984;55(11):629-632.

25. Caton JG, Polson AM. The interdental bleeding index: a simplified procedure for monitoring gingival health. *Compend Contin Educ Dent.* 1985;6(2):88, 90-92.

26. Ramfjord SP. Indices for prevalence and incidence of periodontal disease. *J Periodontol.* 1959;30:51-59.

27. Chattopadhyay A. *Oral Health Epidemiology: Principals and Practice.* Sudbury, MA: Jones and Bartlett; 2011.

28. Lobene RR, Weatherford T, Ross NM, Lamm RA, Menaker L. A modified gingival index for use in clinical trials. *Clin Prev Dent.* 1986;8(1):3-6.

29. U.S. Department of Health and Human Services, Public Health Service, National Institutes of Health. *Oral Health Surveys of the National Institute of Dental Research, Diagnostic Criteria and Procedures.* Bethesda, MD: National Institute of Dental Research; 1991.

30. Klein H, Palmer CE, Knutson JW. Studies on dental caries. I. dental status and dental needs of elementary school children. *Public Health Rep.* 1938;53(19):751-765.

31. Gruebbel AO. A measurement of dental caries prevalence and treatment service for deciduous teeth. *J Dent Res.* 1944;23:163-168.

32. Drury TF, Horowitz AM, Ismail AI, et al. Diagnosing and reporting early childhood caries for research purposes. *J Public Health Dent.* 1999;59(3):192-197.

33. Katz RV. Assessing root caries in populations: the evolution of the root caries index. *J Public Health Dent.* 1980;40(1):7-16.

34. Thylstrup A, Fejerskov O. Clinical appearance of dental fluorosis in permanent teeth in relation to histologic changes. *Community Dent Oral Epidemiol.* 1978;6(6):315-328.

35. Pendrys DG. The fluorosis risk index: a method for investigating risk factors. *J Public Health Dent.* 1990;50(5):291-298.

36. Fédération Dentaire Internationale. An epidemiological index of developmental defects of dental enamel (DDE Index). Commission on Oral Health, Research and Epidemiology. *Int Dent J.* 1982;32(2):159-167.

37. Clarkson J, O'Mullane D. A modified DDE index for use in epidemiological studies of enamel defects. *J Dent Res.* 1989;68(3):445-450.

38. Dean HT. The investigation of physiological effect by the epidemiological method. In: FR Moulton, ed. *Fluorine and Dental Health.* Washington, DC: American Association for the Advancement of Science; 1942:23-71.

39. Horowitz HS, Driscoll WS, Meyers RJ, et al. A new method for assessing the prevalence of dental fluorosis—the tooth surface index of fluorosis. *J Am Dent Assoc.* 1984;109(1):37-41.

Oral Infection Control: Toothbrushes and Toothbrushing

Heather L. Reid, RDH, MS
Linda D. Boyd, RDH, RD, EdD

CHAPTER OUTLINE

LEARNING OBJECTIVES

After studying this chapter, the student will be able to:

1. Identify the characteristics of effective manual and power toothbrushes.
2. Differentiate among manual toothbrushing methods, including limitations and benefits of each.
3. Describe the different modes of action of power toothbrushes.
4. Identify the basis for power toothbrush selection.
5. Describe tongue cleaning and its effect on reducing dental biofilm.
6. Identify adverse effects of improper toothbrushing on hard and soft tissues.

Development of Toothbrushes

The toothbrush has been the principal instrument in general use for oral care and is a necessary part of oral disease control.[1-4] There is a long history of development of toothbrushes since ancient times.

I. Origins of the Toothbrush

- Evidence of toothbrushes has its origins in the Babylonian chew sticks in early 3500 BC.[5]
- The "chew stick," which has been considered the primitive toothbrush, appears in the Chinese literature around 1600 BC.[5]
  - Care of the mouth was associated with religious training and ritual: the Buddhists had a "toothstick," and the Mohammedans used the "miswak" or "siwak."
  - Chew sticks are made from various types of wood by crushing the end of a twig or root and spreading the fibers in a brush-like manner.
  - Miswaks are used in many African and Middle Eastern countries and evidence suggests[4] they have antimicrobial properties.[6]

II. Early Toothbrushes

- It is believed the first toothbrush made of horsehair **bristles** was mentioned in the early Chinese literature around 1000 AD.[5]
- Pierre Fauchard in 1728 in *Le Chirurgien Dentiste* described many aspects of oral health. He was critical of the toothbrush made of horse's hair because it was too soft and advised the use of sponges to vigorously rub the teeth.[7]
- One of the earlier toothbrushes made in England was produced by William Addis around 1780.[8]
  - By the early 19th century, craftsmen in various European countries constructed handles of gold, ivory, or ebony in which replaceable brush heads could be fitted.
  - The first patent for a toothbrush in the United States was issued to HN Wadsworth in 1860.[9]
- In the early 1900s, celluloid began to replace bone handles.
- Nylon bristles were introduced by Dupont De Nemours in 1938.[10]
  - World War II prevented Chinese export of wild boar bristles, so synthetic materials were substituted for natural bristles.
  - Since then, synthetic materials have improved and manufacturers' specifications standardized.

- Most toothbrushes are made exclusively of synthetic materials.
- The first **power toothbrush** to appear in the American market was a Broxodent in 1960.[10]

Manual Toothbrushes

Little evidence exists related to the most effective characteristics of a toothbrush and other aspects of toothbrushing, so clinical experience and individual patient needs will guide recommendations.[11]

I. Characteristics of an Effective Manual Toothbrush

- Conforms to individual patient requirements in size, shape, and texture.
- Easily and efficiently manipulated.
- Readily cleaned and aerated; impervious to moisture.
- Durable and inexpensive.
- Soft bristles.[12]
- Multilevel or angled bristles.[12,13]
- **End-rounded** filaments free of sharp or jagged edges.[12]
- Designed for utility, efficiency, and cleanliness.
- In the United States, look for the ADA (American Dental Association) Seal of Acceptance, and in Canada, look for the CDA (Canadian Dental Association) Seal.

II. General Description

A. Parts (Figure 1)

- Handle: The part grasped in the hand during toothbrushing.
- Head: The working end; consists of **tufts** of **bristles** or **filaments**.
- Shank: The section that connects the head and the handle.

B. Dimensions

- Recommendations in the literature and in different countries seem to vary.

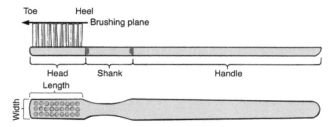

Figure 1 Parts of a Toothbrush

- Generally, the following should be considered in recommending a toothbrush to a patient[13]:
  - Length of the toothbrush head should cover two to three posterior teeth.
  - Width of the **toothbrush head** should cover the intercuspal distance of the first molar.
- General recommendations from the ADA for dimensions include:
  - Total brush length: About 15–19 cm (6–7.5 inches); junior and child sizes are shorter.
  - Head: Length of brushing plane, 25.4–31.8 mm (1–1.25 inches); width, 7.9–9.5 mm (5/16–3/8 inch).
  - Bristle or filament height: 11 mm (7/16 inch).

III. Handle

A. Composition

- Manufacturing specifications: Most often a single type of plastic, or a combination of polymers.
- Properties: Combines durability, imperviousness to moisture, pleasing appearance, low cost, and sufficient maneuverability.

B. Shape

- Preferred characteristics
  - Easy to grasp.
  - Does not slip or rotate during use.
  - No sharp corners or projections.
  - Lightweight, consistent with strength.
- Variations
  - A twist, curve, offset, or angle in the shank with or without thumb rests may assist the patient in adaptation of the brush to difficult-to-reach areas.
  - A handle of larger diameter may be useful for patients with limited dexterity, such as children, aging patients, and those with a disability.

IV. Brush Head

A. Design

- Length: May be 5–12 tufts long and 3–4 rows wide.
- Shape and size: A variety of brush head shapes and sizes from rounded to tapered to angled are available.
- Arrangement of bristle tufts varies in configuration and angulation as shown in **Figure 2**.

B. Brushing Plane (Lateral Profile)

- Length: Range from filaments of equal lengths (flat planes) to those with variable lengths, such as rippled, scalloped, tapered, bi-level, multilevel, and angled (Figure 2).

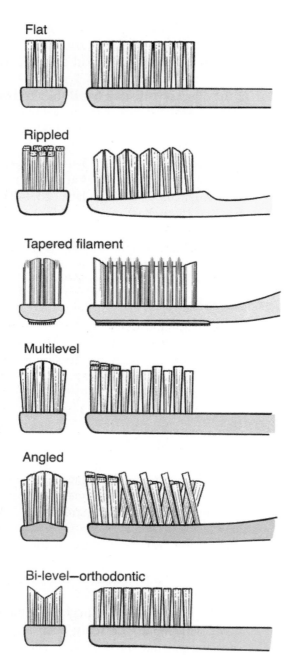

Figure 2 Manual Brush Trim Profiles. A variety of filament profiles are available. In addition to the classic flat planed brush, other trims include the rippled, tapered filaments, bi-level, multilevel, and angled brushes. Brushes for use over orthodontic appliances are made with various bi-level shapes.

- Efficiency in biofilm removal:
  - Research results have demonstrated plaque and gingivitis are better reduced through use of modern bristle technology (i.e., angled, tapered, criss-cross designs versus traditional flat trim designs).[14,15]
  - Ultimately, efficiency in cleaning the hard-to-reach areas, such as extension onto proximal surfaces, malpositioned teeth, or exposed root surfaces, depends on individual patient abilities and understanding.

V. Filaments (or Bristles)

- Most current toothbrushes have nylon filaments.
  - The physical properties of natural bristles cannot be standardized.
  - A comparison of natural bristles and synthetic filaments is reviewed in **Table 1**.
- Many manufacturers of synthetic filaments refer to filaments as "bristles" when communicating with consumers on the toothbrush package and in advertising.
  - Dental professionals need to be aware that most manufacturers of toothbrushes today produce brushes using "synthetic filaments" but still refer to these as "bristles."
- Companies that produce a toothbrush with "natural bristles" may distinguish themselves by using the word "natural" in the product description.
- The **bristle stiffness** depends on the diameter and length of the filament.[4] Brushes designated as soft, medium, or hard may not be consistent among manufacturers.

A. Filament or Bristle Design

- A variety of filament designs are available and may include, but are not limited to, end-rounded, feathered, microfine, and conical shaped.
- Another factor to keep in mind is that the quality of end-rounding varies in both adult and children's toothbrushes depending on the manufacturer.[16] Natural bristles cannot be end-rounded.
- Some evidence suggests end-rounded bristles are less abrasive to gingival damage than bristles that are non-end-rounded (**Figure 3** for examples); however, the overall conclusion by a systematic review found the association of rounding of filaments (or bristles) to gingival recession to be inconclusive.[17]

Power Toothbrushes

Power brushes are also known as power-assisted, automatic, mechanical, or electric brushes. The ADA Council on Scientific Affairs evaluates power brushes for the reduction of dental biofilm and gingivitis.[18]

Table 1 Comparison of Natural Bristles and Synthetic Bristles or Filaments

	Natural Bristles	Bristles/Filaments
Source	Historically made from hog or wild boar hair	Synthetic, plastic materials, primarily nylon
Uniformity	No uniformity of texture. Diameter or wearing properties depending upon the breed of the animal, geographic location, and season in which the bristles were gathered	Uniformity controlled during manufacturing
Diameter	Varies depending on portion of the bristle taken, age, and life of animal	Ranges from extra soft at 0.075 mm (0.003 inch) to hard at 0.3 mm (0.012 inch)
End shape	Deficient, irregular, frequently open ended	End-rounded
Advantages and disadvantages	Cannot be standardized Wear rapidly and irregularly Hollow ends allow microorganisms and debris to collect inside	Rinse clean, dry rapidly Durable and maintained longer End-rounded and closed, repel debris and water More resistant to accumulation of microorganisms

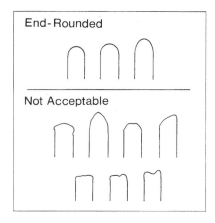

Figure 3 End-Rounded Filaments. Examples of the shape of acceptable end-rounding and of those that are not acceptable are shown.

Data from Silverstone LM, Featherstone MJ. A scanning electron microscope study of the end rounding of bristles in eight toothbrush types. *Quintessence Int.* 1988;19(2):87-107; and Checchi L, Minguzzi S, Franchi M, et al. Toothbrush filaments end-rounding: stereomicroscope analysis. *J Clin Periodontol.* 2001;28(4):360-364.

I. Effectiveness

A. Evolution

- Power toothbrushes have evolved over time due to improved designs and features.
- Power toothbrushes of the 1960–1980 era mimicked the motions of manual brushing.
- Current power brushes move at speeds and motions that often cannot be duplicated by manual brushes.

B. Power Toothbrushes versus Manual Toothbrushes

- There is moderate evidence that power toothbrushes result in a 10% to 20% reduction in plaque and about a 10% reduction in gingivitis when compared to manual toothbrushes.[19]

- Rotating oscillating action power toothbrushes have been shown to be more effective than side-to-side power brushes for reducing plaque and gingivitis.[1]
- Sonic power toothbrushes have not been shown to be more effective than other types of power toothbrushes.[20-25]
- Power toothbrushes, as compared to their manual counterparts, do not damage gingival tissues as much; they may be less damaging because they have mechanisms to alert the patient when they apply excessive force.[4,11] However, when not used properly, power toothbrushes may be more abrasive.[26,27]
- Ultimately, recommendations are based on patient needs and preference.

II. Purposes and Indications

A. Purpose

- Recommended for physically able patients with ineffective manual biofilm removal techniques.
- Facilitate **mechanical dental biofilm control** or removal of food debris from the teeth and the gingiva.
- Reduce calculus and extrinsic dental stain buildup.[28]

B. Indications for Use of Power Toothbrush

Power brushes can be useful for many patients, including:

- Those with a history of failed attempts at more traditional biofilm removal methods.
- Those undergoing orthodontic treatment.

- Those undergoing complex restorative and prosthodontic treatment.
- Aggressive brushers
  - Many models of power toothbrushes will shut off automatically if too much pressure is applied during brushing, which can be a benefit for those who have a tendency to apply too much pressure.[4,11]
- Patients with disabilities or limited dexterity.
  - The large handle of a power brush can be of benefit.
  - Handle weight needs to be considered for these patients.
- When a parent or caregiver must brush for the patient.

III. Description

A. Motion

- The motion of the head of power toothbrushes varies between models and may include one or more of the following (**Table 2**)[12]:
  - Rotation oscillation.
  - Counter oscillation.
  - Sonic or ultrasonic motion.
  - Side to side.
  - Circular.

B. Speeds

- Vary from low to high.
- Generally, power brushes with replaceable batteries move more slowly than those with rechargeable batteries and have been shown to be less effective in plaque biofilm removal.[25,29]
- Movement per minute varies from 3,800 to over 48,000 depending on the manufacturer and type (battery, sonic, or ultrasonic).

C. Brush Head Design

- Adult: The variety of shapes continues to evolve, but a few examples are illustrated in **Figure 4**. They may be small and round, or like traditional manual heads. Trim profiles include flat, bi-level, rippled, or angled.
- Child: A child's power brush head should be specially designed to accommodate a smaller mouth, as shown in **Figure 5**.

D. Filaments or Bristles

- Made of soft, end-rounded nylon.
- Diameters: From extra soft, 0.075 mm (0.003 inch), to soft, 0.15 mm (0.006 inch).

E. Types of Power Source

- Direct
  - Utilizes an electrical outlet.
- Replaceable batteries
  - Relatively inexpensive and convenient.
  - As most batteries lose their power, brush speed is reduced.
  - Advise patients to select a brush that has a water tight handle to avoid corrosion of batteries.

Table 2 Power Toothbrush Motions

Motion	Description
Rotational	Moves in a 360° circular motion.
Counterrotational	Each tuft of filaments moves in rotational motion; each tuft moves counter-directional to the adjacent tuft.
Oscillating	Rotates from center to the left, then to the right; degree of rotation varies from 25° to 55°.
Pulsating	When brush head is on the tooth, pulsations are directed toward the interproximal areas.
Cradle or twist	Side to side with an arc.
Side to side	Side to side perpendicular to the long axis of the brush handle.
Translating	Up and down parallel to the long axis of the brush handle.
Combination	Combination of simultaneous yet different types of movement.
Ultrasonic	Brush head vibrates at ultrasonic frequency (>250 kHz).

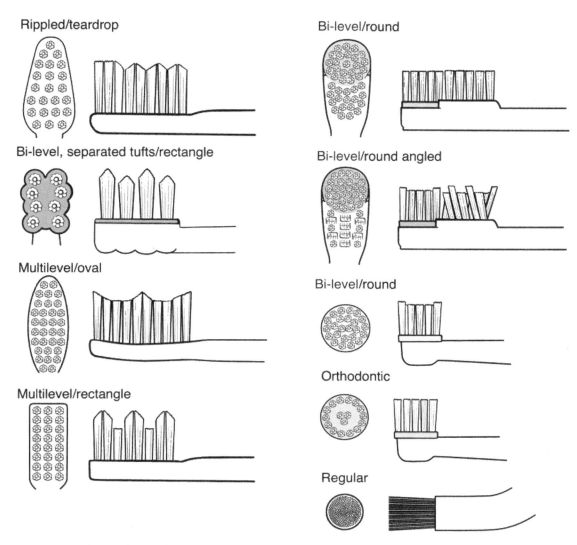

Figure 4 Power Brush Trim Profiles. Power brushes are made in a variety of brush head shapes, such as oval, teardrop, rectangular, and round. Some power brushes have two different-shaped heads on the same brush. In addition, there are a variety of brush head trims on power brushes, including flat, bi-level, and multilevel.

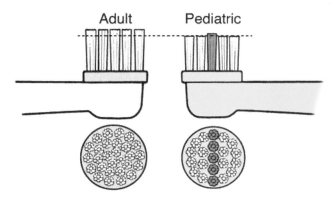

Figure 5 Child Power Brush Profile. Power brushes for children could necessitate smaller head sizes and shorter filaments to allow for access to tight posterior areas. Raised blue filaments allow for better access to occlusal pits and fissures.

- Rechargeable
  - Rechargeable, nonreplaceable battery.
  - Recharges via a stand connected to an electrical outlet.
- Disposable
  - Batteries cannot be replaced or recharged.

Toothbrush Selection for the Patient

Overarching factors in toothbrush selection include the quality of clinical research supporting the efficacy and safety of the brush and the ADA or CDA Seal of Approval, along with the clinical decision making of the clinician regarding what is best for an individual patient.

I. Influencing Factors

Factors influencing the selection of a proper manual or power toothbrush for an individual patient include the following:

A. Patient

- Ability of the patient to use the brush and remove dental biofilm from tooth surfaces without damage to the soft tissue or tooth structure.
- Manual dexterity of the patient.
- The age of the patient and the differences in dentition and dexterity.

B. Gingiva

- Status of gingival and periodontal health.
- Anatomic configurations of the gingiva.

C. Position of Teeth

- Crowded teeth.
- Open contacts.

D. Compliance

- Patient preference may dictate which brush is recommended.
- Patient may have preferences and may resist change.
- Patient may lack motivation, ability, or willingness to follow the prescribed procedure.

E. Specific Factors to Consider for Selection of Power Toothbrush

- Replaceable brush head.
- Features that include a timer and pressure sensor.
- Patient affordability.
  - Battery-operated models are often less expensive and may be a good way for the patient to try out a power toothbrush before investing in a more expensive rechargeable model.

II. Toothbrush Characteristics

- Brush head selection is dependent on the patient's ability to maneuver and adapt the brush correctly to all facial, lingual, palatal, and occlusal surfaces for dental biofilm removal.
- Some research suggests angled tufted designs of manual toothbrush heads and rotating, oscillating round power brush heads are most effective.[14,20,30]

III. Stiffness of Filaments or Bristles

- Toothbrush bristles are typically classified as hard, medium, soft, or extra soft.
  - The same classification for stiffness (i.e., soft) may vary between manufacturers.[31]
- Filaments must have adequate stiffness to remove plaque biofilm and do no harm to oral soft and hard tissues.
- Despite beliefs that a soft toothbrush is more effective, more recent research suggests plaque biofilm removal may be significantly better with a medium toothbrush.[32] However, the ADA recommends a soft bristle toothbrush.[12]
- Research shows that toothbrushes made from thermoplastic elastomer, a rubber-like material, reduce plaque and gingival bleeding, when compared to nylon bristles.[32]
- **Tooth abrasion** and/or **gingival abrasion** and gingival recession are multifactorial even though they are often attributed solely to the failure to use a soft toothbrush.[11]
  - Factors include anatomic features (e.g., tooth position and crowding), toothbrushing technique, frequency, duration, force (pressure), and self-inflicted gingival trauma, which point to the need to individualize recommendations.[33]
- An extra-soft toothbrush may be indicated in conditions such as necrotizing ulcerative gingivitis or following periodontal surgery.

Methods for Manual Toothbrushing

The ideal toothbrushing technique is one that the patient can perform effectively to remove plaque biofilm while avoiding any damage to hard and soft oral tissues. Research on which method is better remains limited (see **Box** 1 for a historical perspective on proper toothbrushing instruction). However, hands-on instruction with the patient leads to improvement in their brushing methods.[34,35]

- Without instruction, normal brushing may consist of vigorous horizontal, vertical, and/or circular strokes.[35]
- Manual toothbrushing methods include the following:
  - Sulcular: Modified Bass.
  - Roll: Rolling stroke, modified Stillman.

- Vibratory: Stillman, Charters, Bass.
- Horizontal (or scrub).
- Circular: Fones.
- Vertical: Leonard.

The Bass and Modified Bass Methods

The Bass and modified Bass methods are widely accepted as effective methods for dental biofilm removal adjacent to and directly beneath the gingival margin (sulcus) despite conflicting evidence.[11,35,36] They are considered to be types of **sulcular brushing**, which may be more effective than other methods, and generally are recommended by the ADA.[12,37] The areas at the gingival margin and in the col are the most significant in the control of gingival and periodontal infections.

I. Purposes and Indications

- Dental biofilm removal adjacent to and directly beneath the gingival margin.
- Open embrasures, cervical areas beneath the height of contour of the enamel, and exposed root surfaces.
- Adaptation to abutment teeth or implants, under the gingival border of a fixed partial denture.

II. Procedure

A. Position the Brush[38]

- Direct the filaments apically (up for maxillary, down for mandibular teeth).
- First, position the sides of the filaments parallel with the long axis of the tooth (**Figure   6A**).
- From that position, turn the brush head toward the gingival margin to make approximately a 45° angle to the long axis of the tooth (**Figure   6B**).
- Direct the filament tips into the gingival sulcus (Figure   6A and B).

B. Strokes[31,38]

- Press lightly so the filament tips enter the gingival sulci and embrasures and cover the gingival margin. Do not bend the filaments with excess pressure.
- Vibrate the brush back and forth with very short strokes without disengaging the tips of the filaments from the sulci (Figure   6C).

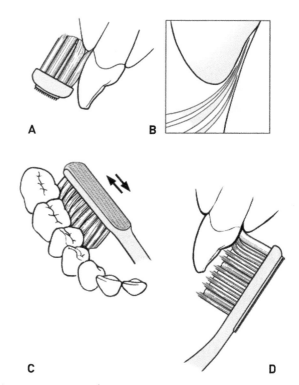

Figure   6 Bass/Modified Bass Method of Brushing. **A:** Filament tips are directed into the gingival sulcus at approximately 45° to the long axis of the tooth. **B:** Brushes designed with tapered filaments reach below the gingival margin with ease. **C:** Brush in position for lingual surfaces of mandibular posterior teeth. **D:** Position for palatal surface of maxillary anterior teeth.

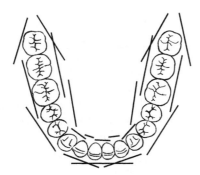

Figure 7 Brushing Positions. Each brush position, as represented by a black line, will overlap the previous position. Note placement at canines, where the distal aspect of the canine is brushed with the premolars and the mesial aspect is brushed with the incisors. Short lines on the lingual anterior aspect indicate a brush placed vertically. The maxillary teeth require a similar number of brushing positions.

- Count at least 10 vibrations.
- In the modified Bass method, the vibratory, sulcular brush stroke is followed by rolling the toothbrush down over the crown of the tooth to clean the rest of the tooth surface.

C. Reposition the Brush

- Apply the brush to the next group of two or three teeth. Take care to overlap placement, as shown in **Figure 7**.

D. Repeat Stroke

- The entire stroke (steps A–C) is repeated at each position around the maxillary and mandibular arches, on both facial and lingual tooth surfaces.

E. Position Brush for Lingual and Palatal Anterior Surfaces

- Tilt the brush handle somewhat vertically for the anterior components (**Figure 6D**).[12] The bristles are directed into the sulci.

III. Limitations

- The toothbrush bristles extend only 0.9 mm below the gingival margin, so plaque removal in the sulcus is limited.[39]
- An individual who is an aggressive brusher may interpret "very short strokes" into a vigorous horizontal scrubbing motion, causing injury to the gingival margin.
- Dexterity requirement for the vibratory stroke may be difficult for certain patients.

The Stillman and Modified Stillman Methods

The modified Stillman method is considered a sulcular brushing technique along with the modified Bass method.

I. Purposes and Indications

- As originally described by Stillman,[40] the method is designed for massage and stimulation, as well as for cleaning the cervical areas. The modified Stillman method adds a rolling stroke to the vibratory stroke to clean the crown of the tooth.[41]
- Dental biofilm removal from cervical areas below the height of contour of the crown and from exposed proximal surfaces.
- General application for cleaning tooth surfaces and massage of the gingiva.

II. Procedure[40]

A. Position the Brush

- Place side of brush on the attached gingiva: The filaments are directed apically (up for maxillary, down for mandibular teeth) in **Figure 8A**. When the plastic portion of the brush head is level with the occlusal or incisal plane, generally the brush is at the proper height, as shown in Figure 7A.
- The brush ends are placed partly on the gingiva and partly on the cervical areas of the tooth and directed slightly apically.

B. Strokes

- Press to flex the filaments: The sides of the filaments are pressed lightly against the gingiva, and blanching of the tissue occurs (**Figure 8B**).
- Angle the filaments: Turn the handle by rotating the wrist so that the filaments are directed at an angle of approximately 45° with the long axis of the tooth.
- Activate the brush: Use a slight rotary motion. Maintain light pressure on the filaments, and keep the tips of the filaments in position on the tooth surface. Count to 10 slowly as the brush is vibrated by a rotary motion of the handle.
- Roll and vibrate the brush: Turn the wrist and work the vibrating brush slowly down over the gingiva and tooth. Make some of the filaments reach interdentally (**Figure 8C**).

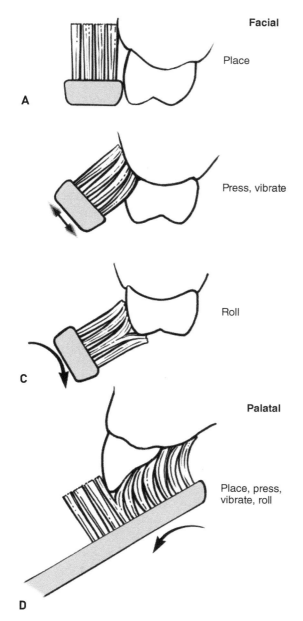

Facial

Place

A

Press, vibrate

B

Roll

C

Palatal

Place, press, vibrate, roll

D

Figure 8 Modified Stillman Method of Brushing. **A:** Initial brush placement with sides of bristles or filaments against the attached gingiva. **B:** The brush is pressed and angled, then vibrated. **C:** Vibrating is continued as the brush is rolled slowly over the crown. **D:** Using the toe of the brush, place the bristles into the gingival sulcus of the maxillary anterior teeth, press lightly, vibrate the bristles, and use a rolling stroke to clean the remainder of the lingual surface. Repeat for each anterior tooth and for the mandibular teeth.

C. Replace Brush for Repeat Stroke

- Reposition the brush by rotating the wrist. Avoid dragging the filaments back over the free gingival margin by holding the brush slightly away from the tooth.

D. Repeat Stroke Five Times or More

- The entire stroke (steps A–C) is repeated at least five times for each tooth or group of teeth. When moving the brush to an adjacent position, overlap the brush position.

E. Position Brush for Anterior Lingual and Palatal Surfaces

- Position the brush somewhat vertically using the toe of the brush head for the anterior components (**Figure 8D**).
- Press and vibrate, roll, and repeat.

III. Limitations

- Careful placement of a brush with end-rounded filaments is necessary to prevent tissue laceration. Light pressure is needed.
- Patient may try to move the brush into the rolling stroke too quickly, and the vibratory aspect may be ineffective for biofilm removal at the gingival margin.

The Roll or Rolling Stroke Method

I. Purposes and Indications

- Removing biofilm, materia alba, and food debris from the teeth without emphasis on gingival sulcus.
  - Used in conjunction with a vibratory technique such as modified Bass, Charters, and Stillman methods.
- Can be particularly helpful when there is a question about the patient's ability to master and practice a more complex method.

II. Procedure[42]

A. Position the Brush

- Filaments: Direct filaments apically (up for maxillary, down for mandibular teeth).
- Place side of brush parallel to and against the attached gingiva: The filaments are directed apically. When the plastic portion of the brush head is in level with the occlusal or incisal plane, generally the brush is at the proper height, as shown in Figure 8A.

B. Strokes

- Press to flex the filaments: The sides of the filaments are pressed lightly against the gingiva. The gingiva will blanch.

- Roll the brush slowly over the teeth: As the brush is rolled, the wrist is turned slightly. The filaments remain flexed and follow the contours of the teeth, thereby permitting cleaning of the cervical areas. Some filaments may reach interdentally.

C. Replace and Repeat Five Times or More

- Repeat the entire stroke: The entire stroke (steps A and B) is repeated at least five times for each tooth or group of teeth.
- Rotate the wrist: When the brush is removed and repositioned, the wrist is rotated.
- Stretch the cheek: The brush is moved away from the teeth, and the cheek is stretched facially with the back of the brush head. Be careful not to drag the filament tips over the gingival margin when the brush is returned to the initial position.

D. Overlap Strokes

- When moving the brush to an adjacent position, overlap the brush position, as shown in Figure 7.

E. Position Brush for Anterior Lingual or Palatal Surfaces

- Tilt the brush slightly vertically and use the toe of the brush head to access the lingual surfaces of the anterior teeth.
- Press (down for maxillary, up for mandibular) until the filaments lie flat against the teeth and gingiva.
- Press and roll (curve up for mandibular, down for maxillary teeth).
- Replace and repeat five times for each brush width.

III. Limitations

- Brushing too high during initial placement can lacerate the alveolar mucosa.
- Minimal plaque removal interproximally or in sulcular areas.
- Tendency to use quick, sweeping strokes results in failure to adequately remove plaque biofilm from the cervical third of the tooth because the brush tips pass over rather than into the area, likewise for the interproximal areas.

Charters Method

Charters strongly believed in prevention and felt dentists were not doing their "full duty" if they were not taking the time to teach patients a system of home care.[43] He advocated for personal demonstration of techniques by the patient. Charters felt particularly strongly about teaching children proper home care and even went so far as to recommend it to be a part of the curriculum in schools.[43]

I. Purposes and Indications

- Loosen debris and dental biofilm.[43]
- Stimulate marginal and interdental gingiva.[43]
- Aid in biofilm removal from proximal tooth surfaces when interproximal tissue is missing creating open embrasures (e.g., following periodontal surgery).[43]
- Remove dental biofilm from abutment teeth and under the gingival border of a fixed partial denture (bridge) or implant-supported bridge or partial denture.

II. Procedure[43]

A. Position the Brush

- Filaments: Direct bristles at 90° angle to the teeth.
- Place side of brush at right angles (90°) to the long axis of the teeth (**Figure 9B**).
- Note the contrast with position for the Stillman method (**Figure 9A**).

B. Strokes

- Press the bristles gently between the teeth, being careful not to injure the gingiva.
- With the bristles between the teeth, use as little pressure as possible and make three to four small rotary movements with the bristles.
  - The sides of the bristles should come into contact with the gingival margin to massage or stimulate them.
- Remove the brush from the interproximal area and move to the next area.

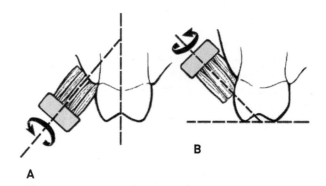

Figure 9 Stillman and Charters Methods Compared. **A:** Stillman: The brush is angled at approximately 45° to the long axis of the tooth. **B:** Charters: The brush is angled at approximately 45° to the occlusal plane, with brush tips directed toward the occlusal or incisal surfaces.

C. Reposition the Brush and Repeat

- Repeat steps for strokes described previously three to four times in each area on the maxillary and mandibular arches.

D. Overlap Strokes

- Move the distance of one embrasure and repeat the process *to overlap strokes.*

III. Limitations

- Brush ends do not engage the gingival sulcus to disturb subgingival bacterial accumulations.
- In some areas, the correct brush placement is limited or impossible; modifications become necessary, consequently adding to the complexity of the procedure.

The Horizontal (or Scrub) Method

I. Purposes and Indications

- Research suggests the horizontal toothbrushing method is appropriate for children younger than 6 years for use on occlusal and lingual surfaces; however, the method should be combined with other techniques.[44]
- Once the child reaches the late mixed dentition stage, modification to another technique can be initiated as the horizontal method has limitations in terms of thorough plaque biofilm removal.

II. Procedure

A. Position the Toothbrush

- Filaments: Direct bristles at right angle to the tooth.
- Place toothbrush head at a 90° angle to the long axis of the teeth on both buccal and lingual posterior surfaces.
- For anterior teeth, the head of the toothbrush is held parallel to the long axis of the tooth and the toe of the brush is used.

B. Stroke

- Bristles are moved in a gentle back and forth motion on the posterior surfaces, buccal, lingual, and occlusal.
- Bristles are moved in an up and down motion on the anterior teeth using the toe of the toothbrush.

III. Limitations

- Although this method can remove plaque biofilm on buccal and lingual surfaces, it does not reach interproximal areas.[33]
- There are also concerns about this method resulting in cervical abrasion if excessive pressure along with an abrasive toothpaste is used in adults.[11]

The Fones (or Circular) Method

I. Purpose and Indications

- This method is easy for children to learn and may be easier than the horizontal method to switch to more appropriate techniques as the child ages.[44]

II. Procedure

- Place toothbrush at 90° to the long axis of the teeth, buccal and lingual, and press bristles gently against the teeth.

A. Stroke

- Bristles are moved in a circular motion several times in each area and then the brush is moved to a new area (**Figure 10**).

III. Limitations

- Efficiency of plaque removal was the lowest as compared to sulcular and horizontal brushing methods.[45,46]

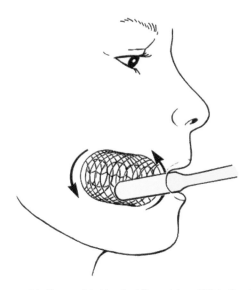

Figure 10 Fones Method of Brushing. With the teeth closed, a circular motion extends from the maxillary gingiva to the mandibular gingiva using light pressure.

Leonard's (or Vertical) Method

I. Purpose and Indication

- May work well for small children.

II. Procedure

- Place toothbrush at 90° to the long axis of the teeth, buccal and lingual, and press bristles gently against the teeth.
- The teeth are edge to edge.

A. Stroke

- Bristles move in an up and down motion with light pressure on the tooth surfaces. Move systematically from area to area around the mouth.

III. Limitations

- Much like the rolling stroke, there is minimal plaque removal interproximally and in the sulcular areas.[47]

Method for Power Toothbrushing

As previously noted, a systematic review found powered toothbrushes reduced plaque biofilm and gingivitis better than a manual toothbrush and may be of benefit for some individuals.[19] However, the type of power supply, mode of action of the powered toothbrush, brushing duration, and method of instruction are factors impacting the effectiveness of biofilm removal.[25]

I. Procedure

Although no clearly defined brushing method has been evaluated, the following was developed by the Swiss Dental Society[31]:

- Place bristles at a 45° to 90° angle to the long axis of the tooth, then turn the brush on.
- Move the brush over the buccal (or lingual) and interproximal surfaces of each tooth (or area depending on the size of the brush head) for about 5 seconds.
- Reposition the brush on the next tooth and repeat both on the buccal and lingual surfaces in a systematic approach.
- Many powered toothbrushes have a built-in 2 minute timer which can signal to the patient the minimum brushing time.

II. Limitations

- Cost for the rechargeable models can be an economic hardship for some patients.
- Some people may not like the sound or vibration of the powered toothbrushes, especially those with oral hyposensitivity. However, desensitization may allow for power toothbrushes to be used and they have been shown to be effective in those with autism.[48]

Supplemental Brushing Methods

I. Occlusal Brushing

A. Purpose

- Loosen food debris and biofilm microorganisms in pits and fissures.
- Remove biofilm from the margins of occlusal restorations.
- Clean pits and fissures to prepare for sealants.

B. Procedure

- Place brush head on the occlusal surfaces of molar teeth with filament tips pointed into the occlusal pits at a right angle.
- Position the handle parallel with the occlusal surface.
- Extend the toe of the brush to cover the distal grooves of the most posterior tooth (**Figure** 11).
- Strokes: The two acceptable strokes include:
  - Vibrate the brush in a slight circular movement while maintaining the filament tips on the occlusal surface throughout a count of 10. Press moderately so filaments do not bend but go straight into the pits and fissures.

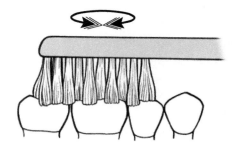

Figure 11 Occlusal Brushing. Small circular or vibrating strokes with light pressure while maintaining filament tips on the occlusal surface permit tips to work their way into pits and fissures.

- Force the filaments against the occlusal surface with sharp, quick strokes; lift the brush off each time to dislodge debris; repeat 10 times.
- Overlap previous stroke by moving the brush to the premolar area. Gradually progress around each maxillary and mandibular arch until all occlusal surfaces have been thoroughly debrided.

II. Brushing Difficult-to-Reach Areas

A. Adaptations

- Hands-on demonstration by the patient is essential so the clinician can assess dexterity and ability of the patient to reach difficult areas. This also allows the clinician to determine if a different oral hygiene aid may be more effective.
- Use of disclosing solution to make biofilm visible to the patient and clinician in difficult-to-reach areas may be useful in order to work with the patient to modify the technique for effective plaque biofilm removal.
- At successive appointments, the difficult-to-reach areas should be monitored with continued refinement of oral self-care techniques.

B. Areas for Special Attention

- Distal surfaces of most posterior teeth (**Figure** 12). At best, the brush may reach only the distal line angles and a single- or end-tufted brush may be necessary. (See Chapter 27.)
- Facially displaced teeth, especially canines and premolars, where the zone of attached gingiva and buccal alveolar bone on the facial surface may be minimal. These areas are at risk for gingival recession and toothbrush abrasion.
- Lingually inclined teeth such as the maxillary anterior teeth.
- Exposed root surfaces: Cemental and dentinal surfaces.
- Overlapped teeth or wide embrasures, which may require use of vertical brush position (**Figure** 13).
- Surfaces of teeth next to edentulous areas.

III. Tongue Cleaning

The dorsum of the tongue is an ideal environment for harboring bacteria and is a key component of the overall oral self-care process.[49]

A. Anatomic Features of the Tongue Conducive to Debris Retention[49]

- Surface papillae: Numerous filiform papillae extend as minute projections, whereas fungiform papillae are not as high and create elevations and depressions that entrap debris and microorganisms. These papillae provide a large surface area for the microflora of the tongue.
- Fissures may be several millimeters deep and also provide a surface for bacterial growth.

B. Microorganisms of the Tongue

- Anaerobic bacteria involved in the production of volatile sulfur compounds related to oral malodor (bad breath) or **halitosis** reside on the tongue.[49]

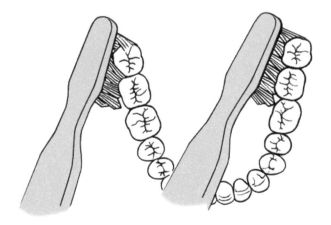

Figure 12 Brushing Problems. Brush placement to remove biofilm from the distal surfaces of the most posterior teeth. The distobuccal surface is approached by stretching the cheek; the distolingual surface is approached by directing the brush across from the canine of the opposite side.

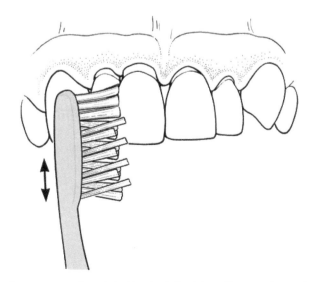

Figure 13 Brush in Vertical Position. For overlapped teeth, open embrasures, and selected areas of recession, the dental biofilm on proximal tooth surfaces can be removed with the brush held in a vertical position.

- Periodontal pathogens such as *Porphyromonas gingivalis*, *Prevotella intermedia*, and *Aggregatibacter actinomycetemcomitans* are also found on the dorsum of the tongue.[49,50]
- Microorganisms in saliva are typically the same as those found on the tongue.

C. Purposes and Indications

- Remove or reduce tongue coating.
  - Tongue coating is a white-brownish layer on the dorsum of the tongue and is made up of desquamated epithelial cells, blood cells and metabolites, food debris, and bacteria.[49]
  - The composition of the coating is affected by factors including periodontal status, salivary flow, age, tobacco use, and oral hygiene.[49]
  - The tongue coating is implicated in halitosis.
- Reduces bacterial load. However, research has not indicated that this reduces the periodontal pathogens on the dorsum of the tongue or in the saliva, so the effect may be primarily on the bacteria producing halitosis.[50]
- Reduces potential for halitosis.[51] Tongue brushing and scraping can be effective in reducing halitosis. According to some research findings, the effect is unclear or may only provide short-term benefit.[3,49]
- Improves taste sensation in smokers and nonsmokers.[52]

D. Brushing Procedure

- Hold the brush handle at a right angle to the midline of the tongue and direct the brush tips toward the throat.
- With the tongue extruded, the sides of the filaments are placed on the posterior part of the tongue surface.
- With light pressure, draw the brush forward and over the tip of the tongue. Repeat three or four times.
- A power brush should only be used for tongue cleaning when the switch is in the "off" position.

E. Types of Tongue Cleaners and Scrapers

As an alternative to brushing the tongue, a tongue cleaner or scraper can be used.

- Tongue cleaners or scrapers are typically made of plastic or a flexible metal strip. A variety of tongue cleaners and scrapers are available and may include the following:

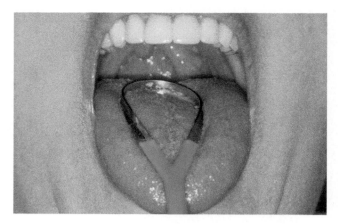

Figure 14 Tongue Cleaners or Scrapers. A variety of plastic or flexible metal cleaners are available to clean the dorsal surface of the tongue.

  - Loop with a single handle (**Figure 14**).
  - Curved with two ends to hold.
  - Raised, textured rubber pad on the back side of the toothbrush head.
- Procedure
  - Place the cleaner toward the most posterior area of the dorsal surface (Figure 14).
  - Press with a light but firm stroke, and pull forward.
  - Repeat several times, covering the entire surface of the tongue.
  - Wash the tongue cleaner under running water to remove debris.

Guidelines for Toothbrushing Instructions

- Comprehensive toothbrushing instruction for a patient involves teaching what, when, where, and how. Hands-on demonstration by the patient is essential. (See Chapter 24 for guidance on effectively educating the patient.)
- In addition to a description of specific toothbrushing methods, the following sections address the grasp, sequence, frequency, duration, and force for toothbrushing.
- Possible detrimental effects from improper toothbrushing and variations for special conditions are described.

I. Toothbrush Grasp

A. Objectives of Instruction on Grasp

- Ability to manipulate the brush for successful removal of dental biofilm.

- A light, controlled grasp accomplishes the following:
  - Control of the brush during all movements.
  - Effective positioning at the beginning of each brushing stroke, follow-through during the complete stroke, and repositioning for the next stroke.
  - Sensitivity to the amount of pressure applied.

B. Procedure

- Grasp the toothbrush handle in the palm of the hand with the thumb against the shank.
  - Grasp the brush near the head so it can be controlled effectively.
  - Do not grasp so close to the head of the brush that manipulation of the brush is hindered or fingers touch the anterior teeth when moving the brush head to molar regions.
- Position according to the brushing method to be used.
- Adapt grasp for the various positions of the brush head on the teeth throughout the procedure; adjust to permit unrestricted movement of the wrist and arm.
- Apply appropriate pressure for removal of the dental biofilm avoiding excessive pressure that results in soft-tissue trauma.

II. Brushing Sequence

- There is no one recommended sequence for brushing. Research suggests similar results irrespective of whether patients begin on the buccal or lingual surfaces.[53]
- The brushing process should be approached in a systematic way to ensure complete coverage for each tooth surface. Technique based on sequence creates habit, which may increase effectiveness.[54]
- Divide the mouth into sextants or quadrants.
- Start brushing from a molar region of one arch around to the midline facial then lingual followed by brushing the occlusal surfaces.
- Repeat in the opposing arch.
- Each brush placement should overlap the previous one for thorough coverage as shown in Figure 7.
- Approaches to address areas where patients may have more difficulty removing plaque biofilm may include:
  - Changing the sequence and starting with areas where the patient misses plaque biofilm, such as the lingual of the mandibular right for a right-handed patient and mandibular left for a left-handed patient.
  - Specific areas with active periodontal disease.

III. Frequency of Brushing

- Brushing a minimum of two times/day has been shown to reduce caries incidence and severity of periodontal disease.[55,56] Research indicates low frequency of toothbrushing as a risk factor for diabetes, dyslipidemia, and cardiovascular disease.[57]
- Regular daily oral self-care is most effective at reducing risk and severity of oral disease. Infrequent brushing results in higher odds for dental caries and more severe periodontal disease.[55,56]
- Failure to adequately disturb plaque biofilm allows for continued maturation, which increases the pathogenic potential of the biofilm. (See Chapter 17.)
- Quality of brushing technique for plaque biofilm removal is equally important as the frequency.

IV. Duration of Brushing

- The average times for brushing range from 60 to 80 seconds in the literature.[58]
- Several factors impact the time required for each individual, including tendency to accumulate plaque, psychomotor skills, position of the teeth, orthodontics, etc.
- Research suggests an increase in plaque biofilm removal with increased brushing time.[59] However, more recent research with power toothbrushes suggests that there is no additional benefit beyond 120 seconds or 2 minutes for brushing duration.[60]

A. The Count System

To ensure thorough coverage with an even distribution of effort in all areas, a system of counting can be useful.

- Count the number of strokes in each area (or 5 or 10, whichever is most appropriate for the particular patient) for modified Stillman or other methods in which a stroke is used.
- Count slowly to 10 for each brush position while the brush is vibrated and filament ends are held in position for the Bass, Charters, or other vibratory method.

B. The Clock System

- For some patients, watching a clock or an egg timer can be helpful to gauge the time they spend brushing.

- However, using a timer does not guarantee thorough biofilm removal, because the easily accessible areas may get more brushing time.

C. Combination
- For many patients, the use of the "count" system in combination with the "clock" system may be most effective.

D. Built-in Timers
- Many power toothbrushes have built-in timers.
- Signals may be set for 30 seconds, 1 or 2 minutes.
- Timers can motivate patients to increase the total time spent brushing.

E. Oral Hygiene Mobile Applications
There are a variety of mobile toothbrushing applications (also known as apps) available for download on a variety of electronic devices, including cell phones and tablets, which provide an interactive brushing experience and reminders, thus enhancing patient oral hygiene.[61-63]

- These applications may include the following features[63]:
  - Educational videos and texts.
  - Goal setting with reminders such as "Time to brush!" set to times designated by the patient.
  - Monitoring of oral hygiene behaviors through reports and graphs of how often a patient brushes or flosses and the duration.
  - Feedback on progress toward goals such as badges for children.
  - Peer support through sharing of progress with friends.
- Research suggests these mobile applications hold promise in terms of improving oral hygiene.
  - In adolescents, use of a mobile app resulted in reductions in gingivitis and plaque compared to verbal oral hygiene instructions.[62] The use of apps also helps to establish good oral health habits.[64]
  - In another study, the majority (>90%) of participants said the app motivated them to brush their teeth longer.[61]

V. Toothbrushing Force
- Toothbrushing force has been evaluated in terms of the impact on gingival recession and tooth abrasion as well as on effectiveness of plaque biofilm removal.[60,65,66]

- Most research suggests plaque removal is improved with force up to a point, beyond which there is no benefit and potential harm.[66]
- Suggested optimal brushing force for plaque removal:
  - Manual toothbrushing: 400 g.[66]
  - Power toothbrushing: 150 g.[60]
- Although force alone does not cause soft- and hard-tissue injury (i.e., gingival recession and tooth abrasion), it is important to provide patient education to avoid aggressive brushing techniques while effectively removing plaque biofilm.[67]
  - Many power toothbrushes have a mechanism to alert the user to excessive force, which may help them to adjust the force applied.[68,69]

VI. General Toothbrushing Instruction

A. Preparation for Instructing Patient
- The dental hygienist must become familiar with an oral self-care product before providing patient education.
- For power toothbrushes, review manufacturer instructions and practice with a toothbrush model, if available, prior to instructing the patient on using it effectively.

B. Patient Education
- Research suggests the most effective teaching strategies for patient education include computer technology, audio and videotapes, written materials, and demonstrations.[70]
  - Verbal instructions alone had only a small effect on patient outcomes (i.e., plaque biofilm removal) and should not be used as a stand-alone educational strategy.
  - Demonstrations had the largest effect on patient outcomes and are an essential component of educating the patient.
  - Multiple educational strategies lead to further improvement in patient outcomes.
- When initially introducing a new power toothbrush or oral self-care aid, a demonstration model and/or video can be helpful to introduce the new product to the patient.
  - Adult learning theory suggests patients come to us with experience, so it is important to understand what the patient already knows prior to beginning patient education.[71]

- Like motivational interviewing, adult learning theory stresses the importance of the adult patient establishing the learning goals. (See Chapter 24.)
- If a patient is familiar with an oral self-care tool such as a toothbrush, allow the patient to demonstrate their technique and help refine it as needed to be effective.
- Disclosing the plaque biofilm in the patient's mouth can be very useful to provide the patient with a way to visualize the biofilm and its removal when practicing brushing and other oral self-care aid techniques. Do not forget to provide the patient with a hand mirror.
  - Disclosing plaque biofilm makes it easy for the patient and clinician to assess whether the techniques have been effective in biofilm removal.
  - In subsequent follow-up appointments, disclosing the plaque biofilm is also a way for the patient and clinical to assess progress toward plaque biofilm removal goals and to identify problem areas requiring further modification of techniques or a different oral self-care aid.
- Observe the patient's technique and refine as needed to show the patient how to adapt the brush head to reach difficult areas.

C. Toothbrushing Procedure

- Select a brush size and shape appropriate for the individual patient.
- Select a dentifrice with minimum abrasiveness.
- Place a small amount of fluoride dentifrice on the brush and spread the dentifrice over the teeth.
- For a manual toothbrush:
  - Place the brush on the most posterior maxillary molar and begin moving around each arch on the buccal and then lingual surfaces using the chosen toothbrushing method until all surfaces are completed.
  - Move the brush to the mandibular teeth and repeat. This sequence may vary depending on the preferences of the patient.
  - Brush the occlusal surfaces of first the maxillary and then the mandibular teeth.
- For a power toothbrush, place the brush in the mouth before turning the power on to prevent splatter.
  - Place the brush on the most posterior maxillary molar and move the brush around all surfaces, including angling into interproximal areas of each tooth if using a small circular brush.

- If using a more typical rectangular brush head, start in the posterior and work on each area individually before moving to the next.
- Carefully angle the brush head to access rotated, crowded, or otherwise displaced teeth.

Toothbrushing for Special Conditions

Prolonged failure to remove plaque biofilm is not indicated because of the association between oral infection and inflammation and many systemic diseases/conditions.[72] Examples of conditions that may require a temporary modification of oral self-care routines may include, but are not limited, to the following conditions.

I. Acute Oral Inflammatory or Traumatic Lesions

When an acute oral condition precludes normal oral self-care, instruct the patient to:

- Brush all areas of the mouth not affected and if tolerable clean the affected area with an extra-soft toothbrush. Reducing the bacterial load is essential to aid in healing.
- Rinse with a warm saline solution to encourage healing and debris removal.
- Consider prescribing an antimicrobial rinse like chlorhexidine to aid in the reduction of bacterial load until normal oral self-care can resume.
- Resume regular biofilm control measures on the affected area as soon as possible.

II. Following Periodontal Surgery

Provide specific instructions concerning brushing while sutures and/or a dressing are in place.

- Perform oral self-care in the areas not involved in the surgery as usual.
- Follow directions provided by the periodontal office for care of the surgical area.
- Rinsing and brushing the surgical area may not be recommended until at least 24 hours after surgery, at which time care should be taken to avoid the gingival areas when brushing.
  - If gingival grafting was done, no brushing may be allowed until the postoperative follow-up appointment.
- An antimicrobial rinse like chlorhexidine may be prescribed to aid with reducing the bacterial load and to aid in healing while the oral self-care process is modified.

III. Following Dental Extraction

- Clean the teeth adjacent to the extraction site the day following surgery.
- Brush areas not involved in the surgery as usual to reduce biofilm and promote healing.
- Beginning 24 hours after surgery, rinse the mouth with a warm, mild saline solution after each meal or snack to help remove food debris from the extraction site.
- Detailed instructions for pre- and post-surgery are found in Chapter 56.

IV. Oral Self-Care of the Neutropenic Patient

Neutropenia or a low white blood cell count (<500 absolute neutrophil count) occurs during treatment such as chemotherapy, radiotherapy, and bone marrow transplant associated with many cancers. Neutropenia puts the patient at increased risk for life-threatening infection. Oral complications can significantly impact the patient's quality of life and ability to recover primarily due to the impact on adequate nutrient intake.[73] (See Chapter 62.)

A. Oral Complications[73]

- **Mucositis** (inflammation and ulceration of the mucous membranes of the mouth and throat).
- Xerostomia (dry mouth).
- **Dysgeusia** (changes in taste).
- Fungal and viral infections such as *Candida* and herpetic lesions.
- **Trismus** (reduce opening of the mouth).
- Diffuse pain.
- Aggravation of existing periodontal diseases.

B. Oral Care Recommendations

- The Joint Task Force of the Multinational Association of Supportive Cancer Care in Cancer/International Society of Oral Oncology (MASCC/ISSOO) and European Society for Blood and Marrow Transplantation developed a protocol for basic oral care for before, during, and after treatment.[73]
- Ongoing interprofessional collaboration with the oncology team by the dental team is essential to maintain the patient's oral health.
- Prevention of infection in the oral cavity is needed to minimize the risk of systemic infection during this immune-compromised state. The

following recommendations have been made by the MASCC/ISSOO guidelines:

- Brush a minimum of two times/day with an extra-soft or soft toothbrush with the bristles softened in hot water.
- If mucositis is present, a topical anesthetic mouthrinse, such as morphine 0.2%, may be necessary for brushing to help minimize oral pain.[74]
- Replace the toothbrush regularly. It is suggested to replace the brush prior to each neutropenic cycle, meaning it should be replaced prior to the beginning of each chemotherapy or radiotherapy treatment cycle.
- Use a fluoride toothpaste; non-mint flavored may be more comfortable if the patient is experiencing mucositis. A prescription fluoride gel, toothpaste, or rinse may also be recommended depending on the patient's caries risk and ability to be compliant with oral self-care.
- The use of chlorhexidine for preventive measures of oral mucositis is not recommended.[74]
- Interproximal cleaning should be done regularly using aids the patient is familiar with to avoid self-injury. (See Chapter 27.)
- Clean the tongue by either brushing or using a tongue cleaner/scraper.
- Any dental prostheses should be cleaned according to instructions found in Chapter 30.

Adverse Effects of Toothbrushing

I. Soft-Tissue Lesions

- Gingival abrasion
  - Evidence of toothbrushing alone resulting in gingival recession is unclear.[17] However, frequency, duration, force, abrasiveness of the dentifrice, and technique may be implicated in recession.[11]
  - Localized gingival abrasion or trauma may occur with vigorous toothbrushing and is most common on the mid-facial aspect on canines, first premolars, or teeth in labioversion or buccoversion.
  - The appearance may be a distinct surface wound where the epithelial tissue has been denuded or it may be punctate lesions that appear as red pinpoint spots.

- To prevent further gingival abrasion, recommend use of a soft toothbrush with end-rounded filaments and observe the patient's toothbrushing technique and modify it as needed.

II. Hard-Tissue Lesions

- Dental abrasion
  - These lesions result from mechanical abrasion and typically appear as wedge-shaped indentations in cervical areas with a smooth, shiny surface. (See Chapter 16.)
  - These lesions are multifactorial and include use of an abrasive dentifrice, stiff toothbrush bristles, occupational causes, and habits such as chewing on pens.[75]
  - Primarily on facial surfaces, especially of canines, premolars, and sometimes first molars, or on any tooth in buccoversion or labioversion, because typically more force is applied to these areas during toothbrushing.
  - When adjacent teeth are involved, the lesions appear in a linear pattern across the quadrant or sextant.
  - Educate the patient about the presence of the abrasion and advise use of a soft toothbrush with end-rounded bristles along with use of a less abrasive dentifrice. The patient should then demonstrate their brushing technique to determine what modifications are necessary.
  - A power toothbrush that alerts the user when too much pressure is applied may be helpful to train the patient not to use excessive force when brushing.

III. Bacteremia

- Evidence suggests daily oral activities including chewing, toothbrushing, and flossing can produce transient bacteremia.[76]
  - The incidence and magnitude of bacteremia are significantly higher in patients with more dental biofilm accumulation and gingival inflammation following toothbrushing.
  - Power toothbrushes cause more bacteremia than manual toothbrushes.[77,78]
- Despite these findings, there is no clear association of transient bacteremia and infective endocarditis.
- However, it suggests the need for patients, especially those who are medically compromised, to maintain meticulous removal of dental biofilm on a daily basis to minimize the magnitude of bacteremia.

Care of Toothbrushes

When discussing the type and features of the toothbrush selected for an individual patient, the number of brushes needed and the frequency of replacement should be included.

I. Supply of Brushes

- Recommend at least two brushes for home use so they can be rotated to ensure they dry thoroughly between brushings. Most people will also want a third toothbrush in a portable container for use at work, school, or travel.
- Purchase of brushes needs to be staggered so that all brushes are not new at the same time and, more importantly, so that they are not old at the same time, thereby resulting in less than optimum biofilm removal.

II. Brush Replacement

Evidence shows toothbrushes with heavy wear are less effective at plaque removal than those with less wear.[12,79]

- There is no ideal timeframe for toothbrush replacement, but a general recommendation is at least every 2–3 months.
- Brushes need to be replaced before filaments become splayed or frayed or lose resiliency.
- The point at which a toothbrush needs replacement is influenced by many factors, including frequency and method of use.

III. Cleaning Toothbrushes

- Clean the toothbrush thoroughly after each use.
- Rinse the brush head with tap water until completely clean of visible debris, dentifrice, and bacteria from between the filaments.[80]
- Allow to dry thoroughly.

A. Toothbrush Contamination

- Toothbrush contamination has been explored in the literature.[81,82] Transmission of bacteria to others in the household has also been suggested, but little evidence exists to support it at this time.

- Toothbrushes become contaminated with pathogenic microorganisms during use as well as the way in which they are stored.[81-83]

B. Toothbrush Disinfection

- Though there is no evidence of harmful effects from the bacteria harbored in toothbrushes, the ADA recognizes individuals may opt for further disinfection.[12]
- Evidence shows toothbrushes soaked in 3% hydrogen peroxide or Listerine mouthwash have 85% less bacterial load.[12,84]
- Individuals with a higher risk for systemic infection, such as those with compromised immune systems, may benefit from the following: [80]
  - Rinse with an antimicrobial mouthrinse prior to brushing to reduce bacterial load.
  - Use of a toothpaste may also reduce bacterial load.[85]
  - Soak the toothbrush in an antimicrobial rinse such as essential oil mouthwash, cetylpyridinium chloride, or chlorhexidine after brushing.[81]
- Toothbrush sanitization using microwaves or ultra violet rays shows a significant reduction in bacteria.[86]

IV. Brush Storage

- Brushes need to be kept in open air with the head in an upright position, apart from contact with other brushes, particularly those of another person to avoid cross contamination.[80]
- Do not store in closed containers. If a portable brush container is used, try to dry the toothbrush prior to putting it in the container. A closed container encourages bacterial growth.[80,81]

Documentation

In the dental chart or record, the documentation for initial toothbrush instruction will include the following:

- Type of toothbrush patient has used to date: manual versus power.
- Recommended changes in type of brush or method of use.
- Description of soft tissue health and/or plaque score with goal(s) for improvement.
- Description of toothbrush education and areas patient has difficulty reaching.
- Tongue cleaning method education provided.
- **Box 2** shows a sample documentation for toothbrush selection and toothbrushing method.

Factors to Teach the Patient

- The effect of dental biofilm formation on the teeth and gingiva.
- Rationale for thorough daily removal of dental biofilm from the teeth, especially before going to sleep.
- The type of brush: manual, power, or both, recommended to maintain optimal oral health for a particular patient.
- Individualized hands-on instruction using an appropriate manual or power brushing method.
- Proper care and maintenance of manual and power brushes.
- Indications for and use of a tongue cleaner.

References

1. Arweiler NB, Auschill TM, Sculean A. Patient self-care of periodontal pocket infections. *Periodontol 2000*. 2018;76(1):164-179.

2. Berchier CE, Slot DE, Haps S, Van der Weijden GA. The efficacy of dental floss in addition to a toothbrush on plaque and parameters of gingival inflammation: a systematic review. *Int J Dent Hyg*. 2008;6(4):265-279.

3. Slot DE, De Geest S, van der Weijden FA, Quirynen M. Treatment of oral malodour. Medium-term efficacy of mechanical and/or chemical agents: a systematic review. *J Clin Periodontol*. 2015;42(suppl 16):S303-S316.

4. Van der Weijden FA, Slot DE. Efficacy of homecare regimens for mechanical plaque removal in managing gingivitis a meta review. *J Clin Periodontol*. 2015;42(suppl 16):S77-S91.

5. Gurudath G, Vijayakumar K, Arun R. Oral hygiene practices: ancient historical review. *J Orofac Res*. 2012;2:225-227.

6. Aumeeruddy MZ, Zengin G, Mahomoodally MF. A review of the traditional and modern uses of *Salvadora persica* L. (Miswak): toothbrush tree of Prophet Muhammad. *J Ethnopharmacol*. 2018;213:409-444.

7. Guerini V. *A History of Dentistry from the Most Ancient Times Until the End of the Eighteenth Century*. Philadelphia, PA: Lea & Febiger; 1909.

8. McCauley HB. Toothbrushes, toothbrush materials and design. *J Am Dent Assoc*. 1946;33(5):283-293.

9. Wadsworth HN. Toothbrush. U.S. Patent US 28,794 A. 1860.

10. Library of Congress. Everyday mysteries: who invented the toothbrush and when was it invented? Published 2019. https://www.loc.gov/rr/scitech/mysteries/tooth.html. Accessed August 8, 2021.

11. Asadoorian J. Canadian Dental Hygienists Association position paper: tooth brushing. *CJDH*. 2006;40(5):232-248.

12. American Dental Association. Oral health topics: toothbrushes. Published 2019. https://www.ada.org/en/member-center/oral-health-topics/toothbrushes. Accessed August 5, 2021.

13. Chun JA, Cho MJ. The standardization of toothbrush form in Korean adult. *Int J Clin Prev Dent*. 2014;10(4):227-236.

14. Slot DE, Wiggelinkhuizen L, Rosema NA, Van der Weijden GA. The efficacy of manual toothbrushes following a brushing exercise: a systematic review. *Int J Dent Hyg*. 2012;10(3):187-197.

15. Xu Z, Cheng X, Conde E, Zou Y, Grender J, Ccahuana-Vasquez RA. Clinical assessment of a manual toothbrush with CrissCross and tapered bristle technology on gingivitis and plaque reduction. *Am J Dent*. 2019;32(3):107-112.

16. Turgut MD, Keceli TI, Tezel B, Cehreli ZC, Dolgun A, Tekcicek M. Number, length and end-rounding quality of bristles in manual child and adult toothbrushes. *Int J Paediatr Dent*. 2011;21(3):232-239.

17. Rajapakse PS, McCracken GI, Gwynnett E, Steen ND, Guentsch A, Heasman PA. Does tooth brushing influence the development and progression of non-inflammatory gingival recession? A systematic review. *J Periodontol*. 2007;34:1046-1061.

18. American Dental Association. Acceptance program: guidelines for toothbrushes. Published 1996. http://www.ada.org/en/science-research/ada-seal-of-acceptance/how-to-earn-the-ada-seal/guidelines-for-product-acceptance. Accessed December 21, 2017.

19. Yaacob M, Worthington HV, Deacon SA, et al. Powered versus manual toothbrushing for oral health. *Cochrane Database Syst Rev*. 2014(6):Cd002281.

20. Deacon SA, Glenny AM, Deery C, et al. Different powered toothbrushes for plaque control and gingival health. *Cochrane Database Syst Rev*. 2010;8:CD004971.

21. Nash DA, Friedman JW, Mathu-Muju KR, et al. A review of the global literature on dental therapists. Community Dent Oral Epidemiol. 2014;42(1):1-10.

22. Grender J, Adam R, Zou Y. The effects of oscillating-rotating electric toothbrushes on plaque and gingival health: A meta-analysis. Am J Dent. 2020;33(1):3-11.

23. van der Sluijs E, Slot DE, Hennequin-Hoenderdos NL, Valkenburg C, van der Weijden F. Dental plaque score reduction with an oscillating-rotating power toothbrush and a high-frequency sonic power toothbrush: a systematic review and meta-analysis of single-brushing exercises. *Int J Dent Hyg*. 2021;19(1):78-92.

24. Grender J, Adam R, Zou Y. The effects of oscillating-rotating electric toothbrushes on plaque and gingival health: a meta-analysis. *Am J Dent*. 2020;33(1):3-11.

25. Erbe C, Jacobs C, Klukowska M, Timm H, Grender J, Wehrbein H. A randomized clinical trial to evaluate the plaque removal efficacy of an oscillating-rotating toothbrush versus a sonic toothbrush in orthodontic patients using digital imaging analysis of the anterior dentition. *Angle Orthod*. 2019;89(3):385-390.

26. Schmickler J, Wurbs S, Wurbs S, et al. The influence of the utilization time of brush heads from different types of power toothbrushes on oral hygiene assessed over a 6-month observation period: a randomized clinical trial. *Am J Dent*. 2016;29(6):307-314.

27. Rosema N, Slot DE, van Palenstein Helderman WH, Wiggelinkhuizen L, Van der Weijden GA. The efficacy of powered toothbrushes following a brushing exercise: a systematic review. *Int J Dent Hyg*. 2016;14(1):29-41.

28. Bizhang M, Schmidt I, Chun YP, Arnold WH, Zimmer S. Toothbrush abrasivity in a long-term simulation on human dentin depends on brushing mode and bristle arrangement. *PLoS One*. 2017;12(2):e0172060.

29. Hamza B, Uka E, Körner P, Attin T, Wegehaupt FJ. Effect of a sonic toothbrush on the abrasive dentine wear using toothpastes with different abrasivity values. *Int J Dent Hyg*. 2021;19(4):407-412.

30. Sharma NC, Galustians HJ, Qaqish J, Cugini M, Warren PR. The effect of two power toothbrushes on calculus and stain formation. *Am J Dent*. 2002;15(2):71-76.

31. van der Sluijs E, Slot DE, Hennequin-Hoenderdos NL, Valkenburg C, van der Weijden F. Dental plaque score reduction with an oscillating-rotating power toothbrush and a high-frequency sonic power toothbrush: a systematic review and meta-analysis of single brushing exercises. *Int J Dent Hyg*. 2021;19(1):78-92.

32. Davidovich E, Ccahuana-Vasquez RA, Timm H, Grender J, Cunningham P, Zini A. Randomised clinical study of plaque removal efficacy of a power toothbrush in a paediatric population. *Int J Paediatr Dent*. 2017;27(6):558-567.

33. Baruah K, Thumpala VK, Khetani P, Baruah Q, Tiwari RV, Dixit H. A review of toothbrushes and toothbrushing methods. *Int J Pharm Sci Invention*. 2017;6(5):29-38.

34. Versteeg PA, Rosema NA, Timmerman MF, Van der Velden U, Van der Weijden GA. Evaluation of two soft manual toothbrushes with different filament designs in relation to gingival abrasion and plaque removing efficacy. *Int J Dent Hyg*. 2008;6:166-173.

35. Litonjua LA, Andreana S, Bush PJ, Cohen RE. Toothbrushing and gingival recession. *Int Dent J*. 2003;53(2):67-72.

36. Brothwell DJ, Jutai DKG, Hawkins RJ. An update of mechanical oral hygiene practices: evidence-based recommendations for disease prevention. *J Can Dent Assoc.* 1998;64(4):295-306.

37. Poyato-Ferrera M, Segura-Egea JJ, Bullon-Fernandez P. Comparison of modified Bass technique with normal tooth-brushing practices for efficacy in supragingival plaque removal. *Int J Dent Hyg.* 2003;1(2):110-114.

38. Smutkeeree A, Rojlakkanawong N, Yimcharoen V. A 6-month comparison of toothbrushing efficacy between the horizontal scrub and modified Bass methods in visually impaired students. *Int J Paediatr Dent.* 2011;21(4):278-283.

39. Ausenda F, Jeong N, Aresenault P, et al. The effect of the Bass intrasulcular toothbrushing technique on the reduction of gingival inflammation: a randomized clinical trial. *J Evid Based Dent Pract.* 2019;19(2):106-114.

40. Bass CC. An effective method of personal oral hygiene, Part II. *J Louisiana State Med Soc.* 1854;106:100-102.

41. Waerhaug J. Effect of toothbrushing on subgingival plaque formation. *J Periodontol.* 1981;52(1):30-34.

42. Stillman PR. A philosophy of the treatment of periodontal disease. *Dent Digest.* 1932;38(9):314.

43. Hirschfeld I. *The Toothbrush: Its Use and Abuse.* Brooklyn, NY: Dental Items of Interest Pubs; 1939.

44. Gibson JA, Wade AB. Plaque removal by the Bass and roll brushing techniques. *J Periodontol.* 1977;48:456-459.

45. Charters W. Home care of the mouth. I. proper home care of the mouth. *J Periodontol.* 1948;19(4):136-137.

46. Bok HJ, Lee CH. Proper tooth-brushing technique according to patient's age and oral status. *Int J Clin Prev Dent.* 2020, 16(4):149-153.

47. Patil SP, Patil PB, Kashetty MV. Effectiveness of different tooth brushing techniques on the removal of dental plaque in 6-8 year old children of Gulbarga. *J Int Soc Prev Community Dent.* 2014;4(2):113-116.

48. Janakiram C, Varghese N, Venkitachalam R, Joseph J, Vineetha K. Comparison of modified Bass, Fones and normal tooth brushing technique for the efficacy of plaque control in young adults: a randomized clinical trial. *J Clin Exp Dent.* 2020;12(2):e123-e129.

49. Shick RA, Ash MM. Evaluation of the vertical method of toothbrushing. *J Periodontol.* 1961;32(4):346-353.

50. Vajawat M, Deepika PC, Kumar V, Rajeshwari P. A clinicomicrobiological study to evaluate the efficacy of manual and powered toothbrushes among autistic patients. *Contemp Clin Dent.* 2015;6(4):500-504.

51. Roldan S, Herrera D, Sanz M. Biofilms and the tongue: therapeutical approaches for the control of halitosis. *Clin Oral Investig.* 2003;7(4):189-197.

52. Laleman I, Koop R, Teughels W, Dekeyser C, Quirynen M. Influence of tongue brushing and scraping on the oral microflora of periodontitis patients. *J Periodontal Res.*2018;53(1): 73-79.

53. Van der Sleen MI, Slot DE, Van Trijffel E, Winkel EG, Van der Weijden GA. Effectiveness of mechanical tongue cleaning on breath odour and tongue coating: a systematic review. *Int J Dent Hyg.* 2010;8(4):258-268.

54. Timmesfeld N, Kunst M, Fondel F, Guildner C, Steinbach S. Mechanical tongue cleaning is a worthwhile procedure to improve the taste sensation. *J Oral Rehabil.* 2021, 48:45-54.

55. Van der Sluijs E, Slot DE, Hennequin-Hoenderdos NL, Van der Weijden GA. A specific brushing sequence and plaque removal efficacy: a randomized split-mouth design. *Int J Dent Hyg.* 2018;16(1):85-91.

56. Nandlal B, Shanbhog, R, Godhi B, Sunila BS. Evaluating the change in skills observed with a novel brushing technique based on sequence learning using video bio-feedback system in children. *Highl Med Medical Sciences.* 2021;14:31-36.

57. Kumar S, Tadakamadla J, Johnson NW. Effect of tooth-brushing frequency on incidence and increment of dental caries: a systematic review and meta-analysis. *J Dent Res.* 2016;95(11):1230-1236.

58. Zimmermann H, Zimmermann N, Hagenfeld D, Veile A, Kim TS, Becher H. Is frequency of tooth brushing a risk factor for periodontitis? A systematic review and meta-analysis. *Community Dent Oral Epidemiol.* 2015;43(2):116-127.

59. Zoraya SI, Azhar AAB. Association between toothbrushing and cardiovascular disease risk factors: a systematic review. *Adv Health Sci Res.* 2019;25:23-29.

60. Gunjalli G, Kumar KN, Jain SK, Reddy SK, Shavi GR, Ajagannanavar SL. Total salivary anti-oxidant levels, dental development and oral health status in childhood obesity. *J Int Oral Health.* 2014;6(4):63-67.

61. Van der Weijden G, Timmerman M, Nijboer A, Lie M, Van der Velden U. A comparative study of electric tooth-brushes for the effectiveness of plaque removal in relation to toothbrushing duration. Timerstudy. *J Clin Periodontol.* 1993;20(7):476-481.

62. McCracken GI, Janssen J, Swan M, Steen N, de Jager M, Heasman PA. Effect of brushing force and time on plaque removal using a powered toothbrush. *J Clin Periodontol.* 2003;30(5):409-413.

63. Underwood B, Birdsall J, Kay E. The use of a mobile app to motivate evidence-based oral hygiene behaviour. *Br Dent J.* 2015;219(4):E2.

64. Alkadhi OH, Zahid MN, Almanea RS, Althaqeb HK, Alharbi TH, Ajwa NM. The effect of using mobile applications for improving oral hygiene in patients with orthodontic fixed appliances: a randomised controlled trial. *J Orthod.* 2017;44(3):157-163.

65. Nolan SL, Giblin-Scanlon LJ, Boyd LD, Rainchuso L. Theory based development and beta testing of a smartphone prototype developed as an oral health promotion tool to influence ECC. *J Dent Hyg.* 2018;92(2):6-14.

66. Lozoya CJS, Giblin-Scanlon L, Boyd LD, Nolen S, Vineyard J. Influence of a smartphone application on the oral health practices and behaviors of parents of preschool children. *J Dent Hyg.* 2019;93(5):6-14.

67. Van der Weijden GA, Timmerman MF, Reijerse E, Snoek CM, van der Velden U. Toothbrushing force in relation to plaque removal. *J Clin Periodontol.* 1996;23(8):724-729.

68. Van der Weijden GA, Timmerman MF, Danser MM, Van der Velden U. Relationship between the plaque removal efficacy of a manual toothbrush and brushing force. *J Clin Periodontol.* 1998;25(5):413-416.

69. Wiegand A, Schlueter N. The role of oral hygiene: does tooth-brushing harm? *Monogr Oral Sci.* 2014;25:215-219.

70. Janusz K, Nelson B, Bartizek RD, Walters PA, Biesbrock AR. Impact of a novel power toothbrush with SmartGuide technology on brushing pressure and thoroughness. *J Contemp Dent Pract.* 2008;9(7):1-8.

71. Van der Weijden FA, Campbell SL, Dorfer CE, Gonzalez-Cabezas C, Slot DE. Safety of oscillating-rotating powered brushes compared to manual toothbrushes: a systematic review. *J Periodontol.* 2011;82(1):5-24.

72. Friedman AJ, Cosby R, Boyko S, Hatton-Bauer J, Turnbull G. Effective teaching strategies and methods of delivery for

patient education: a systematic review and practice guideline recommendations. *J Cancer Educ.* 2011;26(1):12-21.

73. Papadakos CT, Papadakos J, Catton P, Houston P, McKernan P, Jusko Friedman A. From theory to pamphlet: the 3Ws and an H process for the development of meaningful patient education resources. *J Cancer Educ.* 2014;29(2):304-310.

74. Linden GJ, Herzberg MC. Periodontitis and systemic diseases: a record of discussions of working group 4 of the Joint EFP/AAP Workshop on Periodontitis and Systemic Diseases. *J Periodontol.* 2013;84(4 suppl):S20-S23.

75. Elad S, Raber-Durlacher JE, Brennan MT, et al. Basic oral care for hematology-oncology patients and hematopoietic stem cell transplantation recipients: a position paper from the joint task force of the Multinational Association of Supportive Care in Cancer/International Society of Oral Oncology (MASCC/ISOO) and the European Society for Blood and Marrow Transplantation (EBMT). *Support Care Cancer.* 2015;23(1):223-236.

76. Elad S, Kin Fon Cheng K, Lall RV, et al. MASCC/ISOO clinical practice guidelines for the management of mucositis secondary to cancer therapy. *Cancer.* 2020;126(19): 4423-4431.

77. Milosevic A. Abrasion: a common dental problem revisited. *Prim Dent J.* 2017;6(1):32-36.

78. Tomas I, Diz P, Tobias A, Scully C, Donos N. Periodontal health status and bacteraemia from daily oral activities: systematic review/meta-analysis. *J Clin Periodontol.* 2012;39(3):213-228.

79. Misra S, Percival R, Devine D, Duggal M. A pilot study to assess bacteraemia associated with tooth brushing using conventional, electric or ultrasonic toothbrushes. *Eur Arch Paediatr Dent.* 2007;8(1):42-45.

80. Bhanji S, Williams B, Sheller B, Elwood T, Mancl L. Transient bacteremia induced by toothbrushing a comparison of the Sonicare toothbrush with a conventional toothbrush. *Pediatr Dent.* 2002;24(4):295-299.

81. Van Leeuwen MPC, Van der Weijden FA, Slot DE, Rosema MAM. Toothbrush wear in relation to toothbrushing effectiveness. *Int J Dent Hyg.* 2019;17(1):77-84.

82. American Dental Association, Council on Scientific Affairs. Toothbrush care: cleaning, storing and replacement. Updated February 26, 2019. https://www.ada.org/resources/research/science-and-research-institute/oral-health-topics/toothbrushes. Accessed November 11, 2021.

83. Frazelle MR, Munro CL. Toothbrush contamination: a review of the literature. *Nurs Res Pract.* 2012;2012:420630.

84. Ankola AV, Hebbal M, Eshwar S. How clean is the toothbrush that cleans your tooth? *Int J Dent Hyg.* 2009;7(4):237-240.

85. Wetzel WE, Schaumburg C, Ansari F, Kroeger T, Sziegoleit A. Microbial contamination of toothbrushes with different principles of filament anchoring. *J Am Dent Assoc.* 2005;136(6):758-765; quiz 806.

86. Beneduce C, Baxter KA, Bowman J, Haines M, Andreana S. Germicidal activity of antimicrobials and VIOlight Personal Travel Toothbrush sanitizer: an in vitro study. *J Dent* 2010;38(8):621-625.

87. Warren DP, Goldschmidt MC, Thompson MB, Adler-Storthz K, Keene HJ. The effects of toothpastes on the residual microbial contamination of toothbrushes. *J Am Dent Assoc.* 2001;132(9):1241-1245.

88. Agrawal SK, Dahal S, Bhumika TV, Nair NS. Evaluating sanitization of toothbrushes using various decontamination methods: a meta-analysis. *J Nepal Health Res Counc.* 2019;16(41):364-371.

Oral Infection Control: Interdental Care

Lisa J. Moravec, RDH, MSDH

CHAPTER OUTLINE

After studying this chapter, the student will be able to:

1. Review the anatomy of the interdental area and explain why toothbrushing alone cannot remove biofilm adequately for prevention of periodontal infection.
2. Describe embrasure size and patient status of health or disease as factors for evidence-based clinical decision making regarding which interdental device to recommend.
3. Describe the types of interdental brushes and explain why they may be more effective than floss for some patients.
4. Describe the types of dental floss and outline the steps for use of floss or floss loops for biofilm removal from proximal tooth surfaces.
5. Develop a list of the types and purposes of various floss aids, including floss holders and power flossing devices, and provide a rationale for the choice of the best ones to meet a specific patient's needs.
6. Demonstrate and recommend other interdental devices for biofilm removal, including an interdental rubber tip, a toothpick holder, a wooden interdental cleaner, and oral irrigation.

Overview of Interdental Care

Toothbrushing alone cannot accomplish biofilm removal from proximal tooth surfaces and adjacent gingiva to the same degree that it does for the facial, lingual, and palatal aspects. Therefore, interdental biofilm control is essential to complete the patient's oral self-care program.

Interdental cleaning devices ideally should be user-friendly, be effective with plaque removal, and have no deleterious effects on the soft or hard tissues.[1] When the preventive treatment plan is outlined for an individual, assessment is made of the oral condition, the problem areas, and the overall prognosis for improvement or maintenance of gingival health.

- Measures for interdental biofilm control are selected to complement biofilm control by toothbrushing.[2]
- The addition of floss or interdental brushes used with toothbrushing may reduce gingivitis and dental biofilm.[3]
- Daily interdental cleaning is necessary for dental biofilm removal and to reduce gingival inflammation.[2]

The Interdental Area

- In health, the interdental gingiva fills the **interproximal space** and under the contact of the adjacent teeth.
- When the interdental papilla is missing or reduced in height, the shape of the interdental gingiva changes.
- Factors impacting the papilla height include[4]:
  - Shape of the tooth.

- Interproximal bone height.
- Thickness of the gingiva.
- **Figure 1** shows a Class II embrasure from the proximal surface with the **col** and from the facial surface.
- The classification system on papillary height is illustrated in Chapter 18.

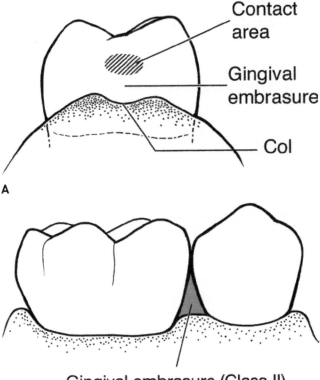

Figure 1 Class II Gingival Embrasure. **A:** Embrasure shown from the proximal surface with the col. **B:** Facial view, with gingival embrasure shown in blue.

I. Anatomy of the Interdental Area

A review of the gingival and dental anatomy of the interdental area can give meaning to and clarify the role and purpose of the various devices available for interdental care.

A. Posterior Teeth

- Between adjacent posterior teeth are two papillae, one facial and one lingual or palatal.
- The papillae are connected by a col, a depressed concave area that follows the shape of the apical border of the contact area (Figure   1).

B. Anterior Teeth

- Between anterior teeth in contact is a single papilla with a pyramidal shape.
- Tip of the papilla may form a small col under the contact area.

C. Epithelium

- The epithelium covering a col is usually thin and not **keratinized epithelium**.
- Col epithelium is less resistant to infection than keratinized surfaces.
- Inflammation in the papilla leads to enlargement; with increased inflammatory cells and edema, the col becomes deeper.
- The col area is inaccessible for ordinary toothbrushing and microorganisms may be harbored in the concave center.
- The incidence of gingivitis is greatest in the interdental tissues.[5]
- Bacteria accumulate in a biofilm on the tooth surface and affect the adjacent periodontal tissue which can lead to periodontal disease.[6]

II. Proximal Tooth Surfaces

- With bacterial infection and loss of attachment, the interdental papillae height is reduced, exposing the proximal tooth surfaces.
- Root concavities, grooves, and furcation areas provide areas for biofilm accumulation and contribute to causation of periodontal disease.[7]
- Irregularities of tooth position, such as rotation or overlapping, and deviations related to malocclusion or tooth loss may also be present.

- The increased root surface and complexity of the root morphology may make removal of bacterial deposits more difficult.

Planning Interdental Care

I. Patient Assessment

A. History of Personal Oral Care

- Self-care history includes type of toothbrush, dentifrice, and adjunct interdental aids currently used (i.e., dental floss, interdental brush, oral irrigation device).[8]
- Frequency and time spent.
- Assess barriers to effective interdental care, including patient preference and compliance.

B. Dental and Gingival Anatomy

- Position of teeth.
- Types and shapes of embrasures: Variation throughout the dentition (i.e., may recommend floss for anterior teeth with tight embrasures and interdental brush for posterior teeth with larger spaces).
- Clinical attachment level: Classification of the periodontal condition.
- Prostheses present: Special interdental care required for fixed and removable prostheses.
- Areas where toothbrush cannot reach.

C. Extent and Location of Dental Biofilm

- Preparation of a biofilm score or biofilm-free score to show the patient the extent of biofilm needing removal on a daily basis. (See Chapter 21.)
- Use of a disclosing agent to show specific sites where biofilm accumulates.
- Evidence of the patient's ability to care for difficult-to-access areas.

D. Personal Factors

- Disability that limits one's ability to carry out needed personal oral hygiene as well as patient compliance with interdental care.
- Oral health literacy about and appreciation for interdental oral care. Clinician should educate patient about the cause of disease, explain biofilm, and teach how to effectively remove biofilm from interdental space.[9]

II. Evidence-Based Clinical Decision Making

- Before selecting an interdental aid, the clinician must clinically assess and make a determination of periodontal health, gingivitis, or periodontitis. Periodontal health is defined by absence of clinically detectable inflammation (no bleeding on probing, erythema, edema, patient symptoms, clinical attachment loss or bone loss).[10]
- Embrasure size and patient status of health or disease are key factors in selection of interdental device.[9]
- Type I Embrasure: Dental floss is indicated for individuals with healthy tissues with high levels of patient compliance. Due to low compliance and/or gingival inflammation, other interdental cleaning devices should be considered.[11,12]
- For individuals with closed embrasures who lack motivation and/or dexterity, the use of easy flossers/floss holders, rubber interdental cleaners/soft picks, oral irrigation, or small interdental brushes are alternatives to traditional dental floss.
- Type II and Type III Embrasure: High quality evidence indicates use of interdental brushes are the most effective interproximal cleaning device for open embrasure spaces[9] and for periodontal maintenance patients.[11,12]

III. Dental Hygiene Care Plan

A. Objectives

- Utilize motivational interviewing to select appropriate interdental aids to help the patient reach optimum oral health. (See Chapter 24.)
- Determine if challenges with compliance exist, including lack of motivation to adhere or patient not remembering instructions for oral self-care.[7]
- Educate the patient on the oral care aids selected.
- The patient must accept responsibility for daily personal care and work as a partner with the oral health team.

B. Initial Care Plan

- Assess oral health behavior to create an individualized care plan that is sustainable and requires minimal reinforcement.[13]
- At first, the simplest procedures are selected for convenience and ease of learning based on the patient's current knowledge, preferences, and oral self-care habits.

- Minimum frequency: Twice daily.
- Keep the daily oral self-care regimen at a realistic level with respect to the time the patient is able or willing to spend.

Selective Interdental Biofilm Removal

I. Relation to Toothbrushing

- Vibratory and sulcular toothbrushing, such as that performed with the Charters, Stillman, and Bass methods, can be successful to some degree in removing dental biofilm near the line angles of the facial and lingual or palatal embrasures.
- Brushing in a vertical position is effective for additional access around line angles onto the proximal surfaces. (See Chapter 26.)

II. Selection of Interdental Aids

- The ideal interdental cleaning aid needs to be user-friendly, remove biofilm effectively, and cause no damage to soft tissues or hard tissues.[1]
- Choices are dependent on oral self-care abilities, embrasure size, disease status, and the risk for future recurrence.
- Flossing is typically recommended for patients with healthy gingiva and normal gingival contour, but is technique sensitive and requires instruction and reinforcement by a dental professional.
- High-quality flossing is a difficult skill for most patients; therefore, other interdental devices may be more effective with higher patient compliance.
- A patient working to control or arrest disease may need more frequent oral self-care than a patient in the maintenance phase.
- With the judicious selection and use of the various methods for interdental care, the dedicated patient can accomplish disease control.
- When gingival inflammation is present, interdental brushes are the preferred interdental cleaning aid.[11,12]
- Periodontal patients who have experienced gingival recession or attachment loss have concave surfaces in the interdental space and furcation areas that require special consideration.
- Stable periodontitis patients remain at higher risk for recurrent disease; therefore, ongoing risk assessment is necessary as part of optimal patient management.[10]

Interdental Brushes

I. Types

A. Small Insert Brushes with Reusable Handle

- Soft nylon filaments are twisted into a fine stainless steel plastic-coated wire. This brush is disposable and inserted into a plastic handle with an angulated shank (**Figure 2A**).
- The small tapered or cylindrical brush heads are of varying sizes, approximately 12–15 mm (1/2 inch) in length and 3–5 mm (1/8–1/4 inch) in diameter.

B. Travel Interdental Brush

- Reuseable travel interdental brushes are also available and may be more convenient for patients when away from home
  - Soft nylon filaments are twisted into a fine stainless steel plastic-coated wire.
  - The wire is continuous with the handle, which is approximately 35–45 mm (1½–1¾ inches) in length (**Figure 2B**).

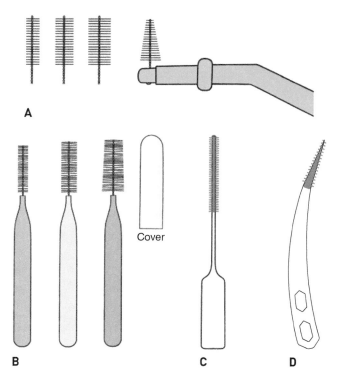

A

B   Cover   **C**   **D**

Figure 2 Interdental Brushes and Cleaners. **A:** Insert brushes for a reusable handle with an angulated shank. **B:** Reusable travel interdental brush with filaments twisted onto a fine plastic-coated wire that ends in a handle and cover. **C:** Disposable interdental cleaner. **D:** Disposable curved interdental cleaner.

- The very short, soft filaments form a narrow brush approximately 30–35 mm (1¼–1½ inches) in length and 5–8 mm (1/4–5/16 inches) in diameter (Figure 2B).

C. Rubber Interdental Cleaners

- Similar to an interdental brush, but do not have a wire. The rubber interdental cleaner or "soft-pick" has small elastomeric fingers that are perpendicular to a plastic core (**Figure 2C** and **D**).[14]
- The soft-pick is effective at biofilm removal and reducing gingival bleeding.[15,16]
- Rubber interdental picks are becoming increasingly popular with patients due to ease of use; patients may find them to be more comfortable than wire interdental brushes during insertion.[17]
- Rubber interdental picks may not remove as much biofilm due to fewer bristles[17] so selection of interdental device to best fit the patients' needs is important.

II. Indications for Use

- It is suggested that interdental brushes should be the first choice for interproximal cleaning.[2]
- Patient preference and anatomy need to be considered when selecting size and style.
  - Interdental brushes have been shown to be easier to use and preferred by patients.[18]
  - Size of the interdental embrasure also determines the choice of interdental brush or cleaner.
- Interdental brushes are more effective in biofilm removal than floss when the brush fills the embrasure.[2,3]

A. For Removal of Dental Biofilm and Debris

- Proximal tooth surfaces adjacent to open embrasures, orthodontic appliances, fixed prostheses, dental implants, periodontal splints, and space maintainers are well suited to interdental brushes and cleaners.
- Concave proximal surfaces are used where dental floss and other interdental aids cannot reach (**Figure 3A**). Floss will not access a concave surface, whereas the interproximal brush can reach and cleanse (**Figure 3B**).[1,8,14,19,20]
  - In patients with open embrasures and moderate to severe attachment loss, the interdental brush is often more effective than floss. However, it is important to choose an interdental

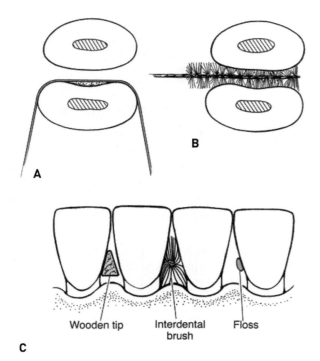

Figure 3 Interdental Care. **A:** Floss positioned on the mesial surface of a maxillary first premolar shows the inability of the floss to remove dental biofilm on a concave proximal tooth surface. **B:** The use of an interdental brush in the same interproximal area to show how dental biofilm can be removed from the proximal surfaces. **C:** Comparison of the access of a wooden tip, an interdental brush, and a piece of dental floss to an open interdental area.

Wooden tip   Interdental brush   Floss

C

brush that fills the embrasure to effectively clean concavities (**Figure 3C**).
- Interdental brushes are a great choice for periodontal patients with larger interdental spaces with recession or root exposure.[2]
• Exposed Class IV furcation areas (see Chapter 20).

B. For Application of Chemotherapeutic Agents

• Fluoride dentifrice, gel, and/or mouthrinse for prevention of dental caries, particularly root surface caries, and for surfaces adjacent to any prosthesis.
• Antimicrobial agents for control of dental biofilm and the prevention of gingivitis.
• Desensitizing agents.

III. Procedure

• Select brush of appropriate diameter to fill the embrasure.
• Insert at an angle in keeping with gingival form; brush in and out.

• For wide embrasures, it is important to remember to apply pressure against the proximal root surfaces to remove the biofilm thoroughly.
  • Insert the interdental brush as shown in Figure 3B–C.
  • Apply pressure toward the mesial proximal surface to remove biofilm.
• Then apply pressure toward the distal proximal surface and remove the biofilm.

IV. Care of Brushes

• Clean the brush during use to remove debris and biofilm by holding under running water.
• Clean thoroughly after use and dry in open air.
• Discard before the filaments become deformed or loosened.

Dental Floss and Tape

Despite daily dental floss along with toothbrushing being recommended to a majority of patients, effectiveness, compliance, and patient dexterity are limitations. High-quality flossing is difficult to achieve and may not confer significant oral health benefits over brushing alone if ineffectively used.[17] Unsupervised flossing does not yield substantial reduction in gingival inflammation when compared to other interdental devices (interdental brushes and water-jets ranked higher).[21]

• Recent studies show only a small reduction in interproximal bleeding in most patients due to low compliance and technique challenges with flossing.[1,2]
• Dental professionals need to determine whether high-quality flossing is an achievable goal when making individualized self-care plans for patients and effectiveness of plaque removal.

I. Types of Floss

• Research has shown no difference in the effectiveness of waxed or unwaxed floss for biofilm removal[22]; however, the effectiveness of flossing for biofilm removal is not supported by evidence.[18,19]

A. Materials

• *Silk*: Historically, floss was made of silk fibers loosely twisted together to form a strand and waxed for proximal surface cleaning.
• *Nylon*: Nylon multifilaments, waxed or unwaxed, have been widely used in circular (floss) or flat (tape) form for biofilm removal from proximal tooth surfaces.

- *Polytetrafluoroethylene (PTFE)*: Monofilament PTFE is used for biofilm removal from proximal tooth surfaces.

B. Features of Waxed Floss

- Smooth surface provided by the wax coating helps the floss slide through the contact area.
- Easing the floss between the teeth may minimize tissue trauma.
- Wax gives strength and durability during application to minimize breakage.

C. Features of Unwaxed Floss

- Thinner floss may be helpful when contact areas are tight.
- Care must be taken to avoid injury when guiding floss through a tight contact area or when moving floss on the tooth surface in an apical direction.
- Unwaxed floss may become frayed due to irregular tooth surface, rough surface of a restoration, or calculus deposit and cause the patient to become frustrated, thereby resulting in lost motivation to floss regularly.

D. Features of PTFE

- Monofilament type resists breakage or shredding when passed over irregular tooth surface, restoration, or calculus deposit.
- Reduces the force required to pass the floss through the contact, which may improve patient compliance with regular flossing and reduce tissue injury or trauma.[23]

E. Enhancements

- Color and flavor have been added to dental floss.
- Therapeutic agents added include fluoride and whitening agents; however, limited research has been published relative to their effectiveness.
- Dental floss that expands in contact with moisture to fill interproximal spaces better.

II. Procedure

- When dental floss is applied with good technique to a flat or convex proximal tooth surface, biofilm can be removed.
- Older biofilm is tenacious and may require more strokes for removal.

- When floss is placed over a concave surface, contact is not possible (Figure 3A), and supplementary devices are needed to remove biofilm completely.

A. Sequence of Flossing

- There is no ideal time to floss, but it may be helpful to floss before brushing to help dislodge food debris and plaque biofilm.

B. Floss Preparation

- **Figure 4** outlines the flossing steps described in detail here in this section.
- Hold a 12- to 15-inch length of floss with the thumb and index finger of each hand; grasp firmly with only 1/2-inch of floss between the fingertips. The ends of the floss may be tucked into the palm and held by the ring and little finger, or the floss may be wrapped around the middle fingers (**Figure 4A** and **B**).
- A circle of floss or "floss loop" may be made by tying the ends together; the circle may be rotated as the floss is used (**Figure 5**).
  - Advantages of creating a floss circle include improved user compliance and easier handling, less waste, and increased floss hygiene and biofilm removal efficacy.[24]

C. Application

- Maxillary teeth: Direct the floss upward by holding the floss over two thumbs or a thumb and an index finger as shown in **Figure 4C**. Rest a side of a finger on the teeth of the opposite side of the maxillary arch to provide balance and a fulcrum.
- Mandibular teeth: Direct the floss down by holding the two index fingers on top of the strand. One index finger holds the floss on the lingual aspect and the other on the facial aspect. The side of the finger on the lingual side is held on the teeth of the opposite side of the mouth to serve as a fulcrum or rest.

D. Insertion

- Hold floss firmly in a diagonal or oblique position.
- Guide the floss past each contact area with a gentle back and forth or sawing motion (**Figure 4D**).
- Control floss to prevent snapping through the contact area into the gingival tissue.

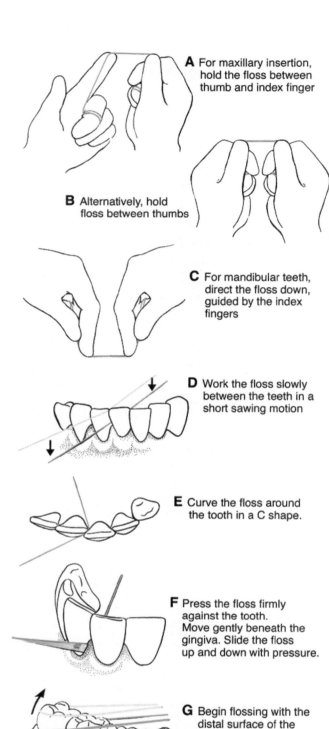

A For maxillary insertion, hold the floss between thumb and index finger

B Alternatively, hold floss between thumbs

C For mandibular teeth, direct the floss down, guided by the index fingers

D Work the floss slowly between the teeth in a short sawing motion

E Curve the floss around the tooth in a C shape.

F Press the floss firmly against the tooth. Move gently beneath the gingiva. Slide the floss up and down with pressure.

G Begin flossing with the distal surface of the most posterior tooth

Figure 4 Use of Dental Floss.

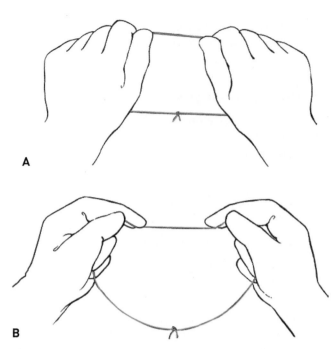

Figure 5 Circle of Floss. The ends of the floss can be tied together for convenient holding. A child may be able to manage floss better with this technique. **A:** Floss held for maxillary teeth. **B:** Floss held for mandibular teeth.

- Pass the floss below the gingival margin, curve to adapt the floss around the tooth, press against the tooth, and slide up and down over the tooth surface several times.
- Move the floss to a new, unused portion for each proximal tooth surfaces.
- Loop the floss over the distal surfaces of the most posterior teeth in each quadrant and the teeth next to edentulous areas (**Figure** 4G). Hold firmly against the tooth and move the floss in an up-and-down motion.

III. Prevention of Flossing Injuries

- Location: **Floss cuts** or **clefts** occur primarily on facial and lingual or palatal surfaces directly beside or in the middle of an interdental papilla. They appear as straight-line cuts beginning at the gingival margin and may result in a floss cleft if the tissue is repeatedly injured.[25]
- Causes
  - Using a piece of floss that is too long between the fingers when held for insertion.
  - Snapping the floss forcefully through the contact area.

E. Cleaning Stroke

- Clean proximal tooth surface separately; for the distal aspect, curve the floss mesially, and for the mesial aspect, curve the floss distally, around the tooth (**Figure** 4E-F).

- Not curving the floss about the tooth adequately and cutting into the gingival margin.

Aids for Flossing

I. Floss Threader

A floss threader is used for biofilm and debris removal around orthodontic appliances or under fixed partial dentures (**Figure   6**).

A. Description
- Floss threaders are flexible plastic and look like a needle with a very large loop at the end through which regular floss is placed.

B. Indication for Use
- Biofilm removal from mesial and distal abutments and under pontic of a fixed partial denture, implant, orthodontic arch wire, or other fixed prosthesis.

C. Procedure
- Individual surface of tooth or implant
  - Take a 12- to 18-inch piece of floss and thread it through the loop on the threader.
  - Put the floss threader under the appliance and pull the floss under the fixed appliance (**Figure   6A**).
  - Then curve the floss in a "C" shape around the proximal surface to remove dental biofilm (**Figure   6B** and **D**).
- Fixed partial denture
  - Thread floss under pontic and apply to distal surface of the mesial abutment and mesial surface of the distal abutment (Figure   6B–D).

II. Tufted Dental Floss

A. Description
Tufted dental floss is regular dental floss alternated with a thickened tufted (spongy) portion. This type of floss is commercially available.

- *Single, precut lengths*
  - Available in pre-cut 2-foot lengths composed of a 5-inch tufted portion adjacent to a 3-inch stiffened end for inserting under a fixed appliance or orthodontic attachment (**Figure   7A**).
- Example: Super Floss.

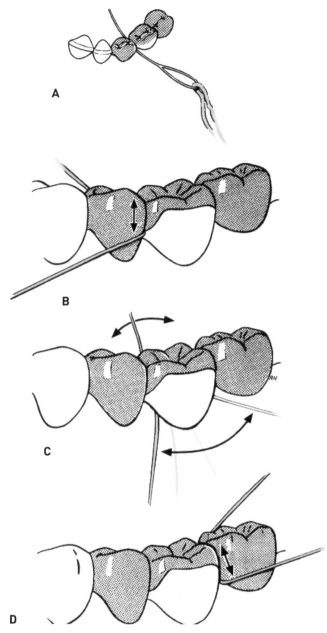

Figure   6 Use of Floss Threader. **A:** Use floss threader to draw the floss between abutment and pontic. **B:** Apply floss to the distal surface of the mesial abutment; pull through 1 or 2 inches. **C:** Slide floss under pontic. Move back and forth several times, as shown by the arrows, to remove dental biofilm from the gingival surface of the pontic. **D:** Apply new section of floss to the mesial surface of the distal abutment.

B. Indication for Use
- Biofilm removal from mesial and distal abutments and under the pontic of a fixed partial denture, implant, or orthodontic appliance. The stiff end of the tufted floss is inserted like a floss threader.

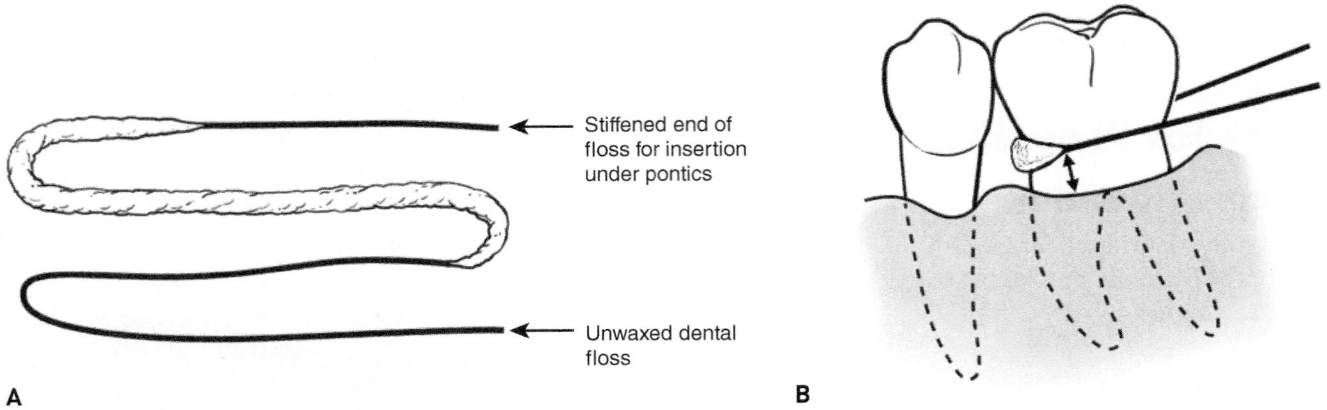

Figure 7 Tufted Dental Floss. A common brand available is called Super Floss, which is available **(A)** in a precut length with a tufted portion and a 3-inch stiffened end for insertion under a fixed prosthesis. **B:** How the tufted part of the floss might be used interproximally to remove biofilm is shown.

C. Procedure

- Individual surface of tooth or implant
  - Curve floss and/or tufted portion around the tooth or implant in a "C" to remove dental biofilm.
  - Move floss horizontally (**Figure 7B**).
- Fixed partial denture
  - Thread tufted floss under pontic and apply to distal surface of the mesial abutment and mesial surface of the distal abutment.

III. Floss Holder

A floss holder can be helpful for a person with a disability or for a parent or caregiver providing oral hygiene care for a child or adult.

- Types
  - Multiuse: Using 12–15 inches of floss, wrapping end around button and threading up across slot on prongs and back down toward button on the other side to keep floss taut (**Figure 8**).
  - Single-use: Disposable floss holder for single use (**Figure 9A-D**). These disposable flossers go by many names, which include, but are not limited to, sword floss, floss picks, or easy flossers.
- Indications for use
  - The mechanical properties, including floss tension and angle, are important considerations when selecting a floss holder.[26]
  - The effectiveness of holders maintaining adequate tension of floss through proximal contacts while not displacing the tissue is crucial for proper use.[26]
  - A novel two-handle flossing system (Gum-chucks) increases control and dexterity, allowing young children to make the "C" shape while flossing,[27] and is an effective alternative to string floss that allows children to floss with greater speed and efficacy (**Figure 10**).[28]
- Procedure
  - Use the same insertion and application procedure as previously described for flossing for use of the floss holder (Figure 9A-D) and single-use flossers such as the dual handle flosser (Figure 10).

IV. Gauze Strip

- Uses
  - For proximal surfaces of widely spaced teeth.
  - For surfaces of teeth next to edentulous areas.
  - For outer mesial and distal surfaces of abutment teeth of a fixed partial denture.
  - For areas under posterior cantilevered section of a fixed appliance, such as the distal portion of a denture supported by implants.
- Procedure
  - Cut 1-inch gauze bandage into a 6- to 8-inch length, and fold in thirds or down the center.
  - Position the fold of the gauze on the cervical area next to the gingival crest and work back and forth several times; hold ends in a distal direction to clean a mesial surface, and in a mesial direction to clean a distal surface (**Figure 11**).

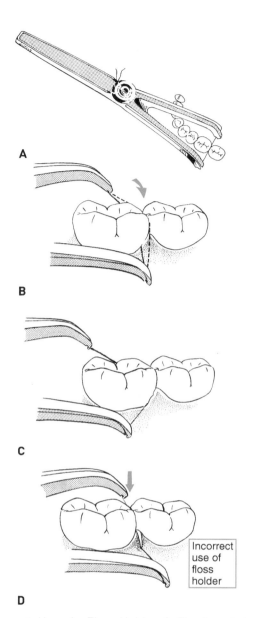

A

B

C

Incorrect use of floss holder

D

Figure 8 Use of a Floss Holder. **A:** The floss is held over the proximal contact for insertion. A hand rest is maintained on the chin to prevent excess pressure. **B:** As the floss is lowered gently and drawn through the contact area, the holder is pulled mesially when the floss is applied to the distal surface and pushed distally when the floss is applied to the mesial surface. **C:** Floss is lowered slightly below the gingival margin. **D:** Floss cut in the papilla when used incorrectly.

Power Flossers

I. Description

- Several types of power flossers are available.
  - One type of power flosser is battery operated and uses a disposable flexible nylon tip for interproximal care (**Figure** **12A**).

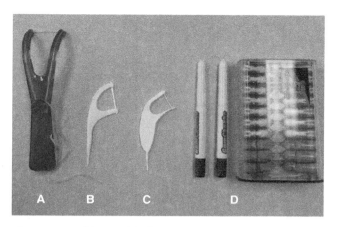

Figure 9 Disposable Single-Use Floss Holders. **A:** Reusable floss holder device. **B:** Disposable floss holder. **C:** Ortho floss holder. **D:** Flossing aid with two handles and disposable tips.

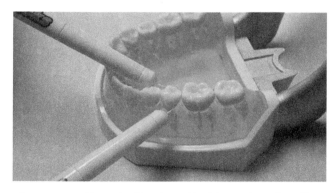

Figure 10 Use of a flossing aid with two handles. The procedure is the same as described for Figure 9.

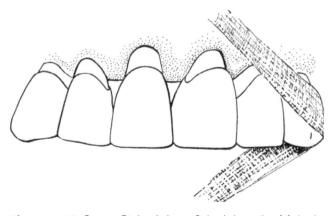

Figure 11 Gauze Strip. A 6- or 8-inch length of 1-inch bandage is folded in thirds and placed around a tooth adjacent to an edentulous area, a tooth with interdental spacing, or the distal surface of the most posterior tooth. A back-and-forth motion is used to clean the dental biofilm from the surface.

- Another type of power flosser is an air flosser, which uses bursts of air and water droplets to disrupt dental biofilm (**Figure 12B**).
- Patient acceptance regarding comfort when compared to dental floss was higher, with the microdroplet device being more effective at reducing biofilm.[29]

II. Indications for Use

- May be helpful for patients who are unable to use regular floss or those with manual dexterity issues.
- A power flosser can also be helpful for those who do not clean interproximally regularly and want to try this tool.

III. Procedure

- If the device has a reservoir, fill it with water.
- Standing near the sink, point the flosser interproximally and activate the device.
- Move systematically through the mouth on the facial and lingual interproximal areas.

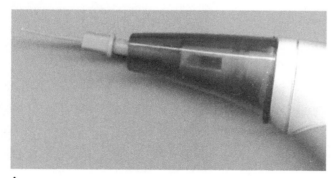

A

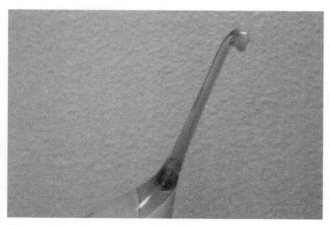

B

Figure 12 Power Dental Flossing Devices. **A.** An example of a powered dental flossing device. **B.** Air flosser.

Single-Tuft Brush (End-Tuft Brush)

I. Description

- The single tuft, or group of small tufts, may be 3–6 mm in diameter and may be flat or tapered (**Figure 13**). The handle may be straight or contra-angled.

II. Indications for Use

- For open interproximal areas
- For fixed dental prostheses
  - The single-tuft brush may be adaptable around and under a fixed partial denture, pontic, orthodontic appliance, precision attachment, or implant abutment.
- For difficult-to-reach areas
  - The lingual surfaces of the mandibular molars, abutment teeth, distal surfaces of the terminal molars, areas of missing teeth, and teeth that are crowded are examples of areas where an end-tuft brush may be of value.

III. Procedure

- Direct the tip of the tuft into the interproximal area and along the gingival margin; go around the distal surfaces from lingual and facial of the most distal teeth in all four quadrants.
- Combine a rotating motion with intermittent pressure, especially in the interproximal areas, to reach as much of the proximal surfaces as possible.
- Use a sulcular brushing stroke.

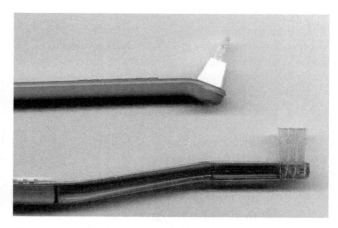

Figure 13 End-Tuft Brushes. End-tuft brushes come in flat and tapered shapes and can be used to clean areas that are difficult to access with a standard toothbrush.

Interdental Tip

The interdental tip may be called a rubber tip or rubber tip stimulator.

I. Composition and Design

- Conical or pyramidal flexible rubber tip may be attached to the end of the handle of a toothbrush or is on a single plastic handle (**Figure 14**).

II. Indications for Use

- For cleaning debris from the interdental area.
- For biofilm removal at and just below the gingival margin.
- The rubber tip is sometimes recommended for stimulation of gingival blood flow, although literature to support this is absent.
- After periodontal surgery, the rubber tip may also be used to shape the interproximal area during healing.

III. Procedure

- Trace along the gingival margin with the tip positioned just beneath the margin (1–2 mm). The adaptation is similar to the toothpick in holder (**Figure 15**).
- Rinse the tip as indicated during use to remove debris, and wash thoroughly at the finish.

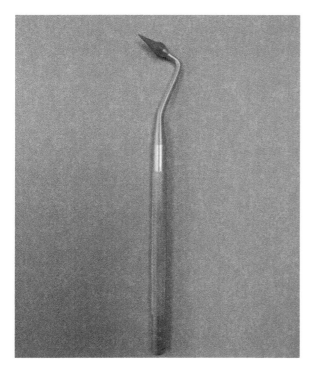

Figure 14 Rubber Tip (Also Called a Rubber Tip Stimulator) with Handle.

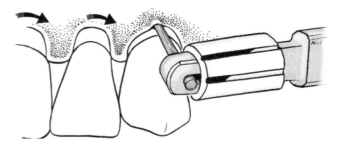

Figure 15 Toothpick in Holder for Dental Biofilm at Gingival Margin. The tip is placed at or just below the gingival margin. Gently trace the gingival margin of each tooth.

Toothpick in Holder

I. Description

A round toothpick is inserted into a plastic handle with contra-angled ends for adaptation to the tooth surface at the gingival margin for biofilm removal. The device is also called a Perio-Aid.

II. Indications for Use

- Patient with periodontitis
  - For biofilm removal at and just under the gingival margin; for interdental cleaning, particularly for concave proximal tooth surfaces; and for exposed furcation area.[30]
- Orthodontic patient
  - For biofilm removal at gingival margin above bands.

III. Procedure

A. Prepare Instrument

- Insert round, tapered toothpick into the end of the holder. One type of holder has angulated ends for use in various positions.
- Twist the toothpick firmly into place. Break off the long end so that sharp edges do not scratch the inner cheek or the tongue during use.

B. Application

- Apply toothpick at the gingival margin.
  - To remove biofilm just below the gingival margin, position the toothpick tip to a 70° angle to the long axis of the tooth and gently trace slightly subgingivally along the gingival margin from one interproximal space to the next[30] (Figure 15).
- For hypersensitive spots, usually at the cervical third of a tooth, the patient can use the tip daily to massage dentifrice for desensitization on the sensitive area.

Wooden Interdental Cleaner

I. Description

- The wooden cleaner is a 2-inch-long device made of wood. It is triangular in cross section, as shown in **Figure 16A**.
- A common brand is Stimudent.

II. Indications for Use

- Application
  - For cleaning proximal tooth surfaces where the tooth surfaces are exposed and interdental gingivae are missing. Space must be adequate, otherwise the gingival tissue can be traumatized.[31]
- Advantages
  - Ease of use.
  - Transported easily and can be used throughout the day.
  - Patients use woodsticks more frequently than dental floss.[31]
  - Although woodsticks do not remove biofilm as effectively as dental floss, research suggests they significantly reduce bleeding and interdental inflammation.[31]
- Limitations
  - As with most interdental devices, the wooden cleaner is advised only for patients who follow instructions carefully.
  - The wooden interdental cleaner cannot access root concavities and irregularities in proximal areas to adequately remove dental biofilm.

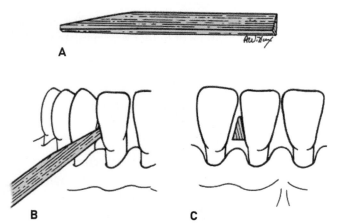

Figure 16 Wooden Interdental Cleaner. **A:** The 2-inch wooden triangular cleaner. **B:** Application on the proximal surface of a tooth with a type III embrasure. The base of the triangle is on the gingival side. **C:** The side of the triangle is rubbed in and out against the proximal surface to remove dental biofilm.

- Difficult to use in posterior areas and from the lingual aspect of the teeth.[31]

III. Procedure

- Fulcrum
  - Teach the patient to use a fulcrum by placing the hand on the cheek or chin or by placing a finger on the gingiva convenient to the place where the tip will be applied.
- Preparation
  - Soften the wood by placing the pointed end in the mouth and moistening with saliva.
- Patient instructions
  - Hold the base of the triangular wedge toward the gingival border of the interdental area and insert with the tip pointed slightly toward the occlusal or incisal surfaces to follow the contour of the embrasure (**Figure 16B–C**).
  - Clean the tooth surfaces by moving the wedge in and out while applying a burnishing stroke with moderate pressure first to one side of the embrasure and then to the other side, about four strokes each.
  - Discard the wooden cleaner as soon as the first signs of splaying are evident.

Oral Irrigation

I. Description

- The oral irrigator was introduced in 1962 and may also be called a water flosser.[32]
- Studies have shown oral irrigators lower bleeding and gingivitis indices, even if plaque levels are not affected.[3, 21,32,33]
- Oral irrigators and interdental brushes are recommended over dental floss for implant maintenance[17] and subjects undergoing orthodontic treatment.[34]
- **Irrigation** is the targeted application of a pulsated or steady stream of water or other **irrigant** for preventive or therapeutic purposes.
  - The purpose of irrigation is to reduce the bacteria and inflammatory mediators that lead to the initiation or progression of periodontal infections.
  - For the patient, irrigation can be a part of routine oral self-care.
- Water flossers use a pulsated stream of water under pressure.[35]
  - The water flossers have been shown to remove supragingival interproximal biofilm and reduce gingival inflammation.[35-40] However, the research has been funded by a single manufacturer, so there is a risk of bias and more

research is needed. Thus, the benefit of oral irrigation is reduction of gingivitis and this effect may not be related to biofilm removal.[18]

- The research on the benefits of **subgingival irrigation** with or without antimicrobial agents in managing microbial and clinical signs of periodontal disease remains inconsistent and more study is needed.[32,41]
  - The oral irrigator does not appear to reduce visible dental biofilm; however, it may have positive effects on gingival health over toothbrushing alone.[18,32]
  - In addition, some research suggests reduced counts of periodontal pathogens.[42]

II. Types of Devices

- Countertop power-driven model has a large reservoir for liquid (**Figure 17A**).
- Cordless model has a large base to serve as a reservoir for liquid and is good for travel (**Figure 17B**).
  - The handle is bulky because of the reservoir and may be too heavy for some patients.
- The shower model attaches to the showerhead or faucet and uses the pressure of the shower water, which may be somewhat lower than the irrigation delivered by the countertop model.

III. Delivery Tips

- A tongue cleaner to remove bacteria and debris (**Figure 18A**).
- A regular brush head is used like a manual toothbrush with water. It has no rotational or vibratory action (**Figure 18B**).

- A filament-type tip can be used in hard to reach areas and around dental implants or bridges (**Figure 18C**).
- An orthodontic tip is available to remove debris and loose dental biofilm from brackets, wires, and bands (**Figure 18D**).
- The subgingival tip is designed for subgingival irrigation with a soft rubber tip (**Figure 18E**) to be placed below the gingival margin.
- Standard jet tip delivers a steady flow of irrigant (**Figure 18F**)

IV. Procedure

These are general instructions for use of an oral irrigator:

- Fill the reservoir with water or other irrigant.
- Choose the appropriate tip.
- Direct the jet tip toward the interdental area until almost touching the tooth surface.
- Hold the tip at a right angle (90°) to the long axis of the tooth for **supragingival irrigation** to remove food debris and loose dental biofilm.
- Lean over the sink to minimize splatter and splashing water on the mirror, countertop, and floor.
- Turn the unit on using low power and increase the water pressure to a rate that is comfortable.
- Use a systematic approach for moving through the mouth such as, maxillary arch first, then the mandibular, facial, palatal, and lingual.
- When done, empty the reservoir to prevent bacterial growth.

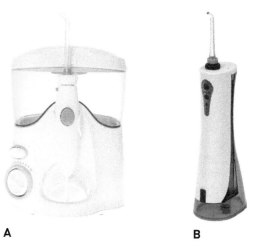

A   B

Figure 17 Water and Air Flossers. **A:** A countertop dental water jet with rechargeable power toothbrush. **B:** A countertop dental water jet.

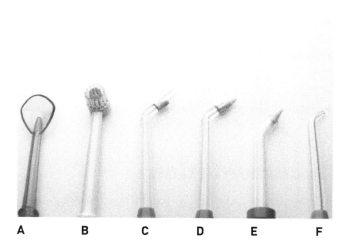

A   B   C   D   E   F

Figure 18 Tips for Water Irrigator. **A.** Tongue cleaner **B.** Toothbrush tip. **C.** Plaque Seeker tip. **D.** Orthodontic tip. E. Pik Pocket tip. **F.** Classic jet tip.

V. Applications for Practice

Regular use of daily personal oral irrigation is beneficial.[32] Use a patient-centered approach to evaluate each patient's needs individually to determine which techniques, products, or devices are appropriate.

A. Reduction of Gingival Inflammation

- The evidence is inconsistent on improving parameters of periodontal health, but there was a positive trend toward improving gingival health.[32]
  - A recent orthodontic study found the powered oral hygiene regimen (electric toothbrush and AirFloss Pro) was significantly more effective than a manual regimen (manual toothbrush and string floss) in reducing plaque on bracketed and nonbracketed teeth, and in reducing gingival bleeding and gingival inflammation in orthodontic subjects.[34]

B. Problem Areas

- Areas that are difficult to access with traditional mechanical methods:
  - Open interdental areas.
  - Malpositioned teeth.
  - Exposed furcations.

C. Special Needs Areas

- Prosthetic replacements such as a bridge with a pontic for a missing tooth and fixed partial dentures.
- Orthodontic appliances.
- Intermaxillary fixation appliances for orthognathic surgery and fractured jaw.
- Complex restorations and other extensive rehabilitation.
- Implant maintenance.
- Ineffective interdental technique due to physical ability or lack of compliance.

Documentation

- Documentation for a patient's interdental care progress needs to include a minimum of the following:
  - All interdental aid recommendations and demonstrations with the patient.
- A sample documentation can be found in **Box 1**.

Box 1 Example Documentation: Recommendations for Daily Interdental Care

- **S**—A 54-year-old male patient presents for routine 3-month continuing care appointment. Patient states, "I do not floss regularly as it is difficult for me, even with the floss holder you gave me last time. Is there another way to clean that area?"
- **O**—Generalized recession and extensive loss of interdental papilla on most posteriors. Observed patient has large hands and limited dexterity when trying to floss. Due to the open embrasure spaces, floss will not be effective in cleaning all surfaces of his teeth.
- **A**—Interdental brush may be a better choice than tufted floss for more thorough cleaning of the wide embrasure spaces in that area of his mouth.
- **P**—Provided instructions for use of two different sizes of interdental brushes with a tapered or cone shape as well as an interdental brush handle with replaceable inserts. The larger size will be used for the patient's posterior teeth with wider embrasures and the smaller size for the anterior areas. Observed patient use of the interdental brushes and worked with him to refine his technique. The patient felt these would do a better job of removing the debris and biofilm and will use these in every space where they fit and is easier for him to use. Samples of the types of interdental brushes were provided and suggestions where he can purchase replacements.

Signed: _____, RDH
Date: _____

Factors to Teach the Patient

- Use of disclosing solution will provide the patient with a visual understanding of the limitation of the toothbrush in accessing and cleaning the interdental area thoroughly.
- Discuss dental biofilm and how it collects on the proximal tooth surfaces when left undisturbed.
- Educate the patient on the reason why the interdental area is more vulnerable to infection.
- Use hands-on demonstrations to show how interdental aids are used to clean the proximal tooth surfaces. It is essential the patient also demonstrates the use of the interdental aids.
- Ensure the patient understands the need to ask the dental professional about new products they see advertised and whether the product meets the patient's individual oral self-care needs.

References

1. Salzer S, Slot DE, Van der FA Weijden, CE. Dorfer efficacy of inter-dental mechanical plaque control in managing gingivitis—a meta-review. *J Clin Periodontol.* 2015;42(suppl 16):S92-S105.

2. Chapple IL, Van der Weijden F, Doerfer C, et al. Primary prevention of periodontitis: managing gingivitis. *J Clin Periodontol.* 2015;42(suppl 16):S71-S76.

3. Worthington HW, MacDonald L, Pericic TP, et al. Home use of interdental cleaning devices, in addition to toothbrushing, for preventing and controlling periodontal diseases and dental caries. *Cochrane Database Syst Rev.* 2019;4(4): CD012018.

4. Joshi K, Baiju CS, Khashu H, Bansal S, Maheswari IB. Clinical assessment of interdental papilla competency parameters in the esthetic zone. *J Esthetic Rest Dent.* 2017;29(4):270-275.

5. Smukler H, Nager MC, Tolmie PC. Interproximal tooth morphology and its effect on plaque removal. *Quintessence Int.* 1989;20(4):249-255.

6. Graves DT, Corrêa JD, Silva TA. The oral microbiota is modified by systemic diseases. *J Dent Res.* 2019;98(2):148-156.

7. Kaur S, Gupta R, Dahiya P, Kumar M. Morphological study of proximal root grooves and their influence on periodontal attachment loss. *J Indian Soc Periodontol.* 2016;20(3):315-319.

8. Drisko CL. Periodontal self-care: evidence-based support. *Periodontol 2000.* 2013;62(1):243-255.

9. Liang P, Ye S, McComas M, Kwon T, Wang CW. Evidence-based strategies for interdental cleaning: a practical decision tree and review of the literature. *Quintessence Int.* 2021;52(1):84-95.

10. Chapple ILC, Mealey BL, Van Dyke TE, et al. Periodontal health and gingival diseases and conditions on an intact and a reduced periodontium: Consensus report of workgroup 1 of the 2017 World Workshop on the Classification of Periodontal and Peri-Implant Diseases and Conditions. *J Periodontol.* 2018;89(Suppl 1):S74-S84.

11. Slot DE, Valkenburg C, Van der Weijden GAF. Mechanical plaque removal of periodontal maintenance patients: a systematic review and network meta-analysis. *J Clin Periodontol.* 2020;47(Suppl 22):107-124.

12. Sanz M, Herrera D, Kebschull M, et al. Treatment of stage I-III periodontitis-the EFP S3 level clinical practice guideline. *J Clin Periodontol.* 2020;47(Suppl 22):4-60.

13. Wilder RS, Bray KS. Improving periodontal outcomes: merging clinical and behavioral science. *Periodontol 2000.* 2016; 71(1):65-81.

14. Graziani F, Palazzolo A, Gennai S, et al. Interdental plaque reduction after use of different devices in young subjects with intact papilla: a randomized clinical trial. *Int J Dent Hyg.* 2018;16(3):389-396.

15. Abouassi T, Woelber JP, Holst K, et al. Clinical efficacy and patients' acceptance of a rubber interdental bristle. A randomized controlled trial. *Clin Oral Investig.* 2014;18(7):1873-1880.

16. Hennequin-Hoenderdos NL, van der Sluijs E, van der Weijden GA, Slot DE. Efficacy of a rubber bristles interdental cleaner compared to an interdental brush on dental plaque, gingival bleeding and gingival abrasion: a randomized clinical trial. *Int J Dent Hyg.* 2018;16(3):380-388.

17. Graetz C, Schoepke K, Rabe J, et al. In vitro comparison of cleaning efficacy and force of cylindric interdental brush versus an interdental rubber pick. *BMC Oral Health.* 2021;21(1):194.

18. Ng E, Lim LP. An overview of different interdental cleaning aids and their effectiveness. *Dent J.* 2019;7(2):56.

19. Berchier CE, Slot DE, Haps S, Van der Weijden GA. The efficacy of dental floss in addition to a toothbrush on plaque and parameters of gingival inflammation: a systematic review. *Int J Dent Hyg.* 2008;6(4):265-279.

20. Larsen HC, Slot DE, Van Zoelen C, Barendregt DS, Van der Weijden GA. The effectiveness of conically shaped compared with cylindrically shaped interdental brushes - a randomized controlled clinical trial. *Int J Dent Hyg.* 2017;15(3):211-218.

21. Kotsakis GA, Lian Q, Ioannou AL, Michalowicz BS, John MT, Chu H. A network meta-analysis of interproximal oral hygiene methods in the reduction of clinical indices of inflammation. *J Periodontol.* 2018;89(5):558-570.

22. Ciancio SG, Shibly O, Farber GA. Clinical evaluation of the effect of two types of dental floss on plaque and gingival health. *Clin Prev Dent.* 1992;14(3):14-18.

23. Dörfer CE, Wündrich D, Staehle HJ, Pioch T. Gliding capacity of different dental flosses. *J Periodontol.* 2001;72(5):672-678.

24. Azcarate-Velázquez F, Garrido-Serrano R, Castillo-Dalí G, Serrera-Figallo MA, Gañán-Calvo A, Torres-Lagares D. Effectiveness of flossing loops in the control of the gingival health. *J Clin Exp Dent.* 2017;9(6):e756-e761.

25. Hallmon WW, Waldrop TC, Houston GD, Hawkins BF. Flossing clefts. Clinical and histologic observations. *J Periodontol.* 1986;57(8):501-504.

26. Wolff A, Staehle HJ. Improving the mechanical properties of multiuse dental floss holders. *Int J Dent Hyg.* 2014;12(4):245-250.

27. Kiran SD, Ghiya K, Makwani D, Bhatt R, Patel M, Srivastava M. Comparison of plaque removal efficacy of a novel flossing agent with the conventional floss: a clinical study. *Int J Clin Pediatr Dent.* 2018;11(6):474-478.

28. Lin J, Dinis M, Tseng CH, et al. Effectiveness of the GumChucks flossing system compared to string floss for interdental plaque removal in children: a randomized clinical trial. *Sci Rep.* 2020;10(1):3052.

29. Stauff I, Derman S, Barbe AG, et al. Efficacy and acceptance of a high-velocity microdroplet device for interdental cleaning in gingivitis patients: a monitored, randomized controlled trial. *Int J Dent Hyg.* 2018;16(2):e31-e37.

30. Lewis MW, Holder-Ballard C, Selders RJ Jr, Scarbecz M, Johnson HG, Turner EW. Comparison of the use of a toothpick holder to dental floss in improvement of gingival health in humans. *J Periodontol.* 2004;75(4):551-556.

31. Hoenderdos NL, Slot DE, Paraskevas S, Van der Weijden GA. The efficacy of woodsticks on plaque and gingival inflammation: a systematic review. *Int J Dent Hyg.* 2008;6(4):280-289.

32. Husseini A, Slot DE, Van der Weijden GA. The efficacy of oral irrigation in addition to a toothbrush on plaque and the clinical parameters of periodontal inflammation: a systematic review. *Int J Dent Hyg.* 2008;6(4):304-314.

33. Bertl K, Edlund Johansson P, Stavropoulos A. Patients' opinion on the use of 2 generations of power-driven water flossers and their impact on gingival inflammation *Clin Exp Dent Res.* 2021;7(6):1089-1095.

34. Nammi K, Starke EM, Ou SS, et al. The effects of use of a powered and a manual home oral hygiene regimen on plaque and gum health in an orthodontic population. *J Clin Dent.* 2019;30(Spec No A):A1-A8.

35. Goyal CR, Lyle DM, Qaqish JG, Schuller R. Efficacy of two interdental cleaning devices on clinical signs of inflammation:

a four-week randomized controlled trial. *J Clin Dent.* 2015;26(2):55-60.

36. Barnes CM, Russell CM, Reinhardt RA, Payne JB, Lyle DM. Comparison of irrigation to floss as an adjunct to tooth brushing: effect on bleeding, gingivitis, and supragingival plaque. *J Clin Dent.* 2005;16(3):71-77.

37. Goyal CR, Lyle DM, Qaqish JG, Schuller R. Evaluation of the plaque removal efficacy of a water flosser compared to string floss in adults after a single use. *J Clin Dent.* 2013;24(2):37-42.

38. Goyal CR, Lyle DM, Qaqish JG, Schuller R. Comparison of water flosser and interdental brush on reduction of gingival bleeding and plaque: a randomized controlled pilot study. *J Clin Dent.* 2016;27(2):61-65.

39. Goyal CR, Lyle DM, Qaqish JG, Schuller R. The addition of a water flosser to power tooth brushing: effect on bleeding, gingivitis, and plaque. *J Clin Dent.* 2012;23(2):57-63.

40. Lyle DM, Goyal CR, Qaqish JG, Schuller R. Comparison of water flosser and interdental brush on plaque removal: a single-use pilot study. *J Clin Dent.* 2016;27(1):23-26.

41. Nagarakanti S, Gunupati S, Chava VK, Reddy BV. Effectiveness of subgingival irrigation as an adjunct to scaling and root planing in the treatment of chronic periodontitis: a systematic review. *J Clin Diagn Res.* 2015;9(7):ZE06-ZE9.

42. Pandya DJ, Manohar B, Mathur LK, Shankarapillai R. Comparative evaluation of two subgingival irrigating solutions in the management of periodontal disease: a clinicomicrobial study. *J Indian Soc Periodontol.* 2016;20(6):597-602.

Dentifrices and Mouthrinses

Amy N. Smith, RDH, MPH, PhD
Kristeen Perry, RDH, MS

CHAPTER OUTLINE

LEARNING OBJECTIVES

After studying this chapter, the student will be able to:

1. Identify and define the active and inactive components in dentifrices and mouthrinses.
2. Explain the mechanism of action for preventive and therapeutic agents in dentifrices and mouthrinses.
3. Explain the purpose and use of dentifrices and mouthrinses.
4. Discuss regulatory agencies for medicines and healthcare products and their purpose.
5. Explain the American Dental Association Seal of Acceptance program or Canadian Dental Association Seal Program and their purpose.

Chemotherapeutics

Recent advances in understanding the pathogenesis of periodontitis have led to alternative therapies that focus on reduction of inflammation in the oral cavity using both mechanical devices and chemotherapeutics.

- Inflammation of periodontal tissues has an impact on the human body beyond the oral cavity.
- Oral inflammation has been linked to several conditions, including diabetes and heart disease.[1,2]
- Increased inflammation associated with diabetes can make a patient more susceptible to periodontal disease.[2,3]
- Oral pathogens can travel to the lungs, causing healthcare-associated pneumonia.[4]
- Either the clinician or the patient can administer chemotherapeutics.

Dentifrices

The benefits of using dentifrices may be preventive, therapeutic, or cosmetic. A dentifrice is a substance applied with a toothbrush or other applicator for:

- Removal of biofilm, stain, and other soft deposits from the gingiva and tooth surfaces.
- Application of therapeutic agents.
- Superficial cosmetic effects.

Preventive and Therapeutic Benefits of Dentifrices

I. Prevention of Dental Caries

- Although fluoride has long been recognized as an anticariogenic agent, the addition of stannous fluoride to a dentifrice was problematic because of lack of compatibility with abrasive agents.[5]
- The first caries-preventive dentifrice contained stannous fluoride (0.4%). It became available commercially in 1955.[6]
- Xylitol, a flavoring agent in some dentifrices, has been shown to provide anticaries benefits.[7]
- Additional information about fluoride dentifrices is described in Chapter 34.

II. Remineralization of Early Noncavitated Dental Caries

- Fluoride enhances remineralization as described in Chapters 25 and 34.

III. Reduction of Biofilm Formation

- Agents used:
  - Zinc citrate.
  - Stannous fluoride.

IV. Reduction of Gingivitis/Inflammation

- An antigingivitis dentifrice can contribute to the improved health of gingival tissue.
- Stannous fluoride has been shown to decrease bleeding sites and reduce the severity of gingivitis.[8,9]
- Dentifrice containing 0.454% stannous fluoride was shown to improve patients' scores on bleeding and gingival indices.[9]
  - Note: Research on the efficacy of this stannous fluoride toothpaste was sponsored by the product manufacturer, which has the potential to introduce bias.

V. Reduction of Dentinal Hypersensitivity

- For in-home treatment of dentinal hypersensitivity, chemical occlusion (potassium nitrate and sodium fluoride) of the dentinal tubules and nerve desensitization are most effective.[10]
- In-home treatment is the first intervention for dentinal hypersensitivity, but if it is not effective, in-office treatments are recommended.[10]
- More information on reducing dentinal hypersensitivity is discussed in Chapter 41.

VI. Reduction of Supragingival Calculus Formation

- "Tartar-control" dentifrices shown to help inhibit supragingival calculus may contain:
  - Pyrophosphate salts.[11]
  - Zinc salts (zinc chloride and zinc citrate).[11]
  - Sodium hexametaphosphate.[12]

Cosmetic Effects of Dentifrices

I. Removal of Extrinsic Stain

- The pigments from foods, tobacco, or chemical agents may become imbedded in the acquired pellicle and dental biofilm.
- Cosmetic results from dentifrice are based on:
  - Mechanical removal of the stained biofilm.
  - Delivery of a bleaching agent.
- Each commercially available product needs to be evaluated individually for efficacy and patient acceptance.
- More information on tooth stains is provided in Chapters 17 and 42.

II. Reduction of Oral Malodor (Halitosis)

- Certain ingredients added to a dentifrice can reduce oral malodor on a temporary basis by inhibiting the production of volatile sulfur compounds (VSCs).
- Chlorhexidine (CHX), cetylpyridinium chloride (CPC), and zinc formulations have a beneficial effect on reducing oral malodor via reduction of VSCs.[13,14]
- Stannous fluoride combined with sodium hexametaphosphate can reduce VSC production.[15]

Basic Components of Dentifrices: Inactives

- Most dentifrices share a common composition of ingredients needed for a stable formulation.
- Dentifrices are sold primarily as pastes and gels. The common ingredients and their function are listed in **Table 1**.
- In addition to the inactive ingredients described in Table 1, a therapeutic dentifrice will have a drug or chemical agent stated as an active ingredient for a specific preventive or therapeutic action.
- The active ingredient represents approximately 1.5% to 2% of the dentifrice's formulation.
- Therapeutic agents are described in **Table 2**.

I. Detergents (Foaming Agents or Surfactants)

- Purposes
  - Lower surface tension.
  - Penetrate and loosen surface deposits.
  - Suspend debris for easy removal by toothbrush.
  - Emulsify/disperse the flavor oils.
  - Contribute to foaming action.

Table 1 Ingredients and Function of Commercially Available Dentifrices

Ingredient	Function	Average Formulation Percentage (%)
Surfactant/detergent	Foaming and cleansing	1–2
Abrasive	Cleaning and polishing	20–40
Binder	Thickening agent and stabilizes formula	1–2
Humectant	Prevents water loss/hardening of dentifrice	20–40
Preservative	Prevents microorganisms from destroying the dentifrice in storage	2–3
Flavoring	Sweetener	1–1.5
Water	Maintains the ingredient in formulation	20–40

Table 2 Therapeutic Active Ingredients in Dentifrices

Benefit	Active Ingredients
Antibiofilm/ antigingivitis	Stannous fluoride, zinc citrate
Anticalculus	Tetrapotassium pyrophosphate, tetra-sodium pyrophosphate, sodium hexa-metaphosphate, zinc compounds
Desensitizer	Potassium nitrate, potassium citrate, potassium chloride, stannous fluoride, strontium chloride
Oral malodor	Essential oils, chlorine dioxide, stannous fluoride/sodium hexametaphosphate

- Substances used
  - Sodium lauryl sulfate USP.
  - Sodium N-lauroyl sarcosinate.

II. Cleaning and Polishing Agents (Abrasives)

- Purposes
  - Cleans well with no damage to tooth surface.
  - A polishing agent is used to produce a smooth tooth surface.
  - A smooth surface can prevent or delay the accumulation of stains and deposits.
- Primary abrasives used[16]:
  - Silica, silicates, and hydrated silica gels.
  - Calcium carbonate.
  - Dicalcium phosphate.
  - Sodium bicarbonate.

III. Binders (Thickeners)

- Purposes
  - Stabilize the formulation.
  - Prevent separation of the solid and liquid ingredients during storage.
- Types used
  - Mineral colloids.
  - Natural gums.
  - Seaweed colloids.
  - Synthetic celluloses.

IV. Humectants (Moisture Stabilizers)

- Purposes
  - Retain moisture.
  - Prevent hardening on exposure to air.

- Substances used
  - Xylitol.
  - Glycerol.
  - Sorbitol.

V. Preservatives

- Purposes
  - Prevent bacterial growth.
  - Prolong shelf life.
- Substances used
  - Alcohol.
  - Benzoates.
  - Dichlorinated phenols.

VI. Flavoring Agents (Sweeteners)

- Purposes
  - Impart a pleasant flavor for increased patient acceptance.
  - Mask other ingredients that may have a less pleasant flavor.
- Substances used
  - Essential oils (peppermint, cinnamon, wintergreen, clove).
  - Artificial noncariogenic sweeteners (xylitol, glycerol, sorbitol).

Active Components of Dentifrices

Dentifrice selections offer a variety of active ingredients that may help prevent caries, dentin hypersensitivity, biofilm formation, gingivitis, calculus formation, and oral malodor.

- The first active ingredient introduced in a dentifrice was fluoride. Major developments in active ingredients have been made since then.
  - Specific active ingredients are summarized in Table 2.

Selection of Dentifrices

I. Prevention or Reduction of Oral Disease

- Dental caries.
- Fluoride-containing dentifrice during remineralization program. (See Chapters 25 and 34.)
- Dentinal hypersensitivity.
- Gingivitis.
- Calculus formation.
- Oral malodor/reduction of VSCs.

II. Considerations for the Pediatric Patient

- Birth to first tooth eruption
  - Caregivers can clean the child's gingiva with a soft infant toothbrush or cloth and water.
- Eruption of first tooth
  - Caregivers can begin to start brushing twice daily using fluoridated toothpaste and a soft, appropriately sized toothbrush.
  - Use a very small "smear" or rice-sized amount of toothpaste to brush the teeth of a child younger than 3 years of age.[17] The small smear of fluoride paste is shown in Chapter 47.
- 2–5 years old
  - The caregiver can dispense a "pea-sized" amount of toothpaste for children over 3 years of age and perform or assist child's tooth brushing.[17] (See Chapter 47 for an illustration of "pea-sized.")
  - Caregivers need to recognize that young children do not have the ability to brush their teeth effectively without help and supervision.
  - Caregivers brushing their own teeth at the same time as the child can provide the child with a role model for brushing habits.
  - Children should be supervised until they are able to adequate remove plaque biofilm, spit out toothpaste, and not swallow excess toothpaste during brushing.

III. Patient-Specific Dentifrice Recommendations

- Dentifrice recommendations are a key part of personal daily care planning and are patient specific.
- Considerations include:
  - Patient's current oral condition.
  - Any patient complaint/concern.
  - Sensitivities or allergies to a specific ingredient.
  - Propensity of staining (stannous fluoride–containing dentifrice).
  - Patient's nontherapeutic/cosmetic choices.
  - Expectation of compliance. When a dentifrice does not appeal in either taste or texture, it will not be used regardless of therapeutic benefits.
  - Personal trial is needed before a recommendation is made. Dental hygienists need firsthand experience with each product they recommend.

Mouthrinses

- Mechanical aids may not be sufficient to maintain optimum oral health for certain patients and may be supplemented with the use of a chemotherapeutic mouthrinse.
- The benefits of using a mouthrinse may be one or more of the following: preventive, cosmetic, and therapeutic.
- Chemotherapeutic rinses may have active ingredients to reduce inflammation.
- Cosmetic rinses can provide some extrinsic stain removal when it is superficial in unattached biofilm.
- **Therapeutic rinses** have healing properties that are delivered by rinsing or irrigation device.
- Delivery: Rinsing can deliver an agent less than 2 mm into the sulcus or pocket and is not a delivery of choice for patients with moderate or deep pockets.[18]
- Functions: A list of general functions of **chemotherapeutic agents** is provided in **Box 1**.

Purposes and Uses of Mouthrinses

I. Before Professional Treatment

- To reduce the numbers of intraoral microorganisms to lower the bacterial load.
- To reduce contamination during aerosol generating procedures such as use of a handpiece or ultrasonic scaler.

II. Self-Care

- As part of personal oral self-care for specific needs.
- Biofilm control.

Box 1 Functions of Chemotherapeutic Agents

- Remineralization: Restore mineral elements.
- Antimicrobial: Bactericidal or bacteriostatic.
  - Biofilm control.
  - Gingival health: Reduction/prevention of gingivitis.
- **Astringent**: Shrink tissues.
- Anodyne: Alleviate pain.
- Buffering: Reduce oral acidity.
- Deodorizing: Neutralize odor.
- Oxygenating: Cleanse.

- Dental caries prevention through remineralization of noncavitated early dental caries.
- Prevention of gingivitis.
- Contribute to malodor control.
- Posttreatment therapy following nonsurgical periodontal therapy:
  - Periodontal surgery.
  - Removal of teeth.

Preventive and Therapeutic Agents of Mouthrinses

I. Fluoride

A. Mechanism of Action

- Stannous fluoride
  - Deposit of fluoride ion on enamel.
  - Tin ion from stannous fluoride interferes with cell metabolism for antimicrobial effect.
- Sodium fluoride:
  - Deposit of fluoride ion on enamel.
  - Cariostatic: Inhibits demineralization and enhances remineralization.

B. Availability and Use

- Available in varying concentrations.
- Uses:
  - Prevention of demineralization.
  - Reduction of hypersensitivity.
  - Reduction of gingivitis.

C. Efficacy

- Reduction in biofilm or dental caries when rinse is used topically by the patient.

D. Considerations

- Stannous: Tooth staining; flavor.
- Instruct patient to expectorate/not to swallow.

II. Chlorhexidine

A. Mechanism of Action

- The mechanisms of action of chlorhexidine (**CHX**) include the following:
  - A cationic bisbiguanide with broad antibacterial activity.
  - Binds to oral hard and soft tissues.
  - Attaches to bacterial cell membrane, thereby damaging the cytoplasm and causing lysis.
  - Binds to pellicle and salivary mucins to prevent biofilm accumulation.
  - Bactericidal and bacteriostatic depending on concentration.
  - Bactericidal concentrations cause cell lysis.
  - Bacteriostatic concentrations interfere with cell wall transport system.
  - The substantivity of CHX: 8–12 hours.
  - Antimicrobial and antigingivitis agent.

B. Availability and Uses

- CHX is the most effective antimicrobial and antigingivitis agent available for clinical use.[19,20]
  - Mouthrinse available by prescription in a 0.12% solution in the United States (higher concentrations are available in other countries); postsurgery for enhanced wound healing (**Figure 1**).
- Recommended uses:
  - Preprocedural rinse to reduce bacterial load before aerosol-producing procedures.
  - Before, during, and after periodontal debridement.
  - Patients who are at a high risk for dental caries.
  - Immunocompromised individuals who are more susceptible to infection.
  - Postsurgery for enhanced wound healing.

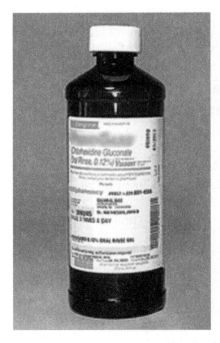

Figure 1 Therapeutic Mouthrinse. Chlorhexidine gluconate mouthrinse aids in plaque biofilm control and requires a prescription for purchase.

Reproduced from Nield-Gehrig J, Willmann D. Foundations of Periodontics for the Dental Hygienist. 3rd ed. Philadelphia, PA: Lippincott Williams & Wilkins; 2011.

C. Efficacy

- CHX is safe and effective in:
  - Preventing and controlling biofilm formation.
  - Reducing viability of existing biofilm.
  - Inhibiting and reducing the development of gingivitis.[20]
  - Reducing mutans streptococci.[20]

D. Considerations

- Low level of toxicity due to poor absorption through mucous membranes.
- Staining of teeth, including smooth surfaces, pits and fissures, restorations, and soft tissues (Figure 2).
- Increase in supragingival calculus formation.
- Altered taste perception.
- Minor irritation to soft tissues, lips, and tongue.

Some research suggests CHX interacts with and is inactivated by sodium lauryl sulfate (a surfactant used in dentifrices) when rinsing is performed immediately after brushing. However, a recent systematic review and meta-analysis indicates that sodium lauryl sulfate does not interfere with the antiplaque effect of CHX.[21]

III. Phenolic-Related Essential Oils

A. Mechanism of Action

- Disrupt cell walls and inhibit bacterial enzymes.
- Decrease pathogenicity of biofilm.
- Antimicrobial and antigingivitis agent.

B. Availability and Uses

- A combination of thymol, eucalyptol, menthol, and methyl salicylate is available as a brand name product and generic product.

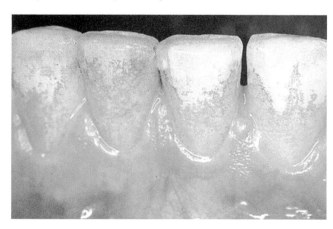

Figure 2 Chlorhexidine Stain

Reproduced from Nield-Gehrig J. *Fundamentals of Periodontal Instrumentation and Advanced Root Instrumentation.* Philadelphia, PA: Lippincott Williams & Wilkins; 2011.

- Recommended uses:
  - Individuals unable to perform adequate brushing and flossing.
  - Initially or periodically to help improve management of dental biofilm.
  - Adjunct for mechanical self-care routines that are not sufficient in reducing biofilm, bleeding, and gingivitis.
  - Preprocedural rinse to reduce bacterial load before instrumentation-producing aerosols.

C. Efficacy

- Significant reduction in the levels of biofilm and gingivitis.[20,22]

D. Considerations

- Burning sensation.
- Bitter taste.
- Poor substantivity.
- Efficacy of individual rinses based on following the manufacturer's instructions and not casual use of the rinse.
- Contraindicated for current or recovering alcoholics due to alcohol content.

IV. Quaternary Ammonium Compounds

A. Mechanism of Action

- The mechanisms of action of quaternary ammonium compounds include[23]:
  - Cationic agents that bind to oral tissues.
  - Rupture the cell wall and alter the cytoplasm.
  - Initial attachment to oral tissue is very strong, but released rapidly.
  - Decreases the ability of bacteria to attach to the pellicle.
  - Low substantivity.

B. Availability and Uses

- The most commonly used agent is CPC, at 0.05% to 0.07%.
- Recommended uses:
  - Reduction in biofilm accumulation.
  - Adjunct for mechanical self-care routines.

C. Efficacy

- Weak evidence for reductions in biofilm and gingivitis and more research is recommended.[24]

- Possible inhibition of calculus formation.[24]
- Preliminary research has shown that CPC inactivated SARS-CoV-2, but the clinical efficacy has not been investigated.[25]

D. Considerations

- Staining of teeth and tongue.[26]
- A burning sensation and occasional desquamation.[26]

V. Oxygenating Agents

A. Mechanism of Action[27]

- Alters bacterial cell membrane, increasing permeability.
- Poor substantivity.

B. Availability and Uses

- The common agents available in commercial rinses are 10% carbamide peroxide and 1.5% hydrogen peroxide.
- Recommended for short-term use to reduce the symptoms of pericoronitis and necrotizing ulcerative gingivitis.[27]

C. Efficacy

- Negligible antimicrobial effect.
- Debriding agent.
- Despite early suggestions of efficacy, hydrogen peroxide has not been proven to inactivate or reduce the viral load of SARS-CoV-2 when used as a mouthrinse.[25]

D. Considerations

- Does not consistently prevent plaque biofilm accumulation short term, but when used long term, some reduction in gingival redness has been noted.[27]
- Occasional reports of erosive changes to oral mucosa.[27]

VI. Oxidizing Agents

A. Mechanism of Action

- Neutralization of VSCs that contribute to oral malodor.

B. Availability and Uses

- Common agents available in commercial rinses are chlorine dioxide (ClO_2) and chlorine dioxide/zinc combination.

C. Efficacy

- Mainly used for management of halitosis.[28]

D. Consideration

- Diluted 0.25% to 0.5% sodium hypochlorite used as a mouthrinse twice per week showed significant reductions in bleeding on probing (BOP), dental biofilm, and gingival inflammation.[29,30]

Commercial Mouthrinse Ingredients

Ingredients and their functions are listed in **Table 3**.

I. Active Ingredients

- Commercial mouthrinses generally contain more than one active ingredient and, therefore, may advertise multiple claims for use.
- Factors that influence how effective an agent may be:
  - Dilution by the saliva.

Table 3 Typical Commercial Mouthrinse Formulation

Ingredient	Function
Alcohol	Enhances flavor impact and contributes to cleansing
Flavor	Used to enhance taste and makes breath temporarily fresh
Humectant	Adds "body" and inhibits crystallization around closure
Surfactant	Solubilizes the flavor and provides foaming action
Water	Major vehicle to carry other ingredients
Preservative	Preserves aqueous formulation
Dyes	Add color
Sweeteners	Contribute to overall flavor perception
Flavor	Makes mouthrinse pleasant to use
Active or functional ingredients	Provide therapeutic and/or benefits

- Length of time the agent is in contact with the tissue or bacteria.
- Evidence supporting the particular product.
- General characteristics of an effective chemotherapeutic agent are shown in **Box 2**.

II. Inactive Ingredients

A. Water

- Makes up the largest percentage by volume.

B. Alcohol

- Use of alcohol in mouthrinses[31]:
  - Increases the solubility of some active ingredients.
  - Acts as a preservative.
  - Percentage varies from 18% to 27%.
  - Enhances flavor.
- No link to oral cancer has been found with regular use of an alcohol-containing mouthrinse.[32]

C. Flavoring

- Essential oils and derivatives (eucalyptus oil, oil of wintergreen).
- Aromatic waters (peppermint, spearmint, wintergreen, or others).
- Artificial noncariogenic sweetener.

III. Patient-Specific Mouthrinse Recommendations

Mouthrinses are formulated for a variety of oral benefits, including mouth freshening, prevention of caries, biofilm control, and control of oral malodor. Several factors are considered when making a mouthrinse recommendation, including:

- Is the patient currently able to control biofilm through other methods?
- Does the patient consider rinsing a substitute for other mechanical procedures such as brushing and interproximal biofilm removal?
- Does the patient's substance abuse history contraindicate recommending an alcohol-containing mouthrinse?
- Could the patient's xerostomia be worsened by the drying effect of an alcohol-containing mouthrinse?

IV. Contraindications

- The use of a mouthrinse can enhance a patient's oral self-care regimen. The patient needs to understand why rinsing is not a substitute for brushing or use of interproximal aids.
- Some agents are contraindicated for children younger than 6 years of age who have a tendency to swallow instead of expectorate.
- Review manufacturer's instructions for age limits as they vary by product.
- Contraindicated in patients with physical or cognitive challenges who cannot follow rinsing instructions.

Procedure for Rinsing

- Many patients, particularly children, must be shown specifically how to rinse. The method can be practiced under supervision.
- **Box 3** suggests steps for teaching a patient to rinse.

Box 2 Characteristics of an Effective Chemotherapeutic Agent

- Nontoxic: The agent does not damage oral tissues or create systemic problems.
- No or limited absorption: The action is confined to the oral cavity.
- Substantivity: The ability of an agent to be bound to the pellicle and tooth surface and be released over a period of time with retention of potency.
- Bacterial specificity: May be broad-spectrum, but with an affinity for the pathogenic organisms of the oral cavity.
- Low-induced drug resistance: Low or no development of resistant organisms to agent.

Box 3 Steps: How to Rinse

- Take a small amount of the fluid into the mouth.
- Close lips; hold teeth slightly apart.
- Force the fluid through the interdental areas with pressure.
- Use the lips, cheeks, and tongue action to force the fluid back and forth between the teeth.
- Balloon the cheeks, then suck them in, alternately several times.
- Divide the mouth into three parts—front, right, and left.
- Concentrate the rinsing first on the front, then on the right, and then on the left side.
- Expectorate.
- Follow manufacturer's directions on amount, length, and frequency of rinsing.

Emerging Alternative Practices

I. Oil Pulling

- The ancient practice of swishing with 10 mL (one tablespoon) of sesame or coconut oil. [33,34]
- Reduction of biofilm. [33,34]
- Reduction of bacteria causing caries, gingivitis, halitosis, and oral thrush. [33,34]

Agencies Regulating Medicine and Healthcare Products

The purpose of the U.S. Food and Drug Administration (FDA) is to ensure the safety and efficacy of medical and dental drugs, equipment, and devices that affect living tissue. All drugs require FDA approval. Rinses and dentifrices are classified by the FDA as cosmetic, **therapeutic**, or a combination of cosmetic and therapeutic. [35]

I. Regulatory Agencies Overview

- Regulatory agencies for oversight of medicine and healthcare products globally include some of the following:
  - United States: Food and Drug Association (FDA)
  - Canada: Health Canada (HC)
  - United Kingdom: Medicines and Healthcare Products Regulatory Agency (MHRA)
  - European Union: European Medicines Agency (EMA)
  - South Africa: South African Health Products Regulatory Authority (SAHPRA)

II. Role of the Regulatory Agencies for Medicines and Healthcare Products

- Regulate safety, quality, and efficacy of drugs, equipment, and devices.
  - Some devices and equipment may be exempt from (dental water jets, power and manual toothbrushes, dental floss) if they have existing or reasonably similar characteristics as previously approved devices of the same type.

III. Dental Product Regulation

- Dental products regulated will vary from agency to agency, but may include:
  - Infection control products.
  - Dental equipment such as ultrasonic instruments.
  - Diagnostic test kits (i.e., dental caries detection devices).
  - Prosthetic and restorative materials such as implants.
  - Surgical and periodontal materials such as guided tissue regeneration membranes, bone-filling material, and growth factors.
  - Prescription drugs, controlled and sustained-release devices, and chemotherapeutics.
  - In the case of dentifrice and mouthrinses, the FDA has reviewed active ingredients under over-the-counter (OTC) monographs, which are regulations that specify the active ingredients and permissible levels of those ingredients, as well as statements required on product labels. [36]

IV. Research Requirements and Documentation

- **Table** 4 outlines the documentation process for a product to receive FDA approval. [37]
  - Regulatory agencies in other countries may have a different process, but rigor in the evidence needed for approval is always a part of this process.

Seal of Acceptance Program

I. American Dental Association Seal of Acceptance

- The American Dental Association (ADA) has promoted safety and effectiveness of dental products for over 92 years. [38]
- The ADA Seal of Acceptance Program, which evaluates OTC products offered to consumers, has been in place since 1931, and is internationally recognized. [38]
- Unlike the FDA, the ADA Seal Program is voluntary, and a company must apply to obtain it by making a product submission. [38]
- Products are awarded the ADA Seal only after the ADA Council on Scientific Affairs has thoroughly

Table 4 Food and Drug Administration Clearance Documentation Process for Oral Care Products

Phase	Study Type	Purpose
Preclinical	Animal studies	Safety/toxicity
I.	Clinical trial with small sample population (20–80)	Determine dosing/safety, how drug is metabolized and excreted, and side effects
II.	Clinical trial with a larger sample population (100–200) who have disease or condition that the product is designed to treat. The test drug is compared to a standard treatment or placebo known as a control	Provides further safety data and preliminary evidence of efficacy
III.	Clinical trial with a large sample population (1,000–3,000) who have a disease or condition to test efficacy, monitor side effects, and identify treatment parameters. The test drug is compared to a standard treatment or placebo known as a control	Identify possible less obvious side effects
IV.	Clinical trials on products that are already approved and on the market	Continue to measure long-term benefits, risks, and optimal protocol

evaluated clinical and laboratory studies on a product and determined that it meets the ADA criteria for safety and effectiveness, when used as directed.[38]

II. Purposes of the Seal Program

The ADA Seal of Acceptance Program is designed to[38]:

- Help the public and dental professionals make informed decisions about consumer dental products.
- Study and evaluate products for safety and efficacy, when used as directed.
- Inform members of the dental team and the public about the safety and efficacy of each product that is accepted.
- Maintain liaisons with regulatory agencies and research and professional organizations.

III. Product Submission and Acceptance Process

A. Information Required from the Company

- A company submitting an application for the ADA Seal must submit the following[38]:
  - Complete ingredient listing.
  - Objective data from clinical and laboratory studies that support the product's safety, and claimed effectiveness, when used as directed.

- Compliance with specific product category; acceptance guidelines if applicable.
- Evidence of good manufacturing processes.

B. Evaluation

- Involves members of the ADA Council on Scientific Affairs, comprising of member dentists from various dental specialities and research scientists.
- Acceptance is for a 5-year period, after which the company can reapply for a new 5-year acceptance.
- Any changes in the product pertaining to composition, manufacturer, claims, etc. need to be communicated to the seal program.

IV. Acceptance and Use of the Seal

- The requirements for use of the seal include the following[38]:
  - Claims of product effectiveness on labeling and in advertising and promotional materials must first be approved by the Council on Scientific Affairs.
  - The use of the ADA Seal (**Figure 3**) on labeling and in promotional materials must be accompanied by an ADA-approved Seal Statement.
  - The Seal Statement tells the consumer what specific claims have been reviewed and approved and indicates why the particular product was accepted.

Content removed due to copyright restrictions

Figure 3 ADA Seal of Acceptance, the American Dental Association, Council on Scientific Affairs. The Seal is awarded to consumer products that meet ADA guidelines for safety and effectiveness.

Reprinted with permission of the ADA Council on Scientific Affairs.

Content removed due to copyright restrictions

Figure 4 CDA Seal of Acceptance, the Canadian Dental Association. The Seal is awarded to consumer products that will deliver oral health benefits validated by CDA and claimed by the manufacturer.

Reproduced from Canadian Dental Association. www.cda-adc.ca/seal.

- A product search can be done on the www.ada.org website to obtain detailed information on each of the accepted products to help consumers and dental professionals select OTC oral care products.[38]
  - Information is included for each product on the basis for acceptance (i.e., the data on which acceptance is based), indications, directions for use, ingredients, label warnings, and company contact information.
  - The Seal website also allows comparisons of the attributes of two to six products in a given product category.
  - This information is printable and can be used to help consumers make informed decisions about the oral care products they use.
  - It can also be useful to dental professionals in recommending OTC oral care products to their patients.
  - Visit www.mouthhealthy.org for preventive oral health resources and ADA Seal product information for patients.
  - Visit www.ada.org/seal for more information on the ADA Seal Program and for access to product information on ADA-accepted products.

Canadian Dental Association Seal Program

- The Canadian Dental Association (CDA) seal (**Figure 4**) validates the claims made by the manufacturer about a specific oral health benefit of a product.[39]

I. Purpose of Seal Program

- Provides assurance a product will improve oral health as claimed.
- For the manufacturer, the seal differentiates the product from others on the market by supporting the oral health benefits of using the product.[39]

II. Product Submission and Acceptance Process

- Participation of manufacturers in applying for the seal is voluntary.
- A completed CDA Seal application is required from the manufacturer and reviewed by a panel of experts.
- Research conducted to support the product is reviewed and the experts may identify additional research needed.
- The oral health benefit claimed must be measurable and clinically significant as it relates to therapeutic, cosmetic, or preventive effects of using the product.

III. Use of the Seal

- Once a CDA Seal is approved, the CDA Seal Statement for the product must specify the oral health benefit(s) verified by the CDA.[39]
- A product search can be done to obtain detailed information on each of the accepted products to help consumers and dental professionals select OTC oral care products.[39]
  - Visit www.cda-adc.ca/en/oral_health/seal /products/seal for more information on the CDA Seal Program and for access to product information on CDA-accepted products.

Documentation

- Information to be documented in the patient's permanent record will include a minimum of the following:

Box   4 Example Documentation: Choosing a Mouthrinse for a Patient with Xerostomia

- **S**—A 76-year-old male presented for a routine maintenance appointment. His chief complaint is a dry mouth. He reports no medication and although he has a history of smoking, he quit 40 years ago. Patient states he eats a lot of apples and other fruits. Patient stated he has been using a "great mouthwash" for the past 25 years. Patient believes it is helping "toughen up his gums" because his mouth is so dry.
- **O**—Extraoral: No significant findings. The intraoral examination reveals decreased salivary flow. The periodontal examination reveals generalized 3- to 4-mm pocket depths with no bleeding on probing present.
- **A**—Patient presents with xerostomia and a history of smoking that increases his risk for caries, oral cancer, and periodontal disease.
- **P**—Discussed xerostomia and probable causes. Discussed the effects of alcohol on the oral cavity and recommended mouthwash that does not contain alcohol to reduce the incidence of dry mouth.

Signed: _____, RDH
Date: _____

- Recommended dentifrice and mouthrinse for daily oral self- care: nonalcohol-containing mouthrinse and antibacterial dentifrice.
- Patient instructed on proper usage, including amount and frequency of use.
- Summary of current oral findings indicating need for recommendations provided.
- Example documentation is provided in Box   4.

Factors to Teach the Patient

- Significance of American Dental Association or Canadian Dental Association Seal, especially that it is a voluntary program and lack of a seal on a product does not signify it is unsafe.
- To ask the dental hygienist and dentist about new dentifrices and mouthrinses, best way to use, and appropriateness for personal needs.
- How to avoid impulse buying with regard to dentifrices, mouthrinses, and other chemical agents. To seek professional advice to avoid contraindications with oral condition and restorations.
- To understand compliance with recommended chemical agent is directly related to expected outcomes (results or improvements).
- Why the use of chemotherapeutics is not a substitute for proper and daily mechanical biofilm removal.
- To check the ingredients of mouthrinses to prevent the purchase of high-alcohol content if xerostomia is a problem.

References

1. Holmlund A, Lampa E, Lind L. Poor response to periodontal treatment may predict future cardiovascular disease. *J Dent Res.* 2017;96(7):768-773.
2. Oberoi SS, Harish Y, Hiremath S, Puranik M. A cross-sectional survey to study the relationship of periodontal disease with cardiovascular disease, respiratory disease, and diabetes mellitus. *J Indian Soc Periodontol.* 2016;20(4):446-452.
3. D'Aiuto F, Gable D, Syed Z, et al. Evidence summary: the relationship between oral diseases and diabetes. *Br Dent J.* 2017;222(12):944-948.
4. Manger D, Walshaw M, Fitzgerald R, et al. Evidence summary: the relationship between oral health and pulmonary disease. *Br Dent J.* 2017;222(7): 527-533.
5. Mellburg JR. Fluoride dentifrices: current status and prospects. *Int Dent J.* 1991;41(1):9-16.
6. Fischman SL. The history of oral hygiene products: how far have we come in 6000 years? *Periodontol 2000.* 1997;15:7-14.
7. Janakiram C, Deepan Kumar CV, Joseph J. Xylitol in preventing dental caries: a systematic review and meta-analyses. *J Natural Sci Biol Med.* 2017;8(1):16-21.
8. Biesbrock A, He T, DiGennaro J, et al. The effects of bioavailable gluconate chelated stannous fluoride dentifrice on gingival bleeding: meta-analysis of eighteen randomized controlled trials. *J Clin Periodontol.* 2019;46(12):1205-1216.
9. Parkinson C, Milleman K, Milleman J. Gingivitis efficacy of a 0.454% w/w stannous fluoride dentifrice: a 24-week randomized controlled trial. *BMC Oral Health.* 2020;20(1):89.
10. Moraschini V, da Costa LS, Dos Santos GO. Effectiveness for dentin hypersensitivity treatment of non-carious cervical lesions: a meta-analysis. *Clin Oral Investig.* 2018;22(2):617-631.

11. Netuveli GS, Sheiham A. A systematic review of the effectiveness of anticalculus dentifrices. *Oral Health Prev Dent.* 2004;2(1):49-58.

12. Winston JL, Fiedler SK, Schiff T, Baker R. An anticalculus dentifrice with sodium hexametaphosphate and stannous fluoride: a six-month study of efficacy. *J Contemp Dent Pract.* 2007;8(5):1-8.

13. Seemann R, Conceicao MD, Filippi A, et al. Halitosis management by the general dental practitioner—results of an international consensus workshop. *J Breath Res.* 2014;8(1):017101.

14. Mendes L, Coimbra J, Pereira A, Resende M, Pinto M. Comparative effect of a new mouthrinse containing chlorhexidine, triclosan and zinc on volatile sulphur compounds: a randomized, crossover, double-blind study. *Int J Dent Hyg.* 2016;14(3):202-208.

15. Farrell S, Barker ML, Gerlach RW. Overnight malodor effect with a 0.454% stabilized stannous fluoride sodium hexametaphosphate dentifrice. *Compend Contin Educ Dent.* 2007;28(12):658-661.

16. Schemehorn BR, Moore MH, Putt MS. Abrasion, polishing, and stain removal characteristics of various commercial dentifrices in vitro. *J Clin Dent.* 2011;22(1):11-18.

17. AAPD Council on Clinical Affairs. Fluoride therapy. *Oral Health Pol Recomm.* 2018;40(6):251-252.

18. Wunderlich RC, Singelton M, O'Brien WJ, Caffesse RG. Subgingival penetration of an applied solution. *Int J Periodontics Restorative Dent.* 1984;4(5):64-71.

19. Van Strydonck DA, Slot DE, Van der Velden U, et al. Effect of a chlorhexidine mouthrinse on plaque, gingival inflammation and staining in gingivitis patients: a systematic review. *J Clin Periodontol.* 2012;39(11):1042-1055.

20. Neely AL. Essential oil mouthwash (EOMW) may be equivalent to chlorhexidine (CHX) for long-term control of gingival inflammation but CHX appears to perform better than EOMW in plaque control. *J Evid Based Dent Pract.* 2012;12(suppl 3):69-72.

21. Elkerbout TA, Slot DE, Bakker EW, Van der Weijden GA. Chlorhexidine mouthwash and sodium lauryl sulphate dentifrice: do they mix effectively or interfere? *Int J Dent Hyg.* 2016;14(1):42-52.

22. Araujo MWB, Charles CA, Weinstein RB, et al. Meta-analysis of the effect of an essential oil-containing mouthrinse on gingivitis and plaque. *J Am Dent Assoc.* 2015;146(8):610-622.

23. Sanz M, Serrano J, Iniesta M, Santa Cruz I, Herrera D. Antiplaque and antigingivitis toothpastes. *Monogr Oral Sci.* 2013;23:27-44.

24. Gunsolley JC. Clinical efficacy of antimicrobial mouthrinses. *J Dent.* 2010;38(suppl 1):S6-S10.

25. Haps S, Slot DE, Berchier CE, Van der Weijden GA. The effect of cetylpyridinium chloride-containing mouth rinses as adjuncts to toothbrushing on plaque and parameters of gingival inflammation: a systematic review. *Int J Dent Hyg.* 2008;6(4):290-303.

26. Carrouel F, Gonçalves L, Conte M, et al. Antiviral activity of reagents in mouth rinses against SARS-CoV-2. *J Dent Res.* 2021;100(2):124-132.

27. Hossainian N, Slot DE, Afennich F, Van der Weijden GA. The effects of hydrogen peroxide mouthwashes on the prevention of plaque and gingival inflammation: a systematic review. *Int J Dent Hyg.* 2011;9(3):171-181.

28. Shinada K, Ueno M, Konishi C, et al. Effects of a mouthwash with chlorine dioxide on oral malodor and salivary bacteria: a randomized placebo-controlled 7-day trial. *Trials.* 2010;11:14.

29. Gonzalez S, Cohen CL, Galván M, Alonaizan FA, Rich SK, Slots J. Gingival bleeding on probing: relationship to change in periodontal pocket depth and effect of sodium hypochlorite oral rinse. *J Periodontal Res.* 2015;50(3):397-402.

30. De Nardo R, Chiappe V, Gómez M, Romanelli H, Slots J. Effects of 0.05% sodium hypochlorite oral rinse on supragingival biofilm and gingival inflammation. *Int Dent J.* 2012;62(4):208-212.

31. Gandini S, Negri E, Boffetta P, La Vecchia C, Boyle P. Mouthwash and oral cancer risk quantitative meta-analysis of epidemiologic studies. *Ann Agric Environ Med.* 2012;19(2):173-180.

32. Naseem M, Khiyani M, Nauman H, et al. Oil pulling and importance of traditional medicine in oral health maintenance. *Int J Health Sci.* 2017;11(4):65-70.

33. Aceves Argemí R, González Navarro B, Ochoa García-Seisdedos P, Estrugo Devesa A, López-López J. Mouthwash with alcohol and oral carcinogenesis: systematic review and meta-analysis. *J Evid Based Dent Pract.* 2020;20(2):101407.

34. Shanbhag VK. Oil pulling for maintaining oral hygiene—a review. *J Tradit Complement Med.* 2017;7(1):106-109.

35. Woolley J, Gibbons T, Patel K, Sacco R. The effect of oil pulling with coconut oil to improve dental hygiene and oral health: a systematic review. *Heliyon.* 2020;6(8):e04789.

36. U.S. Food and Drug Administration. Division of Dermatology and Dental Products (DDDP). https://www.fda.gov/about-fda/center-drug-evaluation-and-research/division-dermatology-and-dental-products-dddp. Accessed August 29, 2021.

37. U.S. Food and Drug Administration. Drug Application Process for Nonprescription Drugs. https://www.fda.gov/drugs/types-applications/drug-applications-over-counter-otc-drugs. Accessed August 29, 2021.

38. American Dental Association. ADA Seal and Acceptance Program and Products. https://www.ada.org/en/science-research/ada-seal-of-acceptance. Accessed August 29, 2021.

39. Canadian Dental Association. CDA Seal Program. https://www.cda-adc.ca/en/oral_health/seal/. Accessed October 11, 2021.

Fluorides

Erin E. Relich, RDH, BSDH, MSA
Lisa F. Mallonee, RDH, RD, LD, MPH

CHAPTER OUTLINE

LEARNING OBJECTIVES

After studying this chapter, the student will be able to:

1. Describe the mechanisms of action of fluoride in the prevention of dental caries.
2. Explain the role of community water fluoridation on the decline of dental caries incidence in a community.
3. Recommend appropriate over-the-counter (OTC) and professionally applied fluoride therapies based on each patient's caries risk assessment.
4. Compare use of fluoride home products (OTC and prescription).
5. Incorporate fluoride into individualized prevention plans for patients of various ages and risk levels.

The use of fluorides provides the most effective method for dental caries prevention and control. Fluoride is necessary for optimum oral health at all ages and is made available at the tooth surface by two general means:

- Systemically, by way of the circulation to developing teeth (pre-eruptive exposure).
- Topically, directly to the exposed surfaces of teeth erupted into the oral cavity[1] (posteruptive exposure).
- Maximum caries inhibiting effect occurs when there is systemic exposure before tooth eruption and frequent topical fluoride exposure throughout life.[2]

Fluoride Metabolism[1,3]

I. Fluoride Intake

- Sources
  - Drinking water that contains fluoride naturally or has been fluoridated.
  - Prescribed dietary supplements.
  - Foods, in small amounts.
  - Foods and beverages prepared at home or processed commercially using water that contains fluoride.
- Varying small amounts ingested from dentifrices, mouthrinses, supplements, and other fluoride products used by the individual.

II. Absorption

A. Gastrointestinal Tract

- Fluoride is rapidly absorbed as hydrogen fluoride through passive diffusion in the stomach.
  - Rate and amount of absorption depend on the solubility of the fluoride compound and gastric acidity.
  - Most is absorbed within 60 minutes.
- Fluoride that is not absorbed in the stomach will be absorbed by the small intestine.
- There is less absorption when the fluoride is taken with milk and other food.

B. Bloodstream

- Plasma carries the fluoride for its distribution throughout the body and to the kidneys for elimination.
- Maximum blood levels are reached within 30 minutes of intake.
- Normal plasma levels are low and rise and fall according to intake.

III. Distribution and Retention

- **Fluoride** is distributed by the plasma to *all* tissues and organs. There is a strong affinity for mineralized tissues.
- Approximately 99% of fluoride in the body is located within the mineralized tissues.
- Concentrations of fluoride are highest at the surfaces next to the tissue fluid supplying the fluoride.
- The fluoride ion (F) is stored as an integral part of the crystal lattice of teeth and bones.
  - Amount stored varies with the intake, the time of exposure, and the age and stage of the development of the individual.
  - The teeth store small amounts, with highest levels on the tooth surface.
- Fluoride that accumulates in bone can be mobilized slowly from the skeleton due to the constant resorption and remodeling of bone.
- Once tooth enamel is fully matured, the fluoride deposited during development can be altered by cavitated dental caries, erosion, or mechanical abrasion.[1]

IV. Excretion

- Most fluoride is excreted through the kidneys in the urine, with a small amount excreted by the sweat glands and the feces.
- There is limited transfer from plasma to breast milk for excretion by that route.[1]

Fluoride and Tooth Development

- Fluoride is a nutrient essential to the formation of teeth and bones, as are calcium, phosphorus, and other elements obtained from food and water.
- A comprehensive review of the histology of tooth development and mineralization is recommended to supplement the information included here.[4,5]

I. Pre-eruptive: Mineralization Stage

- Fluoride is deposited during the formation of the enamel, starting at the dentinoenamel junction, after the enamel matrix has been laid down by the ameloblasts.
  - **Figure 1A** shows the distribution of fluoride in all parts of the teeth during mineralization.

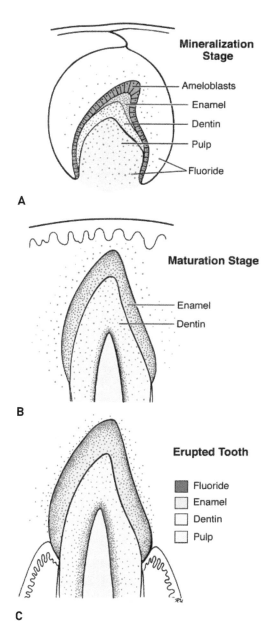

Figure 1 Systemic Fluoride. Green dots represent fluoride ions in the tissues and distributed throughout the tooth. **A:** Developing tooth during mineralization shows fluoride from water and other systemic sources deposited in the enamel and dentin. **B:** Maturation stage before eruption when fluoride is taken up from tissue fluids around the crown. **C:** Erupted tooth continues to take up fluoride on the surface from external sources. Note concentrated fluoride deposition on the enamel surface and on the pulpal surface of the dentin.

- The **hydroxyapatite** crystalline structure becomes **fluorapatite**, which is a less soluble **apatite** crystal.[2]
- Pre-eruptive fluoride may contribute to shallower occlusal grooves and reduce the risk of fissure caries.[2]

- The hard tissue formation of the primary teeth begins in utero. See Chapter 47.
- The first permanent molars begin to mineralize at birth. See Chapter 16.
- Effect of excess fluoride (**fluorosis**)[6,7]
  - Dental fluorosis is a form of hypomineralization that results from systemic ingestion of an excess amount of fluoride during tooth development.
  - During mineralization, the enamel is highly receptive to free fluoride ions.
  - The normal activity of the ameloblasts may be inhibited, and the defective enamel matrix that can form results in discontinuity of crystal growth.
- Dental fluorosis can appear clinically in varying degrees from white flecks or striations to cosmetically objectionable stained pitting. See Chapter 21.
- Chapter 47 lists the weeks in utero when the hard-tissue formation begins for the primary teeth.

II. Pre-eruptive: Maturation Stage

- After mineralization is complete and before eruption, fluoride deposition continues in the surface of the enamel.
  - **Figure** 1B shows fluoride around the crown during **maturation**.
  - Fluoride is taken up from the nutrient tissue fluids surrounding the tooth crown.

III. Posteruptive

- After eruption and throughout the life span of the teeth, the concentration of fluoride on the outermost surface of the enamel is dependent on:
  - Daily topical sources of fluoride to prevent **demineralization** and encourage **remineralization** for prevention of dental caries.
  - Sources for daily topical fluoride include fluoridated drinking water, dentifrices, mouthrinses, and other fluoride preparations used by the patient.
  - The fluoride on the outermost surface is available to inhibit demineralization and enhance remineralization as needed (**Figure** 1C).
  - **Figure** 2A depicts the areas on the tooth that acquire fluoride after eruption.
  - The continuous daily presence of fluoride provided for the tooth surfaces can inhibit the initiation and progression of dental caries.
  - Uptake is most rapid on the enamel surface during the first years after eruption.

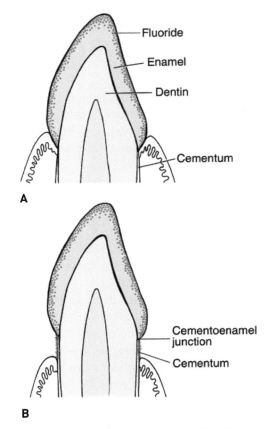

Figure 2 Fluoride Acquisition after Eruption. **A:** Fluoride represented by green dots on the enamel surface is taken up from external sources, including dentifrice, rinse, topical application, and fluoridated drinking water passing over the teeth. **B:** Gingival recession exposes the cementum to external sources of fluoride for the prevention of root caries and the alleviation of sensitivity.

  - Repeated daily intake of drinking water with fluoride provides a topical source as it washes over the teeth throughout life.

Tooth Surface Fluoride

Fluoride concentration is greatest on the surface next to the source of fluoride.

- For the enamel of the erupted tooth, highest concentration is at the outer surface exposed to the oral cavity.
- For the dentin, the highest concentration is at the pulpal surface.
- Periodontal attachment loss or gingival recession can often cause the root surface and cementum to become exposed to the oral cavity and external fluoride sources.

I. Fluoride in Enamel

A. Uptake

- Uptake of fluoride depends on the level of fluoride in the oral environment and the length of time of exposure.
- Hypomineralized enamel absorbs fluoride in greater quantities than sound enamel; it incorporates into the hydroxyapatite crystalline structure to become fluorapatite.[6]
- Demineralized enamel that has been remineralized in the presence of fluoride will have a greater concentration of fluoride than sound enamel.

B. Fluoride in the Enamel Surface

- Fluoride is a natural constituent of enamel.
- The intact outer surface has the highest concentration, which falls sharply toward the interior of the tooth.[8]

II. Fluoride in Dentin[9]

- The fluoride level may be greater in dentin than that in enamel.
- A higher concentration is at the pulpal or inner surface, where exchanges take place.
- Newly formed dentin absorbs fluoride rapidly.

III. Fluoride in Cementum[9]

- The level of fluoride in cementum is high and increases with exposure.
  - With recession of the clinical attachment level, the root surface is exposed to the fluids of the oral cavity.
  - **Figure** 2B shows fluoride acquisition to exposed cementum.
  - Fluoride is then available to the cementum from the saliva and all the sources used by the patient, including drinking water, dentifrice, and mouthrinse.

Demineralization–Remineralization[8]

Figure 3 illustrates the comparative levels of fluoride that may be found in the tooth surface and the sublevel lesion in early dental caries.

I. Fluoride in Biofilm and Saliva

- Saliva and biofilm are reservoirs for fluoride; saliva carries minerals available for remineralization when needed.

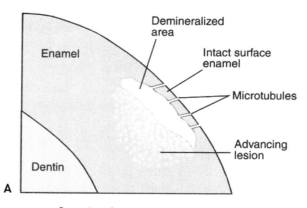

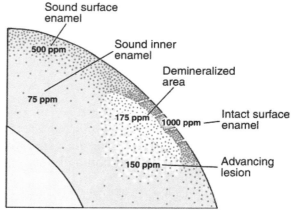

Figure 3 Examples of Enamel Fluoride Content.
A: Early stage of dental caries with an intact surface enamel and subsurface demineralized area.
B: A demineralized area readily takes up available fluoride. As shown, the fluoride content (1000 ppm) of the relatively intact surface over a subsurface demineralized white spot is higher than that of the sound surface enamel (500 ppm). The body of the advancing lesion has a higher fluoride content (150 ppm) than does the sound inner enamel (75 ppm).

- Fluoride helps to inhibit demineralization when it is present at the crystal surface during an acid challenge.
- Fluoride enhances remineralization, forming a condensed layer on the crystal surface, which attracts calcium and phosphate ions.
- High concentrations of fluoride can interfere with the growth and metabolism of bacteria.
- Dental biofilm may contain 5–50 **ppm** fluoride. The content varies greatly and is constantly changing.
- Fluoride may be acquired directly from fluoridated water, dentifrice, and other topical sources and brought by the saliva or by an exchange of fluoride in the biofilm to the demineralizing tooth surface under the biofilm.

II. Summary of Fluoride Action

Having fluoride available topically to the tooth posteruptively is key to its effectiveness.

- Frequent exposure to fluoride, such as from fluoridated water, dentifrice, and mouthrinse, is recommended.
- There are three basic topical effects of fluoride to prevent dental caries[8]:
  - Inhibit demineralization.
  - Enhance remineralization of incipient lesions.
  - Inhibit bacterial activity by inhibiting *enolase*, an enzyme needed by bacteria to metabolize carbohydrates.

Fluoridation

- Fluoridation is the adjustment of the natural fluoride ion content in a municipal water supply to the optimum physiologic concentration to maximize caries prevention and limit enamel fluorosis.[10]
- Fluoridation has been established as the most efficient, effective, reliable, and inexpensive means for improving and maintaining oral health for all who use it.
- Fluoridation was named by the U.S. Centers for Disease Control and Prevention (**CDC**) as one of the 10 most significant public health measures of the 20th century.[10]
- The estimated annual cost per person per year is low, with lower cost per person for communities of more than 20,000 people.[11]
- As of 2018, 63.4% of the total U.S. population received fluoridated water, whereas 73.0% of the population served by public (municipal) water systems received fluoridated water. These percentages vary greatly from state to state.[12]

I. Historical Aspects[13]

A. Mottled Enamel and Dental Caries

- Dr. Frederick S. McKay
  - Early in the 20th century, Dr. McKay began his extensive studies to find the cause of "brown stain," which later was called mottled enamel and now is known as *dental fluorosis*.
  - He observed that people in Colorado Springs, Colorado, with mottled enamel had significantly less dental caries.[14] He associated the condition with the drinking water, but tests were inconclusive.

- H.V. Churchill
  - In 1931, H.V. Churchill, a chemist, pinpointed fluorine as the specific element related to the tooth changes that Dr. McKay had been observing clinically.[15]

B. Background for Fluoridation

- Dr. H. Trendley Dean
  - Epidemiologic studies of the 1930s, sponsored by the U.S. Public Health Service (**USPHS**) and directed by Dr. Dean, led to the conclusion the optimum level of fluoride in the water for dental caries prevention averages 1 ppm in moderate climates.
  - Clinically objectionable dental fluorosis is associated with levels well over 2 ppm.[16]
  - From this knowledge and the fact many healthy people had lived long lives in communities where the fluoride content of the water was much greater than 1 ppm, the concept of adding fluoride to the water developed.
  - It was still necessary to show the benefits from controlled fluoridation could parallel those of natural fluoride.

C. Fluoridation—1945

- The first communities were fluoridated in 1945.
- Research in the communities began before fluoridation was started to obtain baseline information.

D. Control Cities

- Aurora, Illinois, where the natural fluoride level was optimum (1.2 ppm), was used to compare the benefits of natural fluoride in the water supply with those of fluoridation, as well as with a fluoride-free city, Rockford, Illinois.
- Original cities with fluoridation and their control cities in the research are shown in **Box 1**.
- The research conducted in those cities, as well as throughout the world, has documented the influence of fluoride on oral health.

II. Water Supply Adjustment

A. Fluoride Level

- In 2015, the U.S. Department of Health and Human Services updated the recommendation for the optimal concentration of water fluoridation to 0.7 ppm for all communities, regardless of climate.
  - The decision was substantiated by the fact that Americans have access to many more

sources of fluoride today than they did when water fluoridation was first introduced in the United States.[17]

- The change still provides an effective level of fluoride to reduce the incidence of dental caries while minimizing the rate of fluorosis.

B. Chemicals Used

- All fluoride chemicals must conform to the appropriate American Water Works Association standards to ensure the drinking water is safe.[18]
- Sources
  - Compounds from which the fluoride ion is derived are naturally occurring and are mined in various parts of the world.
  - Examples of common sources are fluorspar, cryolite, and apatite.
- Criteria for acceptance of a fluoride compound for fluoridation include:
  - Solubility to permit regular use in a water plant.
  - Relatively inexpensive.
  - Readily available to prevent interruptions in maintaining the proper fluoride level.
- Compounds used:
  - Dry compounds: sodium fluoride (**NaF**) and sodium silicofluoride.
  - Liquid solution: hydrofluorosilicic acid.

Effects and Benefits of Fluoridation

Fluoridated water is a systemic source of fluoride for developing teeth and a topical source of fluoride on the surfaces of erupted teeth throughout life.[19]

I. Appearance of Teeth

- Teeth exposed to an optimum or slightly higher level of fluoride appear white, shiny, opaque, and without blemishes.
  - When the level is slightly more than optimum, teeth may exhibit mild enamel fluorosis seen as white areas in bands or flecks. Without close examination, such spots blend with the overall appearance.
- Today, the majority of fluorosis is mild and not considered an esthetic problem.[10,20]

II. Dental Caries: Permanent Teeth

A. Overall Benefits

- Maximum benefit is seen with continuous use of fluoridated water from birth.
- Estimates have shown the reduction in caries due to water fluoridation alone (factoring out other sources of topical fluoride) among adults of all ages is 27%.[19]
- The effects are similar to communities with optimum levels of natural fluoride in the water.
- Many more individuals are completely caries free when fluoride is in the water.

B. Distribution

- Anterior teeth, particularly maxillary, receive more protection from fluoride than do posterior teeth.[16]
  - Anterior teeth are contacted by the drinking water as it passes into the mouth.

C. Progression

- Not only are the numbers of carious lesions reduced, but the caries rate is slowed.
- Caries progression is also reduced for the surfaces that receive fluoride for the first time after eruption.[21]

III. Root Caries

- Root caries experience in lifelong residents of a naturally fluoridated community is in direct proportion to the fluoride concentration in the water compared with the experience of residents of a fluoride-free community.[22]
- The incidence of root caries is approximately 50% less for lifelong residents of a fluoridated community.[23]

IV. Dental Caries: Primary Teeth

- With fluoridation from birth, the caries incidence is reduced up to 40% in the primary teeth.[10]
- The introduction of fluoridation into a community significantly increases the proportion of caries-free children and reduces the decayed, missing, and filled teeth (**dmft/DMFT**) scores compared to areas that are nonfluoridated over the same time period.[20]

V. Tooth Loss

- Tooth loss due to dental caries is much greater in both primary and permanent teeth without fluoride because of increased dental caries, which progresses more rapidly.[24]

VI. Adults

- When a person resides in a community with fluoride in the drinking water throughout life, benefits continue.[25,26]

VII. Periodontal Health

- Indirect favorable effects of fluoride on periodontal health can be shown.
  - Fluoride functions to decrease dental caries. The presence of carious lesions favors biofilm retention, which can lead to periodontal infection, particularly adjacent to the gingival margin.

Partial Defluoridation

- Water with an excess of natural fluoride does not meet the requirements of the USPHS.
- Several hundred communities in the United States had water supplies that naturally contained more than twice the optimal level of fluoride.
- **Defluoridation** can be accomplished by one of several chemical systems.[27] The **efficacy** of the methods has been shown.
- Examples: The water supply in Britton, South Dakota, has been reduced from almost 7 to 1.5 ppm since 1948, and in Bartlett, Texas, from 8 to 1.8 ppm since 1952. Examinations have shown a significant reduction in the incidence of objectionable fluorosis in children born since defluoridation.[27,28]

School Fluoridation

- To bring the benefits of fluoridation to children living in rural areas without the possibility for community fluoridation, adding fluoride to a school water supply has been an alternative.

- Because of the intermittent use of the school water (only 5 days each week during the 9-month school year), the amount of fluoride added was increased over the usual 1 ppm.
- Example: In the schools of Elk Lake, Pennsylvania, after 12 years with the fluoride level at 5 ppm in the school drinking water, the children experienced a 39% decrease in DMF surfaces compared with those in the control group.[29]
- Example: In the schools of Seagrove, North Carolina, after 12 years with the fluoride level at 6.3 ppm in the school drinking water, the children experienced a 47.5% decrease in DMF surfaces compared with those in the control group.[29]
- Such systems have significance in the long history of fluoridation efforts for all people in the United States.
- School fluoridation has been phased out in several states, and the current extent of this practice is unknown. Operations and maintenance of small fluoridation systems are problematic.[10]

Discontinued Fluoridation

- When fluoride is removed from a community water supply that had dental caries control by fluoridation, the effects can be clearly shown.
- Example: In Antigo, Wisconsin, the action of antifluoridationists in 1960 brought about the discontinuance of fluoridation, which had been installed in 1949.
  - Examinations in the years following 1960 revealed the marked drop in the number of children who were caries free and the steep increase in caries rates.
  - From 1960 to 1966, the number of caries-free children in the second grade decreased by 67%.[30]
  - Fluoridation was reinstated in 1966 by popular demand.

Fluorides in Foods

I. Foods[31]

- Certain foods contain fluoride, but not enough to constitute a significant part of the day's need for caries prevention.
- Examples: Meat, eggs, vegetables, cereals, and fruit have small but measurable amounts, whereas tea and fish have larger amounts.

- Foods cooked in fluoridated water retain fluoride from the cooking water.

II. Salt[32-34]

- Fluoridated salt has not been promoted in the United States, but is widely available and used in Germany, France, and Switzerland along with other European countries where 30% to 80% of the domestic marketed salt is fluoridated.
- Another 30 countries or more use fluoridated salt worldwide for its effectiveness as a community health program.
- Fluoridated salt results in a reduced incidence of dental caries, but there is insufficient evidence for its overall effectiveness.
- Fluoridated salts currently available supply about one-third to one-half of the amount of fluoride ingested daily from 1 ppm fluoridated water.
- Fluoridated salt is recommended by the World Health Organization as an alternative to fluoridated water to target underprivileged groups.

III. Halo/Diffusion Effect

- Foods and beverages that are commercially processed (cooked or reconstituted) in optimally fluoridated cities can be distributed and consumed in nonfluoridated communities.
- The **halo or diffusion effect** can result in increased fluoride intake by individuals living in nonfluoridated communities, providing them some protection against dental caries.[31]

IV. Bottled Water

- Bottled water usually does not contain optimal fluoride unless it has a label indicating that it is fluoridated.
- Patients need to be advised to fill their drinking water bottles from a fluoridated water supply.

V. Water Filters[35]

- Reverse osmosis and water distillation systems remove fluoride from the water, but water softeners do not.
- Carbon filters (for the end of a faucet or in pitchers) vary in their removal of fluoride.
- Carbon filters with activated alumina remove fluoride.
- Patients need to be warned that water filters may remove fluoride from the drinking water and need to be checked with the manufacturer before purchase.

VI. Infant Formula[36-38]

- There has been an increase in breastfeeding in the United States, but infant formula remains a major source of nutrition for many infants.
- Ready-to-feed formulas do not need to be reconstituted, but water is added to powdered and liquid concentrate formulas.
- Breast milk may contain 0.02 ppm fluoride, and all types of infant formula themselves contain a low amount of fluoride (0.11–0.57 ppm).[37]
- The level of fluoride in the water supply used to reconstitute powdered or liquid concentrate formulas determines the total fluoride intake.
- The American Dental Association (**ADA**) recommends continuing to use optimally fluoridated water to reconstitute infant formula while being aware of the possible risk of mild enamel fluorosis in the primary teeth.[38]

Dietary Fluoride Supplements[10,39,40]

- Prescription fluoride supplements were introduced in the late 1940s and are intended to compensate for fluoride-deficient drinking water.
- The current supplementation dosage schedule developed by the ADA and the American Association of Pediatric Dentistry (**AAPD**) and revised in 2010 includes children aged 6 months through 16 years.
  - **Table** 1 contains the daily dosage amounts based on the age of the child and the amount of fluoride in the primary water supply.

Table 1 Fluoride Supplements Dose Schedule (Mg NaF/D)[a]

Content removed due to copyright restrictions

- Clinical recommendations from the ADA Council on Scientific Affairs include the use of fluoride supplements for children:
  - At high risk of developing dental caries.
  - Those whose primary source of drinking water is deficient in fluoride.[41]

I. Assess Possible Need

- Review the patient's history to be certain the child is not receiving other fluoride such as vitamin–fluoride supplements.
- Determine if the fluoride level of all sources of drinking water is below 0.6 ppm.
- Refer to the list of fluoridated communities available from state or local health departments.
- Request water analysis when the fluoride level has not been determined, for example, in private well water.
- Determine if the child's risk for dental caries is high or moderately high before considering the use of fluoride supplements.[39]
- Reassess the caries risk at frequent intervals as the status may be affected by the child's development, personal and family situations, and behavioral factors such as changes in oral hygiene practices.[33,41]

II. Available Forms of Supplements

- NaF supplements are available as tablets; lozenges; and drops in 0.25-, 0.50-, and 1.0-mg dosages.
- Prescribed on an individual patient basis for daily use at home.

A. Tablets and Lozenges

- Tablets are chewed thoroughly, swished/rinsed around in the oral cavity, and forced between the teeth before swallowing.
- Lozenges are dissolved for 1–2 minutes in the mouth to provide both pre-eruptive and poster-uptive benefits.[41]
- Best taken at bedtime after teeth are brushed.
  - Avoid drinking, eating, or rinsing before going to sleep to gain maximum benefit.

B. Drops

- A liquid concentrate with directions that specify the number of drops for the prescription dose daily.
- Primary use for child aged 6 months to 3 years, and patient of any age unable to use other forms that require chewing and swallowing.

III. Prescription Guidelines

- No more than 264 mg NaF (120 mg fluoride ion) to be dispensed per household at one time.
- Take supplements with food to decrease stomach upset.
- Storage
  - Keep products out of reach of children.
  - Keep tablets in the original container, away from heat and direct light, and away from damp places such as a bathroom or kitchen sink area.
- Missed dose
  - Take as soon as remembered.
  - If near time of next dose, take at the next regular time.

IV. Benefits and Limitations

- Prenatal use by pregnant women
  - Administration of prenatal dietary fluoride supplements is not recommended.
  - Some evidence has shown that fluoride crosses the placenta during the fifth and sixth months of pregnancy and may enter the prenatal deciduous enamel.[42]
  - Overall, there is weak evidence to support the use of fluoride supplements to prevent dental caries in primary teeth.
- Daily fluoride supplements offer caries preventive benefits in permanent teeth. School-aged children who chewed, swished, and swallowed 1-mg fluoride tablets daily on school days had significantly lower caries experience than those who did not use fluoride supplements.
- The use of fluoride supplements in children older than 6 years of age shows a 24% decrease in DMF tooth surfaces in permanent teeth compared to no fluoride supplements.[43]
- Consider the child's age, caries risk, and all sources of fluoride exposure before recommending the use of fluoride supplements.[33,41]

Professional Topical Fluoride Applications

Topical fluorides are an essential part of a total preventive program for patients of all ages.

- Fluoridated water and fluoride toothpaste are the primary sources of topical fluoride for patients of all ages and levels of caries risk.

- Additional topical fluoride sources may be professionally applied and/or self-applied by the patient for those at an elevated caries risk.

I. Historical Perspectives

- Professionally applied fluoride has been instrumental in the reduction of dental caries in the United States and other industrialized countries since the early 1940s.
- Dr. Basil G. Bibby conducted the initial topical NaF study using Brockton, Massachusetts schoolchildren.[44]
- More than one-third fewer new carious lesions resulted from a 0.1% aqueous solution applied at 4-month intervals for 2 years by a dental hygienist.
- The research led to extensive studies by Dr. John W. Knutson and others sponsored by the USPHS.
    - The aim was to determine the most effective concentration of NaF, the minimum time required for application, and procedural details.[45,46]

II. Indications

- The professional application of a high-concentration fluoride preventive agent is based on caries risk assessment for the individual patient.
- Indications for a professional fluoride application are outlined in **Box 2**.[47]
- See Chapter 25 for the criteria to determine low, moderate, and high caries risk.

III. Compounds

- **Table 2** provides a summary of the available professional fluoride applications.
    - 2.0% NaF as **gel** or foam delivered in trays.
    - 1.23% acidulated phosphate fluoride (**APF**) as a gel or foam delivered in trays.
    - 5% NaF as a varnish brushed on the teeth.
- 2.0% NaF gel
    - NaF, also called "neutral sodium fluoride" due to its neutral pH of 7.0, contains 9050 ppm fluoride ion.
    - Clinical trials demonstrating the efficacy of neutral NaF are based on a series of four or five applications on a weekly basis.[48]

Box 2 Indications for Professional Topical Fluoride Application[47]

- Patients at an elevated (moderate or high) risk of developing caries. (Refer to Chapter 25.)
- **5% NaF varnish** at least every 3–6 months (for all ages and adult root caries), or
- **1.23% APF gel** 4-minute trays at least every 3–6 months (for 6 years and older and adult root caries).
- Patients at a low risk of developing caries may not benefit from additional topical fluoride other than **OTC**-fluoridated toothpaste and fluoridated water daily.

Data from American Dental Association Council on Scientific Affairs. Topical fluoride for caries prevention: executive summary of updated clinical recommendations and supporting systematic review. *J Am Dent Assoc.* 2013;144(11):1279-1291.

Table 2 Professionally Applied Topical Fluorides

Agent	Form	Concentration	Application Mode/Frequency	Notes
NaF neutral or 7 pH	2% Gel or foam[a]	9050 ppm 0.90% F ion	Tray (4 minutes)/no currently recommended interval	Do not overfill: see Figure 5
Acidulated phosphate 3.5 pH	1.23% Gel or foam[a]	12,300 ppm 1.23% F ion	Tray (4 minutes)/at least every 3–6 months	Do not overfill: see Figure 5
NaF neutral or 7 pH	5% Varnish	22,600 ppm 2.26% F ion	Apply thin layer with a soft brush (1–2 minutes)/at least every 3–6 months depending on caries risk level	Sets up to a hard film
SDF pH 8–10	5.0–5.9% Fluoride	44,800 ppm 4.48% F ion	Apply a thin layer with a microbrush (1 minute and let dry)/apply at least every 6–12 months[67]	Goes on clear, becomes black/gray upon application to cavitated areas

[a]There is limited published clinical evidence supporting the effectiveness of foam.[47]

F, fluoride; NaF, sodium fluoride; ppm, parts per million; SDF, silver diamine fluoride

Data fom Weyant RJ, Tracy SL, Anselmo T, et al. Topical fluoride for caries prevention: executive summary of the updated clinical recommendations and supporting systemic review. J Am Dent Assoc. 2013;144(11):1279-1291; and Horst J, Ellenikiotis H, Milgrom P. UCSF protocol for cariesarrest using silver diamine fluoride: rationale, indications and consent. J Calif Dent Assoc. 2016;44(1):16-28.

- Quarterly or semiannual applications are most common in clinical practice.
- 2.0% NaF foam
  - There is limited clinical evidence to demonstrate foam's effectiveness in caries prevention.
- 1.23% APF gel
  - Contains 12,300 ppm fluoride ion.
  - A 4-minute tray application is recommended at least every 3–6 months per year for individuals aged 6 years and older at an elevated risk for dental caries.[47]
  - Widely used because of its storage stability, acceptable taste, and tissue compatibility.
  - Low pH of 3.5 enhances fluoride uptake, which is greatest during the first 4 minutes.[49]
  - APF may etch porcelain and composite restorative materials, so it is not indicated for patients with porcelain, composite restorations, and sealants.[50]
  - The hydrofluoride component of APF can dissolve the filler particles of the composite resin restorations.
  - Macroinorganic filler particles of composite materials demonstrate noticeable etched patterns generated by APF, whereas many of the more recently available microfilled composites/resins are not as sensitive to the APF.[50]
  - The **prevented fraction** of dental caries ranged from 18% to 41% with the use of APF or NaF gels.[51]
  - In 2018, an expert panel from the ADA recommended the prioritized use of 1.23% APF gel (every 3 to 6 months) or 5% sodium fluoride varnish (every 3 to 6 months) to arrest or reverse noncavitated carious lesions on the facial and lingual surfaces of both primary and permanent teeth.[52]
- 1.23% APF foam
  - There is limited clinical evidence to show the effectiveness of foam in caries prevention.
- 5% NaF varnish
  - Fluoride varnishes (FVs) were developed during the late 1960s and early 1970s to prolong contact time of the fluoride with the tooth surface.[53]
  - Varnishes are safe, effective, fast, and easy to apply, and patient acceptance is good.
  - The use of varnish 2–4 times per year is associated with a 43% decrease in DMFT surfaces in permanent teeth and 37% in primary teeth.[54]
  - Varnish has a higher concentration of fluoride than gel or foam (22,600 ppm fluoride ion),

but an overall less amount of fluoride is used per application (<7 mg varnish vs. 30 mg of gel for a child).
  - Varnish sets quickly and remains on the teeth for up to several hours, releasing fluoride into the pits and fissures, proximal surfaces, and cervical areas of the tooth where it is needed the most.[55]
  - Application is recommended at least every 3–4 months per year for individuals at an elevated risk for dental caries.[47]
  - Varnish is effective in reversing active pit and fissure enamel lesions in the primary dentition[56] and remineralizing enamel lesions, regardless of whether the varnish is applied over or around the demineralizing lesion.[57]
  - Varnish is also effective in reducing demineralization (white areas) around orthodontic brackets.[58]
  - Varnish received approval from the U.S Food and Drug Administration (**FDA**) for use as a cavity liner and for treatment of dentin hypersensitivity.[59] Varnish may be used for dentin hypersensitivity. (See Chapter 41.)
  - Varnish is the only professional topical fluoride to be used for children younger than 6 years.
  - Its use in the United States as a caries preventive agent is considered off-label but has become a standard of care in practice.[55]
  - Fluoride varnish's highest prevented fractions were 21.3% for caries arrest and 55.7% for caries prevention.[60]
  - In 2018, an expert panel from the ADA recommended the prioritized use of sealants and 5% NaF varnish (every 3 to 6 months), 1.23% APF gel (every 3 to 6 months), or 0.2% sodium fluoride mouthrinse (once per week) to arrest or reverse noncavitated carious lesions on the occlusal surfaces of both primary and permanent teeth.[52]
  - As far as the approximal surfaces of primary and permanent teeth, the expert panel suggested 5% sodium varnish application (every 3 to 6 months).[52]
  - Five percent NaF varnish is now offered with different formulations containing mineral enhancements:
    - Complex of casein phosphopeptide and amorphous calcium phosphate (ACP).
    - ACP.
    - Tri-calcium phosphate modified by fumaric acid.

- Calcium and phosphate with xylitol.
  - Calcium sodium phosphosilicate.
  - Sodium trimetaphosphate.
- Some manufacturers are adding mineral additives to the FV formulations with the theory that by making them bioavailable in the saliva, it will increase the overall anticariogenic efficacy.[61]
  - More in vivo research studies with human subjects are needed to determine the efficacy and benefits of mineral enhanced FV formulations.[62]
  - There is no recommendation by the ADA at this time for FV with mineral enhancements.
- Allergic reactions such as contact dermatitis or stomatitis from exposure to the **rosin/colophony**, a sticky secretion typically made from plants or trees contained in FVs, are uncommon, but have been reported in the literature.[59,63-65]
- FV formulations that contain synthetic rosin/colophony are now available on market as an alternative for those patients with a known or suspected allergy to traditional plant-based rosins.
- 38% silver diamine fluoride (SDF)[52,60,66-71]
  - No adverse issues have been reported in Japan since SDF was approved over 80 years ago.
  - 24.4% to 28.8% silver (253,870 ppm Ag—antimicrobial effects)
  - 5.0% to 5.9% fluoride (44,800 ppm F—promotes remineralization)
  - 8% ammonia (stabilizing agent/solvent)
  - pH 8–10, both colorless and tinted (blue) formulations available.
  - FDA cleared in 2015 as a Class II medical device for management of dentinal hypersensitivity.
  - Off-label use is caries arrest and prevention for high caries risk patients.
  - SDF's lowest prevented fractions were 96.1% for caries arrest and 70.3% for caries prevention.[60]
  - In 2017, a panel from the AAPD developed conditional recommendations from the evidence for the use of 38% SDF to arrest the carious lesions of children, adolescents, and those with special needs.[68-70]
  - In 2018, an expert panel from the ADA recommended the prioritized use of 38% SDF twice per year to arrest advanced carious lesions on the coronal surfaces of both primary and permanent teeth over 5% sodium fluoride varnish.[52]
  - Application of SDF biannually is more effective than annual application.[52,71]
  - Anterior teeth have a higher rate of caries arrest after SDF placement than posterior teeth.[69,71]
  - Individual state Dental Hygiene Practice Acts determine whether SDF application is permitted by the registered dental hygienist.

Clinical Procedures: Professional Topical Fluoride

I. Objectives

- Prevention of dental caries
  - Identify special problems, including areas adjacent to restorations, orthodontic appliances, xerostomia, and other risk factors.
  - Box 2 contains indications for the application of a professional fluoride.
  - Examples: active or secondary caries, exposed root surfaces, current orthodontic treatment, low or no fluoride exposure, or xerostomia.
- Remineralization of demineralized areas
  - Demineralized white areas on the cervical third, especially under dental biofilm.
- Desensitization
  - Fluoride aids in blocking dentinal tubules. (See Chapter 41.)
- Varnish covers and protects a sensitive area, and fluoride is slowly released for uptake.

II. Preparation of the Teeth for Topical Application

- General preparation for tray and varnish applications
  - Most patients will receive a professional topical fluoride application following their routine continuing care appointment.
  - When the fluoride application is to be applied at a time other than following scaling and debridement, rubber cup polishing is not routinely necessary because fluoride will penetrate biofilm and provide the same benefits with or without prior polishing.[47,72]
  - Calculus and stain removal are completed first.
  - After calculus removal, apply principles of selective polishing for stain removal.

- Select an appropriate cleaning or polishing agent that will not harm the tooth surface or the restorative material present.
- A fluoride-containing polishing paste is not effective as a fluoride application.[73]
- Preparation and procedure for gel or foam tray application is included in **Table** 3; preparation and procedure for varnish application is described in Table 4.

III. Patient and/or Parent Counseling

- Help patients understand the purposes and benefits as well as the limitations of topical applications.

- Fluoride is one part of the total prevention program that includes daily biofilm control and limitation of cariogenic foods.

IV. Tray Technique: Gel or Foam

- Tray application appointment preparation
  - Prepare the patient for any discomfort, for example, the 4-minute timing when tray application is to be used.
  - Explain the need not to swallow and to expectorate immediately after the tray is removed.
- Tray selection and preparation
  - **Figure** 4 shows tray selection for coverage of all exposed root surfaces.

Table 3 **Procedure for Topical Gel or Foam Professional Tray**

Patient selection	■ Determine need based on caries risk assessment (not to be used for children younger than 6 years of age). ■ Choose the type of fluoride (APF or NaF and gel or foam); data support use of APF gel. ■ Seat upright. ■ Explain procedure including length: 4 minutes. ■ Instruct not to swallow. ■ Tilt head forward slightly.
Tray coverage	■ Choose appropriate size for full coverage. ■ Complete dentition must be covered, including anterior and posterior vertical coverage, distal dam depth, and close fit to teeth. ■ Check for coverage of areas of recession (if unable to cover exposed root surfaces, use varnish application). ■ Proper and improper tray coverage: see Figure 4.
Place gel or foam	■ Use minimum amount of gel or foam in the trays, as shown in Figure 5. ■ Fill tray one-third full with gel; completely fill, but do not overfill with foam.
Dry the teeth	■ Place a saliva ejector in the mouth during the drying procedure ■ Dry the teeth before insertion of trays starting with the maxillary teeth; facial, occlusal, and palatal surfaces and then the mandibular teeth; lingual, occlusal, and facial surfaces.
Insert trays	■ Place both filled trays in mouth. ■ A two-step procedure (one tray at a time) may be required; if so, patient may not rinse but must expectorate after the removal of each tray to prevent swallowing.
Isolation	■ Use a saliva ejector for suction.
Attention	■ Do not leave patient unattended.
Timing	■ Use a timer; do not estimate (4 minutes). ■ Procedure will take 8 minutes when a two-step procedure is used.
Completion	■ Tilt head forward for removal of tray. ■ Instruct patient to expectorate for several minutes; do not allow swallowing. ■ Wipe excess gel or foam from teeth with gauze sponge. ■ Use high-power suction to draw out saliva and gel. ■ Instruct patient that nothing is to be placed in the mouth for 30 minutes; do not rinse, eat, drink, or brush teeth.

APF, acidulated phosphate fluoride; NaF, sodium fluoride.

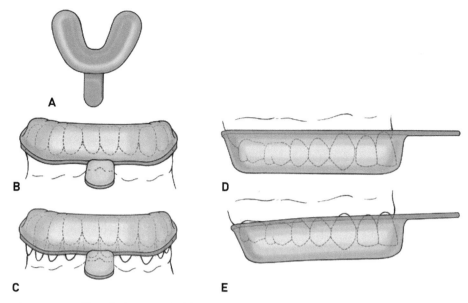

Figure 4 Tray Selection. **A:** Mandibular tray held for try-in. **B:** Tray over teeth is deep enough to cover the entire exposed enamel above the gingiva. **C:** In the patient with recession and areas of root surfaces exposed, the tray may not be deep enough to cover the root surfaces where fluoride is needed for prevention of root caries or hypersensitivity. A custom-made tray is needed. **D:** Tray adequately covers the distal surface of the most posterior tooth. **E:** If the tray does not cover the distal surface of the most posterior tooth or the cervical third of canine and central incisor adequately, the tray may need to be repositioned to cover the distal surface, or a larger stock or custom-made tray is needed.

- Design of trays: maxillary and mandibular trays may be hinged together or separated, are of a natural rounded arch shape to hold the gel and prevent ingestion and are available in various sizes and brands.
- **Figure 5** shows the amount of gel to be placed in each tray.
- Most gels are **thixotropic** to offer better physical and handling characteristics for use in trays.
- Procedures for a professional gel or foam tray fluoride application are listed in Table 3.

V. Varnish Technique[55]

- Varnish application appointment sequence:
    - Dispense varnish: If dispensed from a tube (rather than a single-dose packet), discard any clear varnish because the ingredients have separated and will contain only a fraction of the intended amount of fluoride.[74]
    - Unit-dosed 5% NaF varnish is available in premeasured wells or individual packets of different dosages with an applicator brush to mix the varnish and then apply.

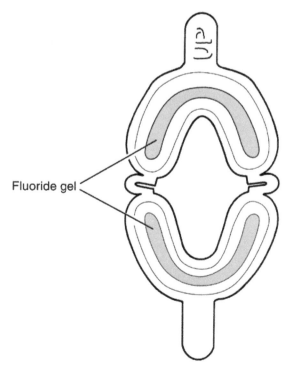

Fluoride gel

Figure 5 Measured Gel in Tray. No more than 2 mL of gel is placed in each tray for children, and no more than 5 mL is placed in each tray for adults. This amount fills each tray size one-third full.

- Unit dosages are generally 0.25, 0.4, or 0.5 mL for the primary, mixed, and permanent dentitions, respectively, and are available in different flavors and colors (yellow, white, and clear).
- Procedures for a professional varnish fluoride application are listed in **Table 4**.

VI. After Application

- Tray application
  - Instruct patients not to rinse, eat, drink, brush, or floss for at least 30 minutes after gel or foam applications.
  - Rinsing immediately after a tray application has been shown to significantly lessen the benefits.[75]
- Varnish application
  - Instruct patients to avoid hot drinks and alcoholic beverages; eating hard, sticky, or crunchy foods; and brushing or flossing the teeth for 4–6 hours after application or until

the next morning to allow fluoride uptake to continue undisturbed.
- Varnish residue is removed by the patient toothbrushing and flossing the next day.

VII. Silver Diamine Fluoride

- Indications[67]
  - Extreme caries risk (xerostomia, severe early childhood caries, or cancer treatments—radiation/chemotherapy).
  - Treatment challenged by behavioral/medical management.
  - Patients with carious lesions that may not all be treated in one visit (stabilize patient).
  - Difficult to treat dental carious lesions.
  - Patients with limited access to dental care (underserved populations).
- Advantages[76]
  - Noninvasive (no needle or drill required).
  - **Cariostatic** agent.
  - Reduces caries risk of adjacent teeth.[66]
  - Reduces dentinal hypersensitivity.

Table 4 Procedure for Varnish Application (5% NaF)	
Patient selection	<ul><li>Determine need based on caries risk assessment (only professional fluoride recommended for children younger than 6 years of age).</li><li>Review the medical history and verify the patient does not have a known rosin/colophony sensitivity or allergy.[59,63-65]</li><li>If there is a suspected or known allergy to rosin/colophony, select a varnish formulation that contains synthetic rosin or utilize an alternative topical fluoride application (tray method with 1.23% APF gel for 6 years and older and adult root caries).</li><li>Explain procedure.</li><li>Seat supine.</li><li>For the infant and toddler, the parent and clinician can sit knee to knee with the child held across the knees.</li><li>Instruct not to swallow during the procedure.</li></ul>
Prepare product	<ul><li>Dispense from a tube or open a single-dose packet.</li><li>Have applicator brush available.</li></ul>
Dry teeth	<ul><li>Varnish sets up in the presence of saliva, but it is recommended to remove excess saliva by wiping the teeth with a gauze square.</li></ul>
Apply varnish	<ul><li>Dip applicator brush in varnish and mix well. Systematically brush a thin layer over all tooth surfaces. For prevention of early childhood caries in the infant, toddler, or very young child, apply to the maxillary anterior teeth first and then proceed to other areas of the dentition if patient is cooperative. For all other patients, use a systematic approach. Begin with mandibular teeth; facial, occlusal, and lingual surfaces and then the maxillary teeth; palatal, occlusal, and facial surfaces. Provide full coverage to all areas of the teeth including areas of recession and the cervical third of facial, lingual, and palatal surfaces and occlusal surfaces. Application time is approximately 1–3 minutes.</li></ul>
Completion	<ul><li>Instruct patient that the teeth will feel like they have a coating or film, but this is not visible if a clear product has been used. Ask the patient to avoid hard foods, drinking hot or alcoholic beverages, brushing, and flossing the teeth until the next day or at least 4–6 hours after application.</li></ul>

- Contraindications[67]
  - Allergy to silver.
  - Pregnancy/breastfeeding.
- Relative contraindications[67,69]
  - Painful sores or raw areas on the gingiva or in the mouth (ulcerative gingivitis or stomatitis).
  - Avoid application on cavitated teeth with suspected pulpal involvement.[69]
- Potential limitations and risks[67]
  - Communicate effectively with the patient/parent/legal guardian/advocate and consider written informed consent form for SDF placement prior to application.
  - Placement of SDF does not eliminate the need for future restorations.
  - SDF needs to be applied one to two times at separate dental hygiene visits for maximum benefit (approximately once every 6–12 months).
  - The affected area of decay will likely stain black/gray permanently upon SDF placement; however, healthy enamel will not stain.
  - If accidentally applied to the skin or gingiva, a brownish stain may appear, which will not wash away immediately (should dissipate within 1–3 weeks).
  - Metallic/bitter taste.
- SDF application appointment sequence[67]
  - Dispense 1 drop in a dappen dish, which will treat up to five surfaces/10 kg per treatment visit, maximum dose 25 µL.

- Protect the clinical environment by covering the unit with plastic and the counter with a tray cover or plastic lined bib.
- Provide a plastic bib and protective eyewear for the patient.
- Isolate the tongue and cheek with gauze/cotton rolls to prevent staining of soft tissues.
- Dry the lesion.
- Immerse microsponge brush in SDF, remove excess on the side of the dappen dish.
- Apply SDF directly to the carious lesion and allow it to absorb for 1–3 minutes; may reapply.
- Allow the area to fully dry for 60 seconds.
- Place gloves, cotton, and microsponge brush in a plastic bag for disposal.
  - Procedures for SDF application are listed in **Table 5**.

Self-Applied Fluorides

- Self-applied fluorides (prescription [**Rx**] and OTC products) are available as dentifrices, mouthrinses, and gels.
- Concentrations of 1500 ppm fluoride or less can be sold OTC.[39] However, some products containing less than 1500 ppm of fluoride are available only by Rx.
- May be applied by toothbrushing, rinsing, or trays that are custom made or disposable.

Table 5 Procedure for SDF Application[67]

Patient selection	▪ Determine indications (e.g., extreme caries risk, xerostomia, severe childhood caries). ▪ Review contraindications/relative contraindications. ▪ Communicate effectively regarding potential limitations and risks with the patient/parent/guardian and consider written informed consent prior to application. ▪ Inform the patient the affected area of decay will likely stain black/gray permanently upon placement of SDF. ▪ Provide protective eyewear and a plastic bib to the patient, and isolate both the tongue and cheek with gauze or cotton rolls to prevent staining.
Prepare operatory and product	▪ To avoid staining, place a tray cover or a plastic lined bib on the counter and ensure operatory unit is adequately protected with plastic. Dispense 1 drop in a dappen dish/10 kg per treatment visit. ▪ Have microsponge brush available.
Dry the carious lesion and apply the SDF	▪ Dry the lesion. Immerse the microsponge in the SDF. Remove any excess product on the side of the dappen dish. Apply directly to the carious lesion and allow it to absorb for 1–3 minutes; may reapply as needed.
Completion	▪ Allow the area to fully dry for 60 seconds. Place microsponge brush, cotton, and gloves into a plastic bag for disposal. ▪ There are no postplacement patient instructions with SDF; however, reevaluation of the area is recommended 2–4 weeks after initial application.[69]

I. Indications

- Patient needs are determined as part of total care planning.
- Indications for use of tray, rinsing, and/or toothbrushing depend on the individual patient prevention needs and caries risk assessment.
- Certain patients need multiple procedures combined with professional applications at their regular continuing care appointments. Special indications are suggested as each method is described in the following sections.

II. Methods

The three methods for self-application are by tray, rinsing, and toothbrushing.

- Tray
  - Custom-made or disposable tray: The tray is selected to fit the individual mouth and completely cover the teeth being treated.
  - Figure 4 shows adequate and inadequate tray coverage on the teeth.
  - Instruction is provided not to overfill the tray.
- Rinsing
  - The patient swishes for 1 minute with a measured amount of a fluoride rinse and expectorates.
  - Certain patients will need to learn how to rinse properly to force the solution between the teeth. Chapter 28 lists steps for teaching how to rinse.
- Toothbrushing
  - A fluoride-containing dentifrice is used for regular brushing after breakfast and before going to bed without further eating.
  - Brush-on gel is used after regular brushing to provide additional benefits.
  - Use an interdental brush to apply fluoride to proximal surfaces or open furcations.

Tray Technique: Home Application

- The original gel tray studies using custom-fitted polyvinyl mouthpieces compared the use of 1.1% APF with plain NaF gel.
- The gel was applied daily over a 2-year period by schoolchildren aged 11–14 years during the school years. Dental caries incidence was reduced up to 80%.[77]

I. Indications for Use

- Rampant enamel or root caries in persons of any age to prevent additional new carious lesions and promote remineralization around existing lesions.
- Xerostomia from any cause, particularly loss of salivary gland function.
- Exposure to radiation therapy.
- Root surface hypersensitivity.

II. Gels Used (Available by Prescription)

- Concentrations[39]
  - 1.1% NaF; 5000 ppm fluoride.
  - 1.1% APF; 5000 ppm fluoride.
- Precautions[39]
  - Dispense small quantities.
  - Maximum adult dose is 16 drops per day (4–8 drops on the inner surface of each custom-made tray).
  - Use neutral sodium preparations on porcelain, composites, titanium, or sealants.
  - Patients with mucositis may experience irritation with the APF due to the high acidity.
- Patient instructions
  - Use the gel tray once each day, preferably just before going to bed without further eating and after toothbrushing and flossing.
  - **Box 3** outlines the procedures for the patient to follow for a home tray application.
  - A printed copy of the instructions is given to the patient.

Fluoride Mouthrinses

- Mouthrinsing is a practical and effective means for self-application of fluoride for individuals at moderate or high caries risk.
- Do not use for patients aged 6 years or younger, or for those unable to rinse for a physical or other reason.[78]
- Rinsing can be part of an individual care plan or can be included in a group program conducted during school attendance.

I. Indications

- Mouthrinsing with a fluoride preparation may be an additional benefit for the following:
  - Young persons during the high-risk preteen and adolescent years.
  - Patients with areas of demineralization.

- Patients with root exposure following recession and periodontal therapy.
- Participants in a school health group program for children older than 6 years.
- Patients with moderate-to-rampant caries risk who live in a fluoridated or nonfluoridated community.
- Patients whose oral health care is complicated by biofilm-retentive appliances, including orthodontics, partial dentures, or space maintainers.
- Patients with xerostomia from any cause, including head and neck radiation and saliva-depressing drug therapy.
- Patients with hypersensitivity of exposed root surfaces.

II. Limitations

- Children younger than 6 years of age and those of any age who cannot rinse because of oral and/or facial musculature problems or other disability.
- Alcohol content:
  - Alcohol-based mouthrinses are not recommended; aqueous solutions are available.
  - Alcohol content of commercial preparations is not advisable for children, especially adolescents.
  - Alcohol-containing preparations are never to be recommended for a person recovering from alcohol use disorder (AUD); however, a history of AUD would not necessarily be known to the clinician.
- Compliance is greater with a daily rinse than with a weekly rinse for at home use.

III. Preparations[39]

- Oral rinses are categorized as low-potency/high-frequency rinses or high-potency/low-frequency rinses.
- Most low-potency rinses may be purchased directly OTC, whereas most high-potency rinses are provided by prescription (Rx).
- **Table 6** contains the compounds, concentration, and recommended frequency of use for currently available self-applied fluoride rinses.

Box 3 Instructions for Home Tray Application

1. One daily application just before bedtime; do not eat or drink until morning. If applied at another time of day, do not eat or drink for at least 30 minutes.
2. Brush and floss before applying tray to remove biofilm and food debris.
3. Use prepared custom-made polyvinyl trays. Disposable trays can be used if the appropriate fit can be obtained.
4. Distribute no more than 4–8 drops or a thin ribbon of the gel on the inner surface of each tray. Each drop is equivalent to 0.1 mL.
5. Expectorate to minimize saliva in the mouth.
6. Apply one tray at a time. Hold head upright.
7. Apply the mandibular tray first; close gently to hold the tray in place.
8. Time by a clock for 4 minutes. Do not swallow.
9. Expectorate several times when the tray is removed to prevent swallowing gel and then prepare the mouth for the other tray.
10. Apply the maxillary tray and follow steps 7–9 as for the mandibular tray.
11. After tray removal, do not eat, drink, or brush teeth for at least 30 minutes.
12. After both trays are removed, rinse the trays under running water and brush them clean.
13. Keep in open air for drying.

Table 6 Patient-Applied Fluoride Mouthrinses (Age 6 Years and Older)

Type/Percentage (RX or OTC)	Concentration in PPM	Frequency of Use (10 mL or 2 Teaspoons Swished for 1 Min)
0.2% NaF (Rx)	905	Once daily or once weekly
0.044% NaF and APF (Rx and OTC)	200	Once daily
0.05% NaF (OTC)	230	Once daily
0.0221% NaF (OTC)	100	Twice daily

APF, acidulated phosphate fluoride; NaF, sodium fluoride; OTC, over-the-counter; Rx, prescription

- Low potency/high frequency (available OTC)
  - Preparations
    - 0.05% NaF; 230 ppm.
    - 0.044% NaF or APF; 200 ppm (available by Rx or OTC depending on the brand).
    - 0.0221% NaF; 100 ppm.
  - Specifications
    - No more than 264 mg NaF (120 mg of fluoride) can be dispensed at one time.
    - A 500-mL bottle of 0.05% NaF rinse contains 100 mg of fluoride.
    - Bottle is required to have a child-proof cap.
    - Rinses are not to be used by children younger than 6 years of age or by children or adults with a disability involving oral and/or facial musculature.
    - Young children do not have sufficient ability to expectorate, and they tend to swallow quickly.
    - The rinse is to be fully expectorated without swallowing.
  - Procedure for use
    - Low-potency rinses are used once or twice daily with 2 teaspoonfuls (10 mL) after brushing and before bedtime. Follow manufacturer's ADA-approved specifications.
    - The adult and pediatric maximum dose is 10 mL of solution.
    - Swish between teeth with lips tightly closed for 60 seconds; spit out.
    - Have the patient practice rinsing at the dental chair.
    - Instruct patient: Do not eat or drink for 30 minutes after rinsing.
- High potency/low frequency (available by Rx)
  - Preparation
    - 0.20% NaF; 905 ppm.
    - Originally recommended as a weekly rinse, but it can be used up to once per day.[47]
  - Procedure for use: the same as for high-frequency/low-potency rinses.

The prevented fraction of dental caries ranges from 30% to 59%, with the use of 0.2% NaF rinse on various rinsing schedules.[51]

IV. Benefits

- Benefits from fluoride mouthrinsing have been documented many times since the original research using various percentages of different fluoride preparations.[79,80]
- Frequent rinsing with low concentrations of fluoride has the following effects:

- Primary teeth present in school-aged children benefit by as much as a 42.5% average reduction in dental caries incidence.[81]
- Greater benefit for smooth surfaces, but some benefit to pits and fissures.
- Greatest benefit to newly erupted teeth.
- The program needs to be continued through the teenage years to benefit the second and third permanent molars.
- Added benefits for a community with water fluoridation.[82]
- Effective in preventing and reversing root caries.[83]

Brush-On Gel

- Brush-on gel has been used as an adjunct to the daily application of fluoride in a dentifrice and as a supplement to periodic professional applications.
- Regular use has been shown to help control demineralization around orthodontic appliances.[84]
- Provides protection against postirradiation caries in conjunction with other fluoride applications.[85]
- In 2018, an expert panel from the ADA recommended the prioritized use of 5000 ppm fluoride (1.1% NaF) toothpaste or gel at least once per day to arrest or reverse noncavitated and cavitated root surfaces or lesions of permanent teeth over other modalities.[52]

I. Preparations

Table 7 contains the type, concentration, and daily usage guidelines for currently available self-applied fluoride gels.

- 1.1% NaF (neutral pH) or 1.1% APF (3.5 pH); 5000 ppm
  - Available as a gel to be used separate from toothbrushing.
- 1.1% neutral NaF is also available as a dentifrice with an **abrasive system** added.
  - The rationale for the dentifrice product is to increase compliance with one step (brushing only) rather than brushing, followed by application of the high-concentration gel with a toothbrush.
  - Requires a prescription.
- Stannous fluoride (**SnF₂**) 0.4% in glycerin base (1000 ppm).
  - Available as a gel to be used separate from toothbrushing.
  - Available OTC.

Table 7 Patient-Applied Fluoride Gels: Brush-On or Use in Custom-Made Trays (Age 6 Years or Older)

Type/Percentage (Rx or OTC)	Concentration in PPM	Daily Usage Guidelines
1.1% NaF gel or paste (Rx)	5000	Brush on teeth, twice per day or 4–8 drops on inner surface of custom-made tray or brush on teeth
1.1% APF (Rx)	5000	Brush on teeth, preferably at night or 4–8 drops on inner surface of custom-made tray
0.4% SnF (OTC)	1000	Brush on teeth, preferably at night

APF, acidulated phosphate fluoride; NaF, sodium fluoride; OTC, over-the-counter; Rx, prescription

II. Procedure

- Teeth are cleaned first with thorough brushing and flossing before gel application with a separate toothbrush.
- Use once a day or more as recommended, preferably at night after toothbrushing and flossing.
- Place about 2 mg of the gel over the brush head and spread over all teeth.
- Brush 1 minute, then swish to force the fluid between the teeth several times before expectorating.
- Do not rinse.

Fluoride Dentifrices

I. Development

- Historically tried with various compounds, including stannous fluoride, NaF, sodium monofluorophosphate, and amine fluoride.
- Early research objectives: to find compatible fluoride, abrasive systems, and formulations containing available fluoride for uptake by the tooth surface.
- In 1960, the first fluoride dentifrice gained approval by the ADA, Council on Dental Therapeutics: 0.4% stannous fluoride.[86]

II. Indications

- Dental caries prevention
  - Fluoride dentifrice approved by the ADA is an integral part of a complete preventive program and is a basic caries prevention intervention for all patients.[86]
  - Recommended for all patients regardless of their caries risk.
  - Toothbrushing that covers all the teeth on all surfaces at least twice per day with fluoridated toothpaste is the foundation for all patients' fluoride regimen.

- Patients with moderate-to-rampant dental caries are advised to brush three or four times each day with a fluoride-containing dentifrice.
- Expectorate, but do not rinse after toothbrushing, to give the fluoride a longer time to be effective.

III. Preparations

Fluoride dentifrices are available as gels or pastes. Amine fluorides are used in other countries, but not available in the United States.

- Current fluoride constituents[87]
  - NaF 0.24% (1100 ppm).
  - Sodium monofluorophosphate (Na_2PO_3 F) 0.76% (1000 ppm).
  - Stannous fluoride (SnF_2) 0.45% (1000 ppm).
- Guidelines for acceptance
  - Look for ADA Seal of Acceptance. The requirements for acceptance of fluoridated toothpaste by the ADA are described in Chapter 28.

IV. Patient Instruction: Recommended Procedures

Advise the patient in the selection of a fluoride dentifrice, the need for frequent use, the method for application to all the tooth surfaces, and the importance of using a fluoride dentifrice to promote oral health.

- Select an ADA-accepted fluoride-containing dentifrice.
- Place recommended amount of dentifrice on the toothbrush.
- Children (younger than 3 years): twice-daily brushing (morning and night) with no more than a "smear" or the size of a grain of rice of fluoride dentifrice spread along the brushing plane.[88,89] Chapter 47 illustrates a small smear.
  - Daily oral care begins with the eruption of the first primary tooth.

- The supervision of oral hygiene by parents or family members with attention to daily biofilm removal by toothbrushing can make a significant impact on the small child's oral health.
- The paste is then spread over all the teeth before starting to brush so that all teeth benefit and large amounts of paste are not available for swallowing. Older child (ages 3–6 years): twice-daily brushing (morning and night) with fluoride toothpaste the size of a small pea.
  - Demonstrate spreading this amount over the ends of the toothbrush and explain that the child is not to swallow excess amounts of dentifrice.[88,89]
- Adults: Use 1/2 inch of fluoride dentifrice twice daily.
  - Spread dentifrice over the teeth with a light touch of the brush.
  - Proceed with correct brushing positions for sulcular removal of dental biofilm. (See Chapter 26.)
  - Do not rinse after brushing to keep fluoride in the oral cavity.[88,90]
- Keep dentifrice container out of reach of children.

V. Benefits

- Twice-daily use has greater benefits than once-daily use.[78]
- Patients at moderate and high caries risk and those who live in a nonfluoridated community benefit from using a dentifrice several times per day to maintain salivary fluoride levels.
- The dentifrice is a continuing source of fluoride for the tooth surface in the control of demineralization and the promotion of remineralization.
- The use of a dentifrice with a fluoride concentration of 1000 ppm and above compared to a dentifrice without fluoride can prevent dental caries up to an average of 23%.[91]

Combined Fluoride Program

- All patients, regardless of caries risk, benefit from at least twice-daily use of a fluoridated dentifrice and consumption of fluoridated water multiple times during each day.
- Patients at moderate-to-high caries risk benefit from additional methods of fluoride exposure.
- Additional caries reduction can be expected when another topical fluoride, such as a mouthrinse or gel tray, is combined with a fluoride dentifrice.[92]

- When self-administered methods are chosen, patient cooperation is a significant factor.
- Age and eruption pattern influence the method selected.
- Continuing care appointments are to be scheduled for frequent professional topical applications for those at moderate and high caries risk and for continuing instruction and motivation regarding daily fluoride use for all patients.

Fluoride Safety

- Fluoride preparations and fluoridated water have wide margins of safety.
- Fluoride is beneficial in small amounts, but it can be injurious if used without attention to correct dosage and frequency.
- All dental personnel need to be familiar with the following:
  - Recommended approved procedures for use of products containing fluoride.
  - Potential toxic effects of fluoride.
  - How to administer general emergency measures when accidental overdoses occur. (See the "Internal Poisoning" section of Chapter 9.)

I. Summary of Fluoride Risk Management

- Use professionally and recommend only approved fluoride preparations for patient use.
  - Products may have approval from the FDA and the ADA in the United States.
  - Read about the programs of the ADA Council on Scientific Affairs and the Seal of Approval of Products in Chapter 28.
- Use only researched, recommended amounts and methods for delivery.
- Know potential toxicity of the various products and be prepared to administer emergency measures for treating an accidental toxic response.
- Instruct patients in proper care of fluoride products.
  - Dentist prescribes no more than 120 mg of fluoride at one time (no more than 480 of the 0.25 mg tablets or 240 of the 0.5 mg tablets).[39] Do not store large quantities in the home.
  - Request parental supervision of a child's brushing or other fluoride administration. Rinses, for example, are not to be used by children younger than 6 years of age.
  - Fluoride products have child-proof caps and are to be kept out of reach of small children

and other persons, such as the intellectually challenged, who may not understand limitations.

- In school health programs, dispensing of the fluoride product is to be supervised by responsible adults. Containers are to be stored under lock and key when not in active use.

II. Toxicity

- Acute toxicity refers to rapid intake of an excess dose over a short time.
  - Acute fluoride poisoning is extremely rare.[93]
- Chronic toxicity applies to long-term ingestion of fluoride in amounts that exceed the approved therapeutic levels.
- Accidental ingestion of a concentrated fluoride preparation can lead to a toxic reaction.
- Certainly lethal dose (CLD)[94]
  - A lethal dose is the amount of a drug likely to cause death if not intercepted by antidotal therapy.
  - Adult CLD: about 5–10 g of NaF taken at one time. The fluoride ion equivalent is 32–64 mg of fluoride per kilogram body weight (mg F/kg; Box 4A).
  - Child CLD: approximately 0.5–1.0 g, variable with size and weight of the child.
- Safely tolerated dose (STD): one-fourth of the CLD
  - Adult STD: about 1.25–2.5 g of NaF (8–16 mg F/kg).
  - Child: Box 4B shows STDs and CLDs for children.
  - Weights given for each selected age are minimal, and calculations for the doses are conservative.
  - As can be noted in Box 5B, less than 1 g (1000 mg) may be fatal for children aged 12 years and younger, and 0.5 g (500 mg) exceeds the STD for all ages shown.
  - For children younger than 6 years of age, however, 500 mg could be lethal.[94]

III. Signs and Symptoms of Acute Toxic Dose

Symptoms begin within 30 minutes of ingestion and may persist for as long as 24 hours.

- Gastrointestinal tract
- Fluoride in the stomach is acted on by the hydrochloric acid to form hydrofluoric acid, an irritant to the stomach lining. Symptoms include:
  - Nausea, vomiting, and diarrhea.

Box 4 Lethal and Safe Doses of Fluoride

A. Lethal and safe doses of fluoride for a 70-kg adult

CLD
5–10 g NaF
Or
32–64 mg F/kg
STD = 1/4 CLD
1.25–2.5 g NaF
Or
8–16 mg F/kg

B. CLDs and STDs of fluoride (mg F/kg) for selected ages

Age (Years)	Weight (lb/kg)	CLD (mg)	STD (mg)
2	22/10	320	80
4	29/13	422	106
6	37/17	538	135
8	45/20	655	164
10	53/24	771	193
12	64/29	931	233
14	83/38	1206	301
16	92/42	1338	334
18	95/43	1382	346

- Abdominal pain.
- Increased salivation and thirst.
- Systemic involvements
  - Blood: calcium may be bound by the circulating fluoride, thus causing symptoms of hypocalcemia.
  - Central nervous system: hyperreflexia, convulsions, and paresthesias.
  - Cardiovascular and respiratory depression: if not treated, may lead to death in a few hours from cardiac failure or respiratory paralysis.

IV. Emergency Treatment

- Induce vomiting
  - Mechanical: digital stimulation at the back of tongue or in the throat.
- Second person
  - Call emergency service; transport to hospital.

- Administer fluoride-binding liquid when patient is not vomiting
  - Milk.
  - Milk of magnesia.
  - Lime water ($CaOH_2$ solution 0.15%).
- Support respiration and circulation
- Additional therapy indicated at emergency room
  - Calcium gluconate for muscle tremors or tetany.
  - Gastric lavage.
  - Cardiac monitoring.
  - Endotracheal intubation.
  - Blood monitoring (calcium, magnesium, potassium, pH).
  - Intravenous feeding to restore blood volume, calcium.

V. Chronic Toxicity

- Skeletal fluorosis[93]
  - Isolated instances of osteosclerosis, an elevation in bone density, can result from chronic toxicity after long-term (10 years or more) ingestion of water with 8–10 ppm fluoride or from inhalation of industrial fumes or dust.
  - Skeletal fluorosis in its early stages is characterized by stiff and painful joints and becomes crippling in its later stages.
  - It has never been a public health concern in the United States, even in communities that naturally have had high levels of fluoride in the water for generations.
  - Is endemic in certain countries such as China and India with high levels of natural fluoride in the water.
  - Predisposing factors, dietary deficiencies, and population differences with regard to fluoride metabolism may play a role in its development in addition to exposure.
  - Methods for defluoridation have been developed, as described in this chapter.
- Dental fluorosis
  - Ingestion of naturally occurring excess fluoride in the drinking water and/or fluoride dental products can produce visible fluorosis only when used during the years of development of the crowns of the teeth, namely, from birth until age 16 or 18 years, or when the crowns of the third permanent molars are completed.
  - No systemic symptoms result from the fluoride, and the individual has protection against dental caries.
  - Scoring system used to describe dental fluorosis is found in Chapter 21.

- Mild fluorosis
  1. Clinical evaluation
     - Mild and very mild forms, dental fluorosis appears as "**white spots**" or **enamel opacities** in the enamel surface.
     - No esthetic or health problem is involved. Many such white spots are not visible, except when scrutinized under a dental light and the surface is dried.
     - Not all white spots in the enamel are related to fluoride intake; distinction can be made by reviewing the patient's dental and fluoride intake history, by noting the location and distribution of the white spots, and by considering the sequence of tooth development.
  2. Relation to fluoride sources
     - Mild fluorosis may result from inadvertent ingestion of excess fluoride by young children during topical procedures, both self-applied and professional.
     - No problem exists when care is taken to follow basic steps, such as those listed in Table 3, Table 4, and Table 5, for professional applications.
     - Mouthrinses are not indicated for children younger than 6 years of age.
     - Small amounts of dentifrice may be swallowed incidentally at each brushing. A child aged 4 years who lives in a nonfluoridated community uses a daily supplement (0.5 mg) and swallows two or three small amounts of dentifrice ingests far less than the STD of 106 mg.

Documentation

A patient receiving a topical fluoride application and/or counseling regarding fluoride needs the following documented in the permanent record:

- Caries risk level (document as low, moderate, high, or very high).
- Current use of fluoride toothpaste and exposure to fluoridated water.
- Type, concentration, mode of delivery, and post-operative instructions if a professional fluoride application is provided.
- Type, amount, and instructions for the use of any Rx or OTC patient-applied fluoride products recommended.
- A sample documentation using the SOAP format is provided in **Box 5**.

Box 5 Example Documentation: Professional Fluoride Application and Prescribing Home Fluoride

- **S**—A 26-year-old male patient presents for a periodic oral examination, radiographs, and dental prophylaxis. Patient states that he drinks high-sucrose beverages on a frequent, daily basis. He also reports using toothpaste with fluoride twice daily and consumes fluoridated water.
- **O**—Patient presents with medication-induced xerostomia. Two proximal cavitated lesions were discovered on bitewing radiographs.
- Patient was classified as being high risk for caries after conducting a caries risk assessment analysis.
- **P**—Applied 5% NaF varnish to the entire dentition and provided postoperative instructions. Prescribed 1.1% NaF gel (two refills) to apply with a separate toothbrush at night. Discussed the need for an additional varnish application in 3 months to help prevent the future onset of dental caries.

Signed: _____, RDH

Date: _____

Factors to Teach the Patient

I. Personal Use of Fluorides

- Purposes, action, and expected benefits relative to the specific forms of fluoride treatment the patient will receive based upon individual caries risk.
- Specific instructions concerning self-applied techniques that will be performed at home.

II. Need for Parental Supervision

- Supervise daily care of child's teeth and mouth with the recommended amount of fluoridated toothpaste to prevent excess ingestion of fluoride.
- Keep fluoride products out of reach of small children.

III. Determine Need for Fluoride Supplements

- Must determine child is at high caries risk and consumes fluoride-deficient drinking water.
- Where to send private water source sample for fluoride analysis.

IV. Fluorides Are Part of the Total Preventive Program

- Emphasize fluoride toothpaste and fluoridated water as the cornerstones for prevention of dental caries.
- Regular professional supervision and care.

V. Fluoridation

- How drinking fluoridated water helps people of all ages and need to advocate to keep in community water supplies.
- How to access the CDC Community Water Fluoridation website to obtain reliable information about fluoridation in the United States.

VII. Bottled Drinking Water/Water Filters

- When bottled water does not have a label indicating that it is fluoridated, recommend filling a water bottle from a fluoridated water supply.
- Check with the water filter manufacturer to be certain the fluoride will not be removed through filtration.
- Distillation and reverse osmosis systems remove fluoride from drinking water, but water softeners do not.

VIII. Infant Formula

- Educate parents that powdered or liquid concentrate infant formula and the water used to reconstitute this formula may contain fluoride.

References

1. Ellwood R, Fejerskov O, Cury JA, Clarkson B. Chapter 18: Fluorides in caries control. In: Fejerskov O, Kidd E, eds. *Dental Caries: The Disease and Its Clinical Management*. 2nd ed. Oxford, England: Blackwell Munksgaard; 2008:293-294.

2. Newbrun E. Systemic benefits of fluoride and fluoridation. *J Public Health Dent*. 2004;64(suppl s1):35-39.

3. Ekstrand J. Chapter 4: Fluoride metabolism. In: Fejerskov O, Ekstrand J, Burt BA, eds. *Fluoride in Dentistry*. 2nd ed. Copenhagen, Denmark: Blackwell Munksgaard; 1996:55-67.

4. Bath-Balough M, Fehrenbach M. *Dental Embryology, Histology, and Anatomy*. 2nd ed. St. Louis, MO: Saunders; 2006: 179-189.

5. Melfi RC, Alley KE. *Permar's Oral Embryology and Microscopic Anatomy*. 10th ed. Philadelphia, PA: Lippincott Williams & Wilkins; 2000:43-87.

6. Levy S. An update on fluorides and fluorosis. *J Can Dent Assoc*. 2003;69(5):286-291.

7. Aoba T, Fejerskov O. Dental fluorosis: chemistry and biology. *Crit Rev Oral Biol Med*. 2002;13(2):155-170.

8. Featherstone JD. The science and practice of caries prevention. *J Am Dent Assoc*. 2000;131(7):887-899.

9. Yoon SH, Brudevold F, Gardner DE, Smith FA. Distribution of fluoride in teeth from areas with different levels of fluoride in the water supply. *J Dent Res*. 1960;39:845-856.

10. Centers for Disease Control and Prevention. Recommendations for using fluoride to prevent and control dental caries in the United States. *MMWR Recomm Rep*. 2001;50(RR-14):1-42.

11. Centers for Disease Control and Prevention. Populations receiving optimally fluoridated public drinking water—United States, 1992–1996. *MWWR Morb Mortal Wkly Rep*. 2008;57(27):737-741.

12. Centers for Disease Control and Prevention. Division of Oral Health, National Center for Chronic Disease Prevention and Health Promotion. Community water fluoridation. Atlanta, GA: Water Fluoridation Statistics; 2018. Page last reviewed September 8, 2020. https://www.cdc.gov/fluoridation/statistics/2018stats.htm. Accessed July 23, 2021.

13. Herschfeld JJ. Classics in dental history: Frederick S. McKay and the "Colorado brown stain." *Bull Hist Dent*. 1978;26(2): 118-126.

14. McKay FS. The relation of mottled enamel to caries. *J Am Dent Assoc*. 1928;15:1429-1437.

15. Churchill HV. Occurrence of fluorides in some waters of United States. *J Ind Eng Chem*. 1931;23:996-998.

16. Dean HT, Arnold FA Jr, Elvove E. Domestic water and dental caries. V. Additional studies of the relation of fluoride domestic waters to dental caries experience in 4425 white children, aged 12 to 14 years, of 13 cities in 4 states. *Public Health Rep*. 1942;57:1155-1179.

17. Department of Health and Human Services. U.S. Public Health Service Recommendation for Fluoride Concentration in Drinking Water for the Prevention of Caries. *Public Health Rep*. 2015;130:1-14. http://www.cdc.gov/fluoridation/index.htm. Accessed October 3, 2022.

18. Centers for Disease Control and Prevention. Engineering and administrative recommendations for water fluoridation, 1995. *MMWR Recomm Rep*. 1995;44(RR-13):1-40.

19. Griffin SO, Regnier E, Griffin PM, Huntley V. Effectiveness of fluoride in preventing caries in adults. *J Dent Res*. 2007;86(5): 410-415.

20. Yeung CA. A systematic review of the efficacy and safety of fluoridation. *Evid Based Dent*. 2008;9(2):39-43.

21. Dirks OB, Houwink B, Kwant GW. Some special features of the caries preventive effect of water fluoridation. *Arch Oral Biol*. 1961;4:187-192.

22. Burt BA, Ismail AI, Eklund SA. Root caries in an optimally fluoridated and a high-fluoride community. *J Dent Res*. 1986; 6(9):1154-1158.

23. Stamm JW, Banting DW, Imrey PB. Adult root caries survey of two similar communities with contrasting natural water fluoride levels. *J Am Dent Assoc*. 1990;120(2):143-149.

24. Ast DB, Fitzgerald B. Effectiveness of water fluoridation. *J Am Dent Assoc*. 1962;65:581-587.

25. Russell AL, Elvove E. Domestic water and dental caries. VII. A study of the fluoride-dental caries relationship in an adult population. *Public Health Rep*. 1951;66(43):1389-1401.

26. Englander HR, Wallace DA. Effects of naturally fluoridated water on dental caries in adults: Aurora-Rockford, Illinois, Study III. *Public Health Rep*. 1962;77(10):887-893.

27. Horowitz HS, Maier FJ, Law FE. Partial defluoridation of a community water supply and dental fluorosis. *Public Health Rep*. 1967;82(11):965-972.

28. Horowitz HS, Heifetz SB. The effect of partial defluoridation of a water supply on dental fluorosis—final results in Bartlett, Texas, after 17 years. *Am J Public Health*. 1972;62(6):767-769.

29. Horowitz HS. Effectiveness of school water fluoridation and dietary fluoride supplements in school-aged children. *J Public Health Dent*. 1989;49(5):290-296.

30. Lemke CW, Doherty JM, Arra MC. Controlled fluoridation: the dental effects of discontinuation in Antigo, Wisconsin. *J Am Dent Assoc*. 1979;80(4):782-786.

31. Jackson RD, Brizendine EJ, Kelly SA, Hinesley R, Stookey GK, Dunipace AJ. The fluoride content of foods and beverages from negligibly and optimally fluoridated communities. *Community Dent Oral Epidemiol*. 2002;30(5):382-391.

32. Burt BA, Marthaler TM. Chapter 16: Fluoride tablets, salt fluoridation, and milk fluoridation. In: Fejerskov O, Ekstrand J, Burt BA, eds. *Fluoride in Dentistry*. 2nd ed. Copenhagen, Denmark: Blackwell Munksgaard; 1996:291-310.

33. Espelid I. Caries preventive effect of fluoride in milk, salt and tablets: a literature review. *Eur Arch Paediatr Dent*. 2009; 10(3):149-156.

34. European Academy of Paediatric Dentistry. Guidelines on the use of fluoride in children: an EAPD policy document. *Eur Arch Paediatr Dent*. 2009;10(3):129-135.

35. American Dental Association. *Fluoridation Facts*. Chicago, IL: American Dental Association; 2005.

36. Hujoel PP, Zina LG, Moimaz SA, Cunha-Cruz J. Infant formula and enamel fluorosis: a systematic review. *J Am Dent Assoc*. 2009;140(7):841-854.

37. Siew C, Strock S, Ristic H, et al. Assessing the potential risk factor for enamel fluorosis: a preliminary evaluation of fluoride content in infant formulas. *J Am Dent Assoc*. 2009; 140(10):1228-1236.

38. Berg J, Gerweck C, Hujoel P, et al. Evidence-based clinical recommendations regarding fluoride intake from reconstituted infant formula and enamel fluorosis. *J Am Dent Assoc*. 2011;142(1):79-87.

39. Burrell KH. Chapter 10: Fluorides. In: Mariotti AJ, Burrell KH, eds. *American Dental Association, Council on*

Scientific Affairs: ADA/PDR Guide to Dental Therapeutics. 5th ed. Chicago, IL: American Dental Association and Thomson PDR; 2009:323-337.

40. Ismail AI, Hasson H. Fluoride supplements, dental caries, and fluorosis: a systematic review. *J Am Dent Assoc.* 2008;139(11): 1457-1468.

41. Rozier RG, Adair S, Graham F, et al. Evidence-based clinical recommendations on the prescription of dietary fluoride supplements for caries prevention. *J Am Dent Assoc.* 2010;141(12):1480-1489.

42. Toyama Y, Nakagaki H, Kato S, et al. Fluoride concentrations at and near the neonatal line in human deciduous tooth enamel obtained from a naturally fluoridated and a non-fluoridated area. *Arch Oral Biol.* 2001;46(2):147-153.

43. Tubert-Jeannin S, Auclair C, Amsallem E, et al. Fluoride supplements (tablets, drops, lozenges or chewing gums) for preventing dental caries in children. *Cochrane Database Syst Rev.* 2011;(12):CD007592.

44. Bibby BG. Use of fluorine in the prevention of dental caries. II. The effects of sodium fluoride applications. *J Am Dent Assoc.* 1944;31:317.

45. Knutson JW. Sodium fluoride solutions: technique for application to the teeth. *J Am Dent Assoc.* 1948;36(1):37-39.

46. Galagan DJ, Knutson JW. The effect of topically applied fluorides on dental caries experience; experiments with sodium fluoride and calcium chloride; widely spaced applications; use of different solution concentrations. *Public Health Rep.* 1948;63(38):1215-1221.

47. Weyant RJ, Tracy SL, Anselmo T, et al. Topical fluoride for caries prevention: executive summary of the updated clinical recommendations and supporting systemic review. *J Am Dent Assoc.* 2013;144(11):1279-1291.

48. Warren DP, Chan JT. Topical fluorides: efficacy, administration, and safety. *Gen Dent.* 1997;45(2):134-140, 142.

49. Ripa LW. An evaluation of the use of professionally (operator applied) topical fluorides. *J Dent Res.* 1990;69(Spec No): 786-796.

50. Soeno K, Matsumura H, Atsuta M, Kawasaki K. Influence of acidulated fluoride agents and effectiveness of subsequent polishing on composite material surfaces. *Oper Dent.* 2002; 27(3):305-310.

51. Poulsen S. Fluoride-containing gels, mouthrinses and varnishes: an update of evidence of efficacy. *Eur Arch Paediatr Dent.* 2009;10(3):157-161.

52. Slayton RL, Urquhart O, Araujo MWB, et al. Evidence-based clinical practice guideline on nonrestorative treatments for carious lesions: a report from the American Dental Association. *J Am Dent Assoc* 2018:149(10):837-849.

53. Beltrán-Aguilar ED, Goldstein JW, Lockwood SA. Fluoride varnishes: a review of their clinical use, cariostatic mechanism, efficacy and safety. *J Am Dent Assoc.* 2000;131(5):589-596.

54. Marinho VC, Worthington HV, Walsh T, Clarkson JE. Fluoride varnishes for preventing dental caries in children and adolescents. *Cochrane Database Syst Rev.* 2013;(7):CD002279.

55. Bawden JW. Fluoride varnish: a useful new tool for public health dentistry. *J Public Health Dent.* 1998;58(4):266-269.

56. Autio-Gold JT, Courts F. Assessing the effect of fluoride varnish on early enamel carious lesions in the primary dentition. *J Am Dent Assoc.* 2001;132(9):1247-1253.

57. Castellano JB, Donly KJ. Potential remineralization of de-mineralized enamel after application of fluoride varnish. *Am J Dent.* 2004;17(6):462-464.

58. Demito CF, Vivaldi-Rodrigues G, Ramos AL, Bowman SJ. The efficacy of fluoride varnish in reducing enamel demineralization adjacent to orthodontic brackets: an in vitro study. *Orthod Craniofac Res.* 2004;7(4):205-210.

59. Association of State and Territorial Dental Directors Fluorides Committee. *Fluoride Varnish: An Evidence-Based Approach Research Brief.* https://astdd.org/docs/fl-varnish-brief-september-2014-amended-05-2016.docx. Accessed September 20, 2022.

60. Rosenblatt A, Stamford TC, Niederman R. Silver diamine fluoride: a caries "silver-fluoride bullet." *J Dent Res.* 2009; 88(2):116-125.

61. Shen P, Bagheri R, Walker GD, et al. Effect of calcium phosphate addition to fluoride containing dental varnishes on enamel demineralization. *Aust Dent J.* 2016;61:357-365. doi:10.111/adj.12385

62. Majithia U, Venkataraghavan K, Choudary P, Trivedi K, Shah S, Virda M. Comparative evaluation of application of different fluoride varnishes on artificial early enamel lesion: an in vitro study. *Indian J Dent Res.* 2016;27:521-527.

63. Bruze M. Systemically induced contact dermatitis from rosin. *Scand J Dentv Res.* 1994;102:376-378.

64. Sharma PR. Allergic contact stomatitis from colophony. *Dent Update.* 2006;33:440-442.

65. Isaksson M, Bruze M, Bjorkner B, Niklasson B. Contact allergy to Duraphat. *Scand J Dent Res.* 1993;101:49-51.

66. Chu CH, Lo ECM. Promoting caries arrest in children with silver diamine fluoride: a review. *Oral Health Prev Dent.* 2008;6(4):315-321.

67. Horst J, Ellenikiotis H, Milgrom P. UCSF protocol for caries arrest using silver diamine fluoride: rationale, indications and consent. *J Calif Dent Assoc.* 2016;44(1):16-28.

68. Crystal, YO, Marghalani AA, Ureles SD, et al. Use of silver diamine fluoride for dental caries management in children and adolescents, including those with special health care needs. *Pediatr Dent.* 2017;39(5):E135-E145.

69. American Academy of Pediatric Dentistry. Chairside guide: Silver diamine fluoride in the management of dental caries lesions. Pediatr Dent 2018;40(6):492-3.

70. American Academy of Pediatric Dentistry. Fluoride therapy. In: *The Reference Manual of Pediatric Dentistry.* Chicago, IL: American Academy of Pediatric Dentistry; 2020:288-291.

71. Crystal YO, Niederman R. Evidence-based dentistry update on silver diamine fluoride. *Dent Clin North Am.* 2019;63(1):45-68.

72. Ripa LW. Need for prior tooth cleaning when performing a professional topical fluoride application: review and recommendations for change. *J Am Dent Assoc.* 1984;109(2):281-285.

73. Vrbic V, Brudevold F, McCann HG. Acquisition of fluoride by enamel from fluoride pumice pastes. *Helv Odontol Acta.* 1967; 11(1):21-26.

74. Shen C, Autio-Gold J. Assessing fluoride concentration uniformity and fluoride release from three varnishes. *J Am Dent Assoc.* 2002;133(2):176-182.

75. Stookey GK, Schemehorn BR, Drook CA, Cheetham BL. The effect of rinsing with water immediately after a professional fluoride gel application on fluoride uptake in demineralized enamel: an in vivo study. *Pediatr Dent.* 1986;8(3):153-157.

76. Castillo J, Rivera S, Aparicio T, et al. The short-term effects of diammine silver fluoride on tooth sensitivity: a randomized controlled trial. *J Dent Res.* 2011;90(2):203-208.

77. Englander HR, Keyes PH, Gestwicki M, Sultz HA. Clinical anticaries effect of repeated topical sodium fluoride applications by mouthpieces. *J Am Dent Assoc.* 1967;75(3):638-644.

78. Adair SM. Evidence-based use of fluoride in contemporary pediatric dental practice. *Pediatr Dent.* 2006;28(2):133-142.

79. Torell P, Ericsson Y. The potential benefits derived from fluoride mouthrinses. In: Forrester DJ, Schulz EM, eds. *International Workshop on Fluorides and Dental Caries Reductions.* Baltimore, MD: University of Maryland School of Dentistry; 1974:114-176.

80. Birkeland JM, Torell P. Caries-preventive fluoride mouth-rinses. *Caries Res.* 1978;12(suppl 1):38-51.

81. Ripa LW, Leske GS, Varma A. Effect of mouthrinsing with a 0.2 percent neutral NaF solution on the deciduous dentition of first to third grade school children. *Pediatr Dent.* 1984;6(2):93-97.

82. Driscoll WS, Swango PA, Horowitz AM, Kingman A. Caries-preventive effects of daily and weekly fluoride mouthrinsing in a fluoridated community: final results after 30 months. *J Am Dent Assoc.* 1982;105(6):1010-1013.

83. Heijnsbroek M, Paraskevas S, Vav der Weijden GA. Fluoride interventions for root caries: a review. *Oral Health Prev Dent.* 2007;5(2):145-152.

84. Stratemann MW, Shannon IL. Control of decalcification in orthodontic patients by daily self-administered application of a water-free 0.4 percent stannous fluoride gel. *Am J Orthod.* 1974;66(3):273-279.

85. Wescott WB, Starcke EN, Shannon IL. Chemical protection against postirradiation dental caries. *Oral Surg Oral Med Oral Pathol.* 1975;40(6):709-719.

86. American Dental Association, Council on Dental Therapeutics. Evaluation of Crest toothpaste. *J Am Dent Assoc.* 1960;61:272.

87. Mariotti MJ, Burrell K. Mouthrinses and dentifrices. In: *American Dental Association, Council on Scientific Affairs: ADA/PDR Guide to Dental Therapeutics.* 5th ed. Chicago, IL: American Dental Association and Thomson PDR; 2009: 305-321.

88. American Academy of Pediatric Dentistry Liaison with Other Groups Committee; and American Academy on Pediatric Dentistry Council on Scientific Affairs. Guideline on fluoride therapy. *Pediatr Dent.* 2013;36:171-174.

89. American Dental Association Council on Scientific Affairs. Fluoride toothpaste use for young children. *J Am Dent Assoc.* 2014;145(2):190-191.

90. Sjogren K, Melin NH. The influence of rinsing routines on fluoride retention after toothbrushing. *Gerodontology.* 2001; 18(1):15-20.

91. Walsh T, Worthington HV, Glenny AM, Appelbe P, Marinho VC, Shi X. Fluoride toothpastes of different concentrations for preventing dental caries in children and adolescents. *Cochrane Database Syst Rev.* 2010;(1):CD007868.

92. Marinho VC. Cochrane reviews of randomized trials of fluoride therapies for preventing dental caries. *Eur Arch Paediatr Dent.* 2009;10(3):183-191.

93. Whitford GM. Acute and chronic fluoride toxicity. *J Dent Res.* 1992;71(5):1249-1254.

Dentinal Hypersensitivity

Amy N. Smith, RDH, MPH, PhD

CHAPTER OUTLINE

LEARNING OBJECTIVES

After studying this chapter, the student will be able to:

1. Describe stimuli and pain characteristics specific to hypersensitivity and explain how this relates to differential diagnosis.
2. Describe the factors that contribute to dentin exposure and behavioral changes that could decrease hypersensitivity.
3. Explain the steps in the hydrodynamic theory.
4. Describe two mechanisms of desensitization and their associated treatment interventions for managing dentin hypersensitivity.

The dental hygienist is often the first oral health professional to become aware of the presence of hypersensitive teeth when a patient presents for care. Individuals who have hypersensitivity may be uncomfortable during dental hygiene treatment, since exposure to stimuli such as a cold water spray or contact with metal instruments can elicit the pain of hypersensitive teeth.

- Patients often report activities of daily living such as eating or drinking cold foods or beverages cause pain and request information about causes and treatment for their discomfort.
- Hypersensitivity is often difficult to diagnose because the presenting symptoms can be confused with other types of dental pain with a different etiology.
- Management of hypersensitivity can be a challenge because there are numerous treatment approaches with varying degrees of efficacy.
- Knowledge of the predisposing factors that lead to gingival recession and loss of enamel or cementum and dentin can assist patients in preventing conditions that cause or exacerbate hypersensitivity.

Hypersensitivity Defined

A definitive characteristic associated with **dentinal hypersensitivity** is pain elicited by a stimulus and alleviated upon its removal. Numerous types of stimuli can lead to pain response in individuals with exposed dentin surfaces.

I. Stimuli That Elicit Pain Reaction

- Tactile: contact with toothbrush and other oral hygiene devices, eating utensils, dental instruments, and friction from prosthetic devices such as denture clasps.
- Thermal: temperature change caused by hot and/or cold foods and beverages, and cold air as it contacts the teeth. Cold is the most common stimulus for pain.
- Evaporative: dehydration of oral fluids as from high-volume evacuation or application of air to dry teeth during intraoral procedures.
- **Osmotic**: alteration of pressure in dentinal tubules due to solubility changes in the dentinal fluid.
- Chemical: acids in foods and beverages such as citrus fruits, condiments, spices, wine, and carbonated beverages; acids produced by acidogenic

bacteria following carbohydrate exposure; acids from gastroesophageal reflux or vomiting; acidic formulation of whitening agents.

II. Characteristics of Pain from Hypersensitivity

- Sharp, short, or transient pain with rapid onset.
- Cessation of pain upon removal of stimulus.
- Presents as a chronic condition with acute episodes.
- Pain in response to a stimulus that would not normally cause pain or discomfort.
- Discomfort that cannot be ascribed to any other dental defect or pathology.[1]

Etiology of Dentinal Hypersensitivity

A review of tooth anatomy facilitates an understanding of the mechanism of hypersensitivity.

I. Anatomy of Tooth Structures

A. Dentin

- The portion of the tooth covered by enamel on the crown and cementum on the root.
- Composed of fluid-filled dentinal tubules that narrow and branch as they extend from the pulp to the dentinoenamel junction or from the pulp to the dentinocemental junction (**Figure 1**).
- Only the portions of the dentinal tubules closest to the pulp are potentially innervated with nerve fiber endings from the pulp chamber.[2]

B. Pulp

- Highly innervated with nerve cell fiber endings that extend just beyond the dentinopulpal interface of the dentinal tubules.[3]
- Body portions of odontoblasts (dentin-producing cells) located within the pulp wall extend their processes from the dentinopulpal junction a short way into each dentinal tubule (Figure 1).

C. Nerves

- Nerve fiber endings extend just beyond the dentinopulpal junction and wind around the odontoblastic processes as shown in Figure 1.[4] However, not all dentinal tubules contain nerve fiber endings.
- Nerves react via the same **neural depolarization mechanism (sodium-potassium pump)**, which characterizes the response of any nerve to a stimulus.

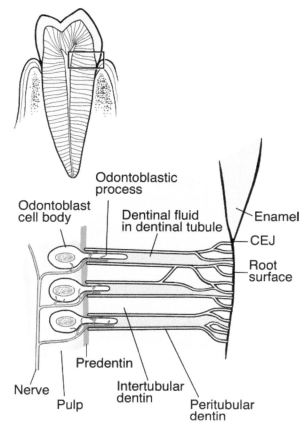

Figure 1 Relationship of Dentinal Tubules and Pulpal Nerve Endings. Nerve endings from the pulp wrap themselves around the odontoblasts that extend only a short distance into the tubule. Fluid-filled dentinal tubules transmit fluid disturbances through the mechanism known as hydraulic conductance. CEJ, cementoenamel junction.

II. Mechanisms of Dentin Exposure

- The sequential events of gingival recession, loss of cementum or enamel, and subsequent dentin exposure, as seen in **Figure 2**, can result in hypersensitivity.
- Loss of enamel or cementum can expose dentin gradually or suddenly as in tooth fracture.
- As a result of the lower mineral content of cementum and dentin compared with enamel, demineralization occurs more rapidly and at a lower critical pH.
- Acute hypersensitivity may occur with sudden dentin exposure since gradual exposure allows for the development of natural desensitization mechanisms such as **smear layer** or sclerosis. After many years, secondary or **tertiary/reparative dentin** may form, which also protects the pulp.

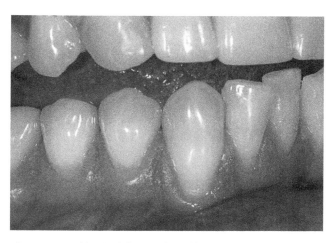

Figure 2 Gingival Recession. Note recession from the mandibular right central incisor to the second premolar. If the thin cemental layer of the exposed root surface is lost, dentin hypersensitivity can develop.

A. Factors Contributing to Gingival Recession and Subsequent Root Exposure

The occurrence of gingival recession has a multifactorial etiology. Potential causes include:

- Effects of improper oral self-care:
  - Use of a medium or hard-bristle toothbrush.
  - Frequent, long-term aggressive use of the toothbrush and/or other oral hygiene devices.
- An anatomically narrow zone of attached gingiva is more susceptible to abrasion.
- Facial orientation of one or more teeth.
- A tight and short labial or buccal frenum attachment that pulls on gingival tissues.
- Subgingival instrumentation involving excessive scaling and debridement in shallow sulci.[5]
- Tissue alteration due to apical migration of junctional epithelium from periodontal diseases.
- Periodontal surgical procedures can alter the architecture of gingival tissues resulting in recession.
- Surgical procedures such as crown lengthening, repositioning of gingival tissues, or tooth extractions can affect gingival coverage of adjacent teeth.
- Orthodontic tooth movement may result in loss of periodontal attachment.
- Restorative procedures, such as crown preparation, that abrade marginal gingival tissues.
- Metal jewelry used in an oral piercing of the lip or tongue that repeatedly traumatizes the adjacent facial or lingual gingival tissue.

B. Factors Contributing to Loss of Enamel and Cementum

- Loss of tooth structure rarely develops from a single cause but rather from a combination of contributing factors.
- Cementum at the cervical area is thin and easily abrades when exposed.
- Enamel and cementum do not meet at the cementoenamel junction in about 5–10% of teeth, leaving an area of exposed dentin.

C. Attrition, Abrasion, and Erosion

- Attrition can occur due to parafunctional habits such as bruxing.
- Abrasion to sound enamel due to increased toothbrushing forces has not been supported in recent research.[6,7]
- Effects of attrition and abrasion are exacerbated when acid erodes the tooth surface or when the tooth is brushed immediately after consumption of acidic foods and beverages.
- Hypersensitivity may be a clinical outcome of erosion.[8]
- Erosion can occur from dietary acids, such as citrus fruits/juices, wine, and carbonated drinks.[9]
- Dietary acid intake results in an immediate drop in oral pH; after normal salivary neutralization, a physiologic pH of 7 reestablishes within minutes.
- Frequent acid consumption is a critical factor, holding or "swilling" of acidic agents, holding low-pH foods such as citrus fruits against teeth, or continual snacking increases erosion risk.
- Gastric acids from conditions such as gastric reflux, morning sickness, or self-induced vomiting (bulimia) repeatedly expose teeth to a highly acidic environment.

D. Abfraction

- Abfraction, a wedge-shaped cervical lesion, has a questionable etiology.[10-13]
- A cervical lesion caused by lateral/occlusal stresses or tooth flexure from bruxing.
- Microscopic portions of the enamel rods chip away from the cervical area of the tooth, resulting in loss of tooth structure (**Figure 3**).
- Lesion appears as a wedge or V-shaped cervical notch.
- A cofactor with abrasion for loss of tooth structure and potential sensitivity.

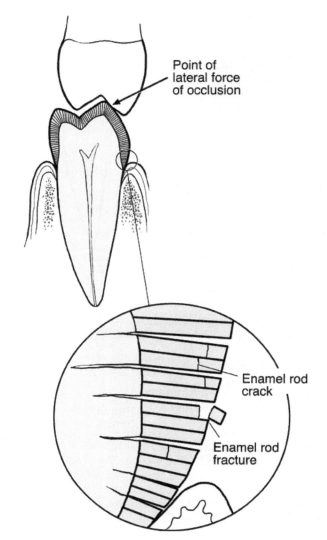

Figure 3 Process of Abfraction. Lateral occlusal forces stress the enamel rods at the cervical area, resulting in enamel rod fracture over time. In an advanced stage, a wedge- or V-shaped cervical lesion is visible. Although minute cracks in the enamel rods may not be clinically evident, the tooth can exhibit hypersensitivity.

E. Other Factors

- Crown preparation procedures that remove enamel or cementum can expose dentin at the cervical area.
- Instrumentation during scaling or root debridement procedures on thinning cementum.
- Frequent or improper stain-removal techniques, in which abrasive particles wear away the cementum and dentin.
- Root surface carious lesions.
- Removal of proximal enamel using a sandpaper disk or strip to create additional space for orthodontic movement of crowded teeth, also known as "enamel stripping."

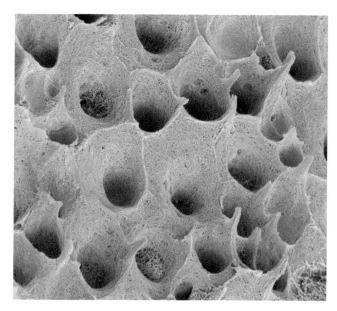

Figure 4 Open Dentin Tubules. A scanning electron micrograph (SEM) of dentinal tubules.

© STEVE GSCHMEISSNER/SCIENCE PHOTO LIBRARY/Getty Images.

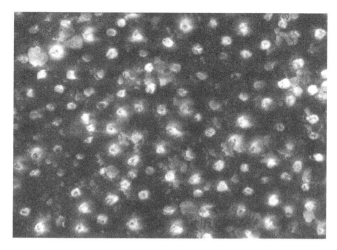

Figure 5 Partially Occluded Dentin Tubules. These dentin tubules are nearly filled.

Fraunhofer Institute for Mechanics of Materials, Freiburg, Germany. Authors: Vanessa Sternitzke, Maria Morawietz, Andreas Kiesow. Reprinted with permission.

III. Hydrodynamic Theory

Hydrodynamic theory is a currently accepted explanation for transmission of stimuli from the outer surface of the dentin to the pulp.

- Described in the 1960s by Brännström, who theorized that a stimulus at the outer aspect of dentin will cause fluid movement within the dentinal tubules.[14]
- Fluid movement creates pressure on the nerve endings within the dentinal tubule, which transmits the pain impulse by stimulating the nerves in the pulp.
- Credibility for this theory is supported by the greater number of widened dentin tubules seen in hypersensitive teeth compared with nonsensitive teeth.[2] **Figure** 4 depicts open dentinal tubules at the microscopic level. **Figure** 5 depicts partially occluded dentinal tubules.

Natural Desensitization

- Hypersensitivity can decrease naturally over time, even without treatment interventions.
- These mechanisms include those listed here.

I. Sclerosis of Dentin

- Occurs by mineral deposition within tubules as a result of traumatic stimuli, such as attrition or dental caries.

- Creates a thicker, highly mineralized layer of **intratubular or peritubular dentin** (deposited within the periphery of the tubules).
- Results in a smaller-diameter tubule that is less able to transmit stimuli through the dentinal fluid to the nerve fibers at the dentinopulpal interface.

II. Secondary Dentin

- Deposited gradually on the floor and roof of the pulp chamber after the apical foramen is completed.
- Formed more slowly than primary dentin; both types of dentin are created by odontoblasts.
- Creates a "walling off" effect between the dentinal tubules and the pulp to insulate the pulp from dentin fluid disturbances caused by a stimulus such as dental caries.
- With aging, **secondary dentin** accumulates, resulting in a smaller pulp chamber with fewer nerve endings and less sensitivity.

III. Smear Layer

- Consists of organic and inorganic debris that covers the dentinal surface and the tubules.[15]
- Accumulates following scaling and root instrumentation, use of toothpaste (abrasive particles), cutting with a bur, attrition, or abrasion.
- Occludes the dentinal tubule orifices, forming a "smear plug" or a natural "bandage" that blocks stimuli.

- The nature of the smear layer changes constantly since it is subject to effects such as mechanical disruption from ultrasonic debridement, or dissolution from acid exposure.

IV. Calculus

- Provides a protective coating to shield exposed dentin from stimuli.
- Postdebridement sensitivity can occur after removal of heavy calculus deposits; dentinal tubules may become exposed as calculus is removed.

The Pain of Dentin Hypersensitivity

Individuals react differently to pain based on factors such as age, gender, situation and context, previous experiences, pain expectations, and other psychological and physiologic parameters.

I. Patient Profile

The prevalence of reported hypersensitivity varies due to differences in the stimulus, and whether data are gathered by patient report or standardized clinical examination. Patient accounts may not represent true hypersensitivity since the pain can be confused with other conditions.

A. Prevalence of Hypersensitivity

- Current systematic review articles reveal a global prevalence of dental hypersensitivity to be between 3% and 65% with most populations ranging from 10% to 30%.[16-18]
- Most commonly found among 30- to 40-year-olds.[16,17]
- Higher prevalence has been reported in periodontally involved populations.[16,18]
- Incidence and severity decline with advancing age due to the effects of sclerosis and secondary dentin.[16]
- Gingival recession is more prevalent with aging.[19] However, dentinal hypersensitivity is not more prevalent with aging.
- Hypersensitivity, when measured objectively, occurs more often in women.[16,20]

B. Teeth Affected

- Hypersensitivity has been reported to occur primarily at the cervical one-third of the facial surfaces of premolars and mandibular anterior teeth,[21] or on premolars and molars.[16]
- Can occur on any tooth exhibiting predisposing factors.

II. Pain Experience

A. Neural Activity

- Stimuli that affect the fluid flow within the dentinal tubules can activate the terminal nerve endings near to or surrounding the dentinal tubules; activation of these nerve fibers elicits the pain response.
- Occurs via the depolarization/neural discharge mechanism that characterizes all nerve activity.
- The sodium–potassium pump depolarizes the nerve as potassium leaves the nerve cell and sodium enters it.

B. Pain Perception

- The degree of pain is not always proportional to the amount of recession, the percentage of tooth structure loss, or to the quality or quantity of stimulus.
- Individuals experience the subjective phenomenon of pain differently. Many diverse variables such as stress, fatigue, and health beliefs can impact pain perception.

C. Impact of Pain

- Hypersensitivity can manifest as acute or chronic pain; acute pain may result in anxiety, whereas chronic pain may contribute to depression.
- Stress may exacerbate the pain response.
- Persistent discomfort from dentin hypersensitivity may affect quality of life.

Differential Diagnosis

- Etiology of pain can be systemic, pulpal, periapical, restorative, degenerative, or neoplastic.
- A differential diagnosis can rule out other causes of pain before treating for hypersensitivity.
- Skilled interviewing and diagnostics contribute to the differential diagnosis.
- Components to consider in the differential diagnosis of tooth pain are detailed in **Table   1.**

I. Differentiation of Pain

- Hypersensitivity pain elicited by a nonnoxious stimulus, such as cold water, can mimic pain elicited by a noxious agent, such as cavitated dental caries.

Table 1 Differential Diagnosis of Tooth Pain

Condition	Signs and Symptoms	Clinical Assessment
Dentinal hypersensitivity	Thermal, mechanical, evaporative, osmotic, chemical sensitivity Sharp, sudden, transient pain	Clinical examination: gingival recession and loss of tooth structure
Caries extending into dentin	Thermal sensitivity Pain on pressure Pain with sweets	Clinical examination Radiographic examination
Pulpal caries	Thermal sensitivity Severe, intermittent, or throbbing pain Pain on chewing	Clinical examination Radiographic examination
Fractured restoration	Thermal sensitivity Pain on pressure	Clinical examination
Fractured tooth	Thermal sensitivity Pain on pressure	Occlusal examination Transillumination
Recently placed restoration	Thermal sensitivity Pain on pressure	Dental history Clinical examination Occlusal examination
Occlusal trauma	Chemical sensitivity Thermal sensitivity Pain on pressure Mobility	Occlusal examination
Pulpitis	Severe, intermittent, throbbing pain	Thermal and electric pulp tests Percussion
Sinus infection	"Nondescript" tooth pain Nasal congestion (drainage) Sinus pressure Headache	Clinical examination, including extraoral sinus palpation Radiographic examination
Galvanic pain	Sudden, sharp stabbing pain on tooth-to-tooth contact	Examination for contact between restoration of dissimilar nonprecious metals
Periodontal ligament inflammation	Pain on chewing Clinical examination, including palpation for apical tenderness	Percussion
Abfraction	"Cratered" areas of enamel or dentin at cementoenamel junction in the shape of a wedge or V-shaped notch	Clinical examination Occlusal examination

- The pain of hypersensitivity subsides when the stimulus is removed.
- It is difficult to distinguish between the pain of hypersensitivity and other causes of dental pain when both are in the mild-to-moderate range. Many types of dental pain can be intensified by thermal, sweet, and sour stimuli.
- Chewing pain (occlusal pressure) can be indicative of pulpal pathology.
- Pulpal pain is severe, intermittent, and throbbing. The pain results from deep dental caries, pulpal inflammation, vertical tooth fracture, or infection, and may occur without provocation and persist after stimulus is removed.

II. Data Collection by Interview

- Utilize direct, open-ended, and nonleading questions.
  - Establish the location, degree of pain, onset/duration, source of stimulus, intensity, and alleviating factors related to the painful

response; patients may have difficulty characterizing the pain.

- Ask trigger questions as suggested in **Box   1** to elicit detailed information to characterize the pain and assist in the dental hygiene diagnosis.
- Establish rapport, combined with effective listening and counseling skills, to develop collaborative treatment/management strategies.
- Record a thorough dental history, including pain chronology, nature, location, aggravating and alleviating factors, and history of dental treatment/restorations.

III. Diagnostic Techniques and Tests

When patients have difficulty describing and localizing their pain, the following diagnostic techniques and tests can aid in differentiating among the numerous causes of tooth pain.

- Visual assessment of tooth integrity and surrounding tissues.
- Palpation of extra and intraoral soft tissues.
- Evaluation of nasal congestion, drainage, or sinus expressed as tooth pain.
- Occlusal examination with use of marking paper to detect a premature contact or hyperfunction following placement of a new restoration.

- Radiographic assessment to determine signs of pulpal pathology, vertical tooth fracture, or other irregularities of the teeth or surrounding structures.
- Percussion with use of an instrument handle to lightly tap on each tooth. A pain response may indicate pulpitis.
- Mobility testing may detect trauma or periodontal pathology.
- Pain from biting pressure with use of a bite stick to assess pain indicative of tooth fracture.
- Transillumination with a high-intensity, focused light to enhance visualization of a cracked tooth; dye may also indicate a fracture line.
- Pulpal pathology assessment with thermal or electric pulp tests.

Hypersensitivity Management

When the differential diagnosis indicates dentinal hypersensitivity, the dental hygiene care plan includes further assessment and patient counseling combined with treatment interventions.

I. Assessment Components

- Determine extent and severity of pain.
  - Solicit a self-report of symptoms, including the eliciting stimuli.
  - Quantify and record the baseline pain intensity using objective measures such as the visual analog scale (VAS) and/or the verbal rating scale (VRS), as described in **Box   2**.
- Determine if oral self-care procedures contribute to loss of gingival attachment or tooth structure.
- Use a diet analysis to assess the frequency of acidic food and beverage intake; correlate intake with timing of toothbrushing.
- Explore parafunctional habits, such as bruxing, that may contribute to abfraction and attrition.

II. Educational Considerations

- Provide education regarding etiology and contributing factors. Explain the natural mechanisms for resolution of hypersensitivity over time.
- Discuss realistic oral self-care measures that the patient is likely to maintain and include technique demonstrations.
- Utilize effective communication and motivational interviewing skills to promote compliance and to decrease patient anxiety. (See Chapter 24.)

Name: _____
Date: _____
Teeth: _____

VAS—Visual Analog Scale
Please place an "X" on the line at a position between the two extremes to represent the level of pain that you experience.

No Discomfort		Severe Discomfort

Discomfort Scale

VRS—Verbal Rating Scale
0 = No discomfort/pain, but aware of stimulus
1 = Slight discomfort/pain
2 = Significant discomfort/pain
3 = Significant discomfort/pain that lasted more than 10 seconds

III. Treatment Hierarchy

- There are two basic treatment goals:
  - Pain relief.
  - Modification or elimination of contributing factors.
- Address mild-to-moderate pain with conservative approaches or agents; more severe pain may require an aggressive approach.
- Sequence treatment approaches from the most conservative and least invasive measures to more aggressive modalities.
- Prognosis of pain resolution is difficult to predict due to variable success with different treatment options among individuals.
  - Historically, a vast array of treatment approaches have been utilized with varying degrees of success; no one best method has been identified due to lack of quality **randomized controlled trial** (RCT) data, difficulties inherent in dentin hypersensitivity research design, and a significant placebo effect.
  - A trial-and-error approach may be necessary to determine the most effective treatment option.
  - Characteristics of an ideal desensitizing agent are listed in **Box   3** and can be useful evaluation criteria when selecting a desensitizing agent.
- Treatment options that include both oral self-care measures and professional interventions with the same objective of reducing hypersensitivity have a synergistic effect.

- Minimal application time.
- Easy application procedure.
- Does not endanger the soft tissues.
- Acceptable cost.
- Requires few dental appointments.
- Does not cause pulpal irritation or pain.
- Rapid and lasting effect.
- Causes no staining.
- Consistently effective.
- Acceptable taste.

IV. Reassessment

- Evaluate treatment interventions.
  - Allow sufficient time to elapse (2–4 weeks) to evaluate effectiveness of treatment recommendations; assess and reinforce behavioral changes.
  - Repeat the VAS and/or the VRS to compare changes in pain perceptions from baseline.
- If pain persists, a different option may provide relief.

Oral Hygiene Care and Treatment Interventions

I. Mechanisms of Desensitization

- Desensitization agents and oral self-care measures disrupt the pain transmission as described by the hydrodynamic theory in one of two ways[17]:
- Prevent nerve depolarization that interrupts the neural transmission to the pulp. This physiologic process is the mechanism of action for potassium-based products.[22]
- Prevent a stimulus from moving the tubule fluid by occlusion of dentin tubule orifices or reduction in tubule lumen diameter.

II. Behavioral Changes

- Encourage habits that allow tubules to remain occluded or that occlude **patent** tubules.
- Use a motivational interviewing approach to help the patient commit to appropriate oral self-care and dietary habits before or in conjunction with self-applied or professionally applied desensitizing agents. (Motivational interviewing is discussed in Chapter 24.)
- Educate the patient that some products may take 2–4 weeks to decrease sensitivity.

A. Dietary Modifications

- Have patient analyze acidic food and beverage habits that incite pain from dissolution of the smear layer, which covered open dentinal tubules.[23] Examples include citrus fruits and juices, acidic carbonated beverages, sharp flavors and spices, pickled foods, wines, and ciders.
- Counsel patient regarding change in dietary habits.
- Help patient determine if brushing is sequenced immediately after consuming acidic foods and beverages. Advise altering sequence to eliminate combined effects of erosion and abrasion, which can accelerate tooth structure loss.[24]
- Guide patient toward mouthrinses with a non-acidic formulation.
- Provide professional treatment referrals for patients with eating disorders such as bulimia or systemic conditions such as acid reflux that repeatedly create an acidic oral environment.
- The acidic environment created by bulimia and acid reflux can be neutralized by rinsing with water (particularly fluoridated water) or an alkaline rinse such as bicarbonate of soda in water.
- Counsel patient to eliminate or reduce extremes of hot and cold foods and beverages to avoid discomfort.

B. Dental Biofilm Control

- In the presence of dental biofilm, the dentinal tubule orifices increase to three times the original size; with reestablishment of biofilm control measures, there is a 20% decrease in size.[25]
- The presence/amount of dental biofilm on exposed root surfaces does not directly correlate with the degree of dentin sensitivity,[20] suggesting biofilm composition may be a factor.

C. Eliminate Parafunctional Habits

- Help patient evaluate bruxing and clenching behaviors and whether additional treatment is indicated.
- Determine need for occlusal adjustments to reduce destructive forces.
- Coach patient to monitor occurrence of subconscious parafunctional behaviors and levels of stress. Identify whether stress reduction protocols are needed.
- Introduce behavior modification techniques and refer when needed.

D. Toothbrush Type and Technique

- Brush one or two teeth at a time with a soft or ultrasoft toothbrush, rather than using long, horizontal strokes over several teeth to prevent further recession and loss of tooth structure.
- Identify brushing sequence and adjust by beginning in least sensitive areas and ending with more sensitive areas. In the initial phases of brushing, toothbrush filaments are stiffer and brushing is more aggressive.
- Help patient investigate current toothbrush grip. Adjust to a modified pen grasp rather than a traditional palm grasp to reduce the amount of pressure applied.
- Explore receptivity to use of a power toothbrush because it removes dental biofilm effectively with less than half the pressure of a manual toothbrush; an individual using a manual toothbrush typically exerts 200–400 g of pressure; 70–150 g of pressure is usually exerted with a power toothbrush.[26] Some power toothbrushes have a self-limiting mechanism to reduce filament action if too much pressure is applied.
- Recommend and demonstrate dental biofilm control measures that are meticulous, yet gentle, and do not contribute to further abrasion of hard or soft tissues.

III. Desensitizing Agents

- There are study design challenges when researching desensitization due to subjectivity of the pain response, the strong placebo effect, and the process of natural desensitization.
- Despite widespread professional recommendation and use, there is little in vivo scientific evidence validating the efficacy and mechanisms of action of desensitizing agents.
- RCTs are needed to support professional recommendation and treatment. The exception is fluoride, with a substantial body of knowledge validating its usefulness as a desensitizing agent.
- Desensitizing agents can be categorized according to their mechanisms of action, either depolarization of the nerve or occlusion of the dentinal tubule. Potassium salts are the only agents that are theorized to work by depolarization.

A. Potassium Salts

- Formulations containing potassium chloride, potassium nitrate, potassium citrate, or potassium oxalate reduce depolarization of the nerve cell membrane and transmission of the nerve impulse.[24]

- Potassium nitrate dentifrices containing fluoride are widely used[22] and readily available over the counter.

B. Fluorides

- Precipitate calcium fluoride (CaF_2) crystals within the dentinal tubule to decrease the lumen diameter.[24]
- Create a barrier by precipitating CaF_2 at the exposed dentin surface to block open dental tubules.[27]
  - Fluoride varnishes are Food and Drug Administration (FDA)-approved for tooth desensitization and a cavity liner, although they are frequently used "off-label" for dental caries prevention.
  - Fluoride gels and varnishes are most commonly used and are a successful treatment modalilty.[28,29]

C. Oxalates

- Block open dental tubules.[30]
- Oxalate salts such as potassium oxalate and ferric oxalate precipitate calcium oxalate crystals to decrease the lumen diameter.[30]

D. Glutaraldehyde

- Coagulates proteins and amino acids within the dentinal tubule to decrease the dentinal tubule lumen diameter.[30]
- Can be combined with hydroxyethylmethacrylate, a hydrophilic resin, which seals tubules.[30]
- Creates calcium crystals within the dentinal tubule to decrease the lumen diameter.[31]

E. Calcium Phosphate Technology

- Advocated for use as a caries control agent to reduce demineralization and increase remineralization by releasing calcium and phosphate ions into saliva for deposition of new tooth mineral (hydroxyapatite).[32]
  - Calcium phosphates can compromise the bioavailability of fluorides since calcium and fluoride react to form calcium fluoride.[33]
  - May be effective for patients with poor salivary flow and consequent deficient calcium phosphate levels.[34]
- Agents that support remineralization may lessen dentinal hypersensitivity by occluding dentinal tubule openings.

- Most studies in support of calcium phosphate technology are animal, in vitro, or in situ models designed to analyze remineralization rather than hypersensitivity.
  - One in vivo study found a reduction in bleaching-induced sensitivity at days 5 and 14 when amorphous calcium phosphate (ACP) was added to a bleaching gel.[35]
  - Additional research related to calcium phosphate technologies is needed.[36]
- ACP
  - Theorized to plug dentinal tubules with calcium and phosphate *precipitate*; promotes an ACP reservoir within the saliva.
  - Enhances fluoride delivery in calcium and phosphate-deficient saliva.[34]
  - May remineralize areas of acid erosion and abrasion and reduce hypersensitivity.[35]
- Calcium sodium phosphosilicate (CSP)
  - Contains sodium and silica in addition to calcium and phosphorus.
  - Delivered in solid bioactive glass particles that react in the presence of saliva and water to release calcium and phosphate ions and create a calcium phosphate layer that crystallizes to hydroxyapatite.
  - Reacts with saliva; sodium buffers the acid, and calcium and phosphate saturate saliva to fill demineralized areas with new hydroxyapatite.
  - Claims include remineralizing enamel and dentin, positive impact on acid erosion and abrasion, a bactericidal effect, and reduction in hypersensitivity.
  - RCT comparing a CSP and a potassium nitrate toothpaste found, using a VAS, that CSP paste was significantly better at reducing dentin hypersensitivity.[37]
- Casein phosphopeptide (CPP)–ACP
  - CPP is a milk-derived protein that stabilizes ACP and allows it to be released during acidic challenges.
  - Researchers are exploring benefits such as remineralization of acid erosion, caries inhibition, and reduction of dentinal hypersensitivity.
- Tricalcium phosphate (TCP)
  - Developed in an effort to create a calcium material that can coexist with fluoride to provide greater efficacy than fluoride alone.[34] Additional components are added to β-TCP to "functionalize" it. Increased remineralization has been demonstrated in vitro[38]; in vivo evidence is needed.

IV. Self-Applied Measures

A. Dentifrices

- In many OTC sensitivity-reducing dentifrices, 5% potassium nitrate, sodium fluoride, or stannous fluoride separately or in combination are the active desensitizing agents. Studies have suggested that some of the desensitizing effects of dentifrices may be due to the blocking action of the abrasive particles.[24]
- Tartar control dentifrices may contribute to increased tooth sensitivity for some individuals, although the mechanism is unclear.
- Dentifrices containing highly concentrated fluoride (5000 ppm fluoride) combined with an abrasive to facilitate extrinsic stain control are available by prescription. This formulation is also available with the addition of potassium nitrate.

B. Gels

- Gels containing 5000 ppm fluoride are a prescription product brushed on for generalized hypersensitivity or burnished into localized areas of sensitivity.
- Contain no abrasive agents for biofilm and stain control.
- Can be self-applied with custom or commercially available fluoride or whitening trays.

C. Mouthrinses

- Mouthrinse containing 0.63% stannous fluoride can be prescribed for daily use to treat hypersensitivity.
- Short-term use (2–4 weeks) will limit staining concerns.

V. Professionally Applied Measures

A. Tray-Delivered Fluoride Agents

- A tray delivery system can be used to apply a 2% neutral sodium fluoride solution.
- Select trays of adequate height and fill with sufficient fluoride agent to cover the cervical areas of each tooth.

B. Fluoride Varnish

- A 5% sodium fluoride varnish maintains prolonged contact with the tooth surface by serving as a reservoir to release fluoride ions in response to pH changes in saliva and biofilm.[39]
- Does not require a dry tooth surface, which is advantageous since drying the tooth can be a painful procedure for a patient with dentin hypersensitivity.
- Use a microbrush to apply the varnish to the exposed dentin surface.
- Instruct the patient to avoid oral hygiene self-care for several hours to allow the fluoride to stay in contact with the tooth surface for as long as possible, preferably overnight.

C. 5% Glutaraldehyde

- Use a microbrush to apply to the affected tooth surface.
- Prevent excess flow into soft tissues with cotton roll isolation since contact with soft tissues may cause gingival irritation.

D. Oxalates

- Oxalate preparations are applied (burnished) to a dried tooth surface.
- May provide immediate and short-term relief, rather than long-term relief.

E. Unfilled or Partially Filled Resins

- Used to cover patent dentinal tubules.
- Resins are applied following an acid etch step that may remove the smear layer and cause discomfort.
- The tooth surface must be dehydrated before resin application, which can create discomfort.
- Use of local anesthetic may facilitate patient comfort during this procedure.

F. Dentin-Bonding Agents

- Obturates the tubule opening and does not require use of acid etch or dehydration; a single application may protect against further erosion for 3–6 months.
- Methylmethacrylate polymer is a common dentin sealer.

G. Glass Ionomer Sealants/Restorative Materials

- Glass ionomer may be placed in the presence of moisture, which eliminates the need for drying the tooth.

- In addition to the glass ionomer restoration physically blocking the dentinal tubule, there is an added benefit of slow fluoride release.

H. Soft-Tissue Grafts

- Surgical placement of soft-tissue grafts to cover a sensitive dentinal surface.

I. Lasers

- Nd:YAG laser treatment can obliterate dentinal tubules through a process called "melting and resolidification." When used with an appropriate protocol, there is no resulting damage to the pulp or dentin surface cracking.[40,41]
- Low-level diode laser treatments have shown a reduction in dentinal hypersensitivity, but the exact mechanism of action is unclear.[42]
- Diode laser treatments combined with sodium fluoride varnish application have shown an immediate decrease in sensitivity.[43]
- A recent meta-analysis of laser use for dentinal hypersensitivity concluded that diode and YAG lasers both produced immediate and long-term desensitizing effects when compared to the control treatments.[44]
- Long term, in vivo studies are needed to establish safety and efficacy of laser treatment for dentin hypersensitivity. The FDA has not approved these devices for this therapeutic modality.

VI. Additional Considerations

A. Periodontal Debridement Considerations

- Preprocedure
  - Explain potential for sensitivity resulting from calculus removal and/or instrumentation of teeth with areas of exposed cementum or dentin.
  - Patients are likely to respond more favorably to treatment when prepared for what might occur.
  - When multiple teeth in the same treatment area are hypersensitive during scaling and root instrumentation procedures, local anesthetics and/or nitrous oxide analgesia can be utilized.
  - Desensitizing agents that are marketed for immediate relief from severe hypersensitivity can be used.

- Postprocedure
  - Professionally applied desensitization agents can be used.
  - Patient is instructed in daily oral self-care behavior changes and use of self-applied desensitizing agents.

B. Tooth Whitening-Induced Sensitivity

Tooth whitening agents, such as hydrogen peroxide and carbamide peroxide, may contribute to increased dentinal hypersensitivity.

- Thought to result from by-products of 10% carbamide peroxide (3% hydrogen peroxide and 7% urea) readily passing through the enamel and dentin into the pulp; the reversible pulpitis is caused from the dentin fluid flow and pulpal contact of the hydrogen peroxide without apparent harm to the pulp.[45]
- Hypersensitivity may dissipate over time, lasting from a few days to several months.
- Exposed dentin and preexisting dentin hypersensitivity increase hypersensitivity risk secondary to whitening.
- Some whitening products contain fluoride or potassium nitrate to eliminate or minimize the effects of sensitivity.
- Recommendations to prevent or reduce tooth whitening–induced sensitivity include[45]:
  - Use of a potassium nitrate, fluoride, or other desensitization product starting 2 weeks before or concurrently with whitening.
  - Some at-home whitening gels incorporate 5% potassium nitrate, fluoride, and ACP.
  - Home-use whitening products are usually less concentrated than professionally applied in-office treatment options, with less hypersensitivity risk.
  - Allow for a "recovery period" between whitening sessions during which desensitizing agents are used. Decrease frequency of use by whitening every second or third day. (See Chapter 43 for more information.)

C. Research Developments

- The search for the ideal desensitizing agent is ongoing.
- Evidence-based scientific research indicated as new products are developed; in vivo research protocols are needed to support clinical application.

Documentation

The permanent record for a patient with a history of tooth sensitivity needs to include at least the following information:

- Medical and dental history, vital signs, extra and intraoral examinations, consultations, and individual progress notes for each appointment and maintenance appointments.

- For dentin hypersensitivity: identify teeth involved (including measurements of recession, attached gingiva, abfractions, and attrition), differential diagnosis, and all treatments, along with patient instruction for ideal oral self-care, diet, and other for preventive recommendations.
- Outcomes and posttreatment directions.
- A progress note example for the patient with hypersensitive dentin may be reviewed in **Box   4**.

Factors to Teach the Patient

- Etiology and prevention of gingival recession.
- Factors contributing to dentin hypersensitivity.
- Mechanisms of dentin tubule exposure, which can allow various stimuli to trigger pain response.
- Natural desensitization mechanisms that may lessen sensitivity over time.
- Appropriate oral hygiene self-care techniques, such as using a soft toothbrush and avoiding a vigorous brushing technique that may exacerbate current gingival recession and subsequent abrasion of root surfaces.
- Connection between an acidic diet and dentin sensitivity; need to eliminate specific foods and beverages that can trigger sensitivity.
- Toothbrushing is not recommended immediately after consumption of acidic foods or beverages.
- Behavior modifications or treatments for eliminating parafunctional habits.
- The challenges of managing hypersensitivity, hierarchy of treatment measures, and variable effect of treatment options.

References

1. Addy M. Etiology and clinical implications of dentine hypersensitivity. *Dent Clin North Am*. 1990;34(3):503-514.
2. Absi EG, Addy M, Adams D. Dentine hypersensitivity: the development and evaluation of a replica technique to study sensitive and non-sensitive cervical dentine. *J Clin Periodontol*. 1989;16(3):190-195.
3. Frank RM. Attachment sites between the odontoblast process and the intradental nerve fibre. *Arch Oral Biol*. 1968;13(7): 833-834.
4. Thomas HF, Carella P. Correlation of scanning and transmission electron microscopy of human dentinal tubules. *Arch Oral Biol*. 1984;29(8):641-646.
5. Dufour LA, Bissell HS. Periodontal attachment loss induced by mechanical subgingival instrumentation in shallow sulci. *J Dent Hyg*. 2002;76(3):207-212.
6. Wiegand A, Burkhard JP, Eggmann F, Attin T. Brushing force of manual and sonic toothbrushes affects dental hard tissue abrasion. *Clin Oral Investig*. 2013;17(3):815-822.

7. Heasman PA, Holliday R, Bryant A, Preshaw PM. Evidence for the occurrence of gingival recession and non-carious cervical lesions as a consequence of traumatic toothbrushing. *J Clin Periodontol*. 2015;42(Suppl 16):S237-S255.

8. Absi EG, Addy M, Adams D. Dentine hypersensitivity: the effect of toothbrushing and dietary compounds on dentine in vitro. *J Oral Rehabil*. 1992;19(2):101-110.

9. Prati C, Montebugnoli L, Suppa P, Valdrè G, Mongiorgi R. Permeability and morphology of dentin after erosion induced by acidic drinks. *J Periodontol*. 2003;74(4):428-436.

10. Staninec M, Nalla RK, Hilton JF, et al. Dentin erosion simulation by cantilever beam fatigue and pH change. *J Dent Res*. 2005;84(4):371-375.

11. Litonjua LA, Andreana S, Bush OJ, et al. Wedged cervical lesions produced by toothbrushing. *Am J Dent*. 2004;17(4):237-240.

12. Estafan A, Furnari PC, Goldstein G, et al. In vivo correlation of noncarious cervical lesions and occlusal wear. *J Prosthet Dent*. 2005;93(3):221-226.

13. Sarode GS, Sarode CS. Abfraction: a review. *J Oral Maxillofac Pathol*. 2013;17(2):222-227.

14. Brännström M, Linden LA, Astrom A. The hydrodynamics of the dental tubule and of pulp fluid: a discussion of its significance in relation to dentinal sensitivity. *Caries Res*. 1967;1(4):310-317.

15. Eldarrat AH, High AS, Kale GM. In vitro analysis of "smear layer" on human dentine using ac-impedance spectroscopy. *J Dent*. 2004;32(7):547-554.

16. Splieth CH, Tachou A. Epidemiology of dentin hypersensitivity. *Clin Oral Invest*. 2013;17(suppl 1):S3-S8.

17. Shiau HJ. Dentin hypersensitivity. *J Evid Base Pract*. 2012;12(suppl 1):220-228.

18. Kim JW, Park JC. Dentin hypersensitivity and emerging concepts for treatments. *J Oral Bio*. 2017;59(4):211-217.

19. Mantzourani M, Sharma D. Dentine sensitivity: past, present, and future. *J Dent*. 2013;41(suppl 4):S3-S17.

20. Kassaba MM, Cohen RE. The etiology and prevalence of gingival recession. *J Am Dent Assoc*. 2003;134(2):220-225.

21. Gillam DG, Aris A, Bulman JS, et al. Dentine hypersensitivity in subjects recruited for clinical trials: clinical evaluation, prevalence and intraoral distribution. *J Oral Rehabil*. 2002;29(3):226-231.

22. Orchardson R, Gillam DG. The efficacy of potassium salts as agents for treating dentin hypersensitivity. *J Orofac Pain*. 2000;14(1):9-19.

23. Correa FO, Sampaio JE, Rossa C, et al. Influence of natural fruit juices in removing the smear layer from root surfaces—an in vitro study. *J Can Dent Assoc*. 2004;70(10):697-702.

24. Orchardson R, Gilla DC. Managing dentin hypersensitivity. *J Am Dent Assoc*. 2006;137(7):990-998.

25. Kawasaki A, Ishikawa K, Suge T, et al. Effects of plaque control on the patency and occlusion of dentine tubules in situ. *J Oral Rehabil*. 2001;28(5):439-449.

26. Van Der Weijden GA, Timmerman MF, Reijerse E, et al. Toothbrushing force in relation to plaque removal. *J Clin Periodontol*. 1996;23(8):724-729.

27. Suge T, Ishikowa K, Kawasaki A, et al. Effects of fluoride on the calcium phosphate precipitation method for dentinal tubule occlusion. *J Dent Res*. 1995;74(4):1079-1085.

28. Ritter AV, de L Dias W, Miguez P, et al. Treating cervical dentin hypersensitivity with fluoride varnish: a randomized clinical study. *J Am Dent Assoc*. 2006;137(7):1013-1020.

29. Cunha-Cruz J, Wataha JC, Zhou L, et al. Treating dentin hypersensitivity, therapeutic choices made by dentists of the Northwest PRECEDENT network. *J Am Dent Assoc*. 2010;141(9):1097-1105.

30. Haywood VB. Dentine hypersensitivity: bleaching and restorative considerations for successful management. *Int Dent J*. 2002;52(suppl 1):376.

31. Pashley DH, Kalathoor S, Burnham D. The effects of calcium hydroxide on dentin permeability. *J Dent Res*. 1986;65(3):417-420.

32. Featherstone JD. The continuum of dental caries-evidence for a dynamic disease process. *J Dent Res*. 2004;83(Spec No C):C39-C42.

33. Karlinsey RL, Mackey AC, Walker ER, et al. Surfactant-modified B-TCP: structure, properties, and in vitro remineralization of subsurface enamel lesions. *J Mater Sci Mater Med*. 2010;21(4):2009-2020.

34. Chow L, Wefel JS. The dynamics of de- and remineralization. *Dimensions Dent Hyg*. 2009;7(2):42-46.

35. Giniger M, MacDonald J, Ziemba S, et al. The clinical performance of professionally dispensed bleaching gel with added amorphous calcium phosphate. *J Am Dent Assoc*. 2005;136(3):383-392.

36. Yengopal V, Mickenautsch S. Caries-preventive effect of casein phosphopeptide-amorphous calcium phosphate (CPP-ACP): a meta-analysis. *Acta Odontol Scand*. 2009;21:1-12.

37. Pradeep AR, Sharma A. Comparison of clinical efficacy of a dentifrice containing calcium sodium phosphosilicate to a dentifrice containing potassium nitrate and to a placebo on dentinal hypersensitivity: a randomized clinical trial. *J Periodontol*. 2010;81(8):1167-1173.

38. Karlinsey RL, Mackey AC, Walker ER, et al. Preparation, characterization and in vitro efficacy of an acid-modified β-TCP material for dental hard-tissue remineralization. *Acta Biomater*. 2010;6(3):969-978.

39. Shen C, Autio-Gold J. Assessing fluoride concentration uniformity and fluoride release from 3 varnishes. *J Am Dent Assoc*. 2002;133(2):176-182.

40. Kara C, Orbak R. Comparative evaluation of Nd:YAG laser and fluoride varnish for the treatment of dentinal hypersensitivity. *J Endod*. 2009;35(7):971-974.

41. Lopes AO, Aranha ACC. Comparative evaluation of the effects of Nd:YAG laser and a desensitizer agent on the treatment of dentin hypersensitivity: a clinical study. *Photomed Laser Surg*. 2013;31(3):132-138.

42. Yilmaz H, Kurtulmus-Yilmaz S, Cengiz E. Long-term effect of diode laser irradiation compared to sodium fluoride varnish in the treatment of dentine hypersensitivity in periodontal maintenance patients: a randomized controlled clinical study. *Photomed Laser Surg*. 2011;29(11):721-725.

43. Corona S, Nascimento T, Catirse A, Lizarelli R, Dinelli W, Palma-Dibb R. Clinical evaluation of low-level laser therapy and fluoride varnish for treating cervical dentinal hypersensitivity. *J Oral Rehabil*. 2003;30(12):1183-1189.

44. Hu ML, Zheng G, Han JM, Yang M, Zhang YD, Lin H. Effect of lasers on dentine hypersensitivity: evidence from a meta-analysis. *J Evid Based Dent Pract*. 2019;19(2):115-130.

45. Haywood VB, Sword RJ. Tray bleaching status and insights. *J Esthet Restor Dent*. 2021;33(1):27-38.

169

Extrinsic Stain Removal

Heather Doucette, DipDH, BSc, MEd
Linda D. Boyd, RDH, RD, EdD

CHAPTER OUTLINE

LEARNING OBJECTIVES

After studying this chapter, the student will be able to:

1. Describe the difference between a cleaning agent and a polishing agent.
2. Explain the basis for selection of the grit of polishing paste for each individual patient.

3. Discuss the rationale for avoiding polishing procedures on areas of demineralization.
4. Explain the effect abrasive particle shape, size, and hardness have on the abrasive qualities of a polishing paste.
5. Explain the types of powdered polishing agents available and their use in the removal of tooth stains.
6. Explain patient conditions that contraindicate the use of air-powder polishing.

Introduction

After treatment by scaling, root debridement, and other dental hygiene care, the teeth are assessed for the presence of remaining dental stains.

- The cleaning or **polishing agents** used must be selected based on the patient's individual needs such as the type, location, and amount of stain present.
- Preliminary examination of each tooth will reveal the surfaces to be treated, which may be tooth structure (enamel, or in the case of recession, cementum, or dentin) or when restored, a variety of dental materials (metal or esthetic, tooth-color restorations).
- Preservation of the surfaces of both the teeth and the restorations is of primary importance during all cleaning and **polishing** procedures.
- Stain removal requires the use of polishing agents with various **abrasive** grits. The smallest, least abrasive **grit** is used.
- Some patients will not consider their teeth "cleaned" unless they have been polished. For this situation when no extrinsic stain is present, use a **cleaning agent** to avoid abrasion of the dental hard tissues and remove dental biofilm.
- Incorrect selection of a prophylaxis paste can worsen hypersensitivity.
- The longevity, esthetic appearance, and smooth surfaces of dental restorations depend on appropriate care by the dental hygienist and the daily oral self-care by the patient.

Purposes for Stain Removal

Stains on the teeth are not etiologic factors for oral disease.

- The removal of stains is for esthetic, not for therapeutic or health, reasons.
- The American Dental Hygienists' Association and the Academy of Periodontology include tooth polishing in their definitions of the term "oral prophylaxis."[1,2]

Science of Polishing

- Polishing is intended to produce intentional, selective and controlled wear. Within the science of **tribology**, polishing is considered to be **two-body abrasion** or **three-body abrasion**.[3]
  - Two-body abrasive polishing involves the abrasive particles attached to a medium, such as a rubber cup impregnated with abrasive particles and does not require a polishing paste.
  - Three-body abrasive polishing is the type most commonly used by dental hygienists, in which loose abrasive particles (like those in prophy polishing paste) form a slurry between the tooth surface and the polishing application device (rubber cup or brush).[3]

Effects of Cleaning and Polishing

Attention must be given to the positive and negative effects of polishing so evidence-based decisions can be made for the treatment of each patient.

I. Precautions

- As with all gingival manipulation, including oral self-care with a toothbrush,[4] bacteremia can be created during the use of power-driven stain removal instruments.
- A thorough medical history is essential before all treatment and must be reviewed and updated at each succeeding appointment.
- Patients at risk due to existing medical conditions may require antibiotic prophylaxis as specified by the patient's medical provider. (See Chapter 11.)

II. Environmental Factors

A. Aerosol Production

- Aerosols, droplets, and spatter are created during the use of some dental instruments, including a slow-speed handpiece with a rubber cup to hold polishing paste, the air-water syringe, and air polishing.[5]

- Polishing with a slow-speed handpiece is considered moderate risk for contamination while air polishing and use of an air-water syringe is high risk.[5]
- The biologic contaminants of aerosols can stay suspended for long periods and contaminate surfaces, particularly the clinician's torso and arm, and the patient's body.[5]
  - These aerosols may provide a means for possible disease transmission to dental personnel, as well as to other patients, but further research is needed.[5]
- Use of aerosol-generating procedures (AGPs) must be avoided if possible when a patient is known to have an infectious disease.[6]
  - AGPs may need to be avoided or limited for those with a chronic respiratory disease or who are immunocompromised.
- Centers for Disease Control and Prevention (CDC), Occupational Safety and Health Administration (OSHA), and local guidelines should be followed during all dental care, including AGPs. (See Chapter 6 and 7.)

B. Spatter

- Serious eye damage and infection have occurred because of spatter from polishing paste or from other dental instruments.[7]

III. Effect on Teeth

A. Removal of Tooth Structure

- The fluoride-rich outer surface of the enamel is necessary for protection against dental caries and care must be taken to preserve it.
- Excessive abrasion from coarse polishing paste results in a surface with more scratches prone to extrinsic stain reformation and retention of plaque biofilm.[8]
- The least abrasive prophylaxis paste or cleaning agents should be used to minimize removal of tooth surface.[8]

B. Areas of Demineralization

- Demineralization: Polishing demineralized white spots of enamel is contraindicated. More surface enamel is lost from abrasive polishing over demineralized white spots than over intact enamel.[8]
- Remineralization: Demineralized areas of enamel can remineralize with exposure to fluoride from saliva, water, dentifrices, and professional fluoride

applications along with remineralization agents (e.g., CPP-ACP [casein phosphopeptide-amorphous calcium phosphate]).[9] Polishing procedures can interrupt enamel surface remineralization.

C. Areas of Thin Enamel, Cementum, or Dentin

- Areas of thin enamel are contraindicated for polishing and include:
  - Enamel hypoplasia.
  - Hypomineralization.
  - Amelogenesis imperfecta. (See Chapter 16.)
- Exposed dentin and cementum
  - Exposure of dentinal tubules: Cementum and dentin are softer and more porous than enamel, so greater amounts of their surfaces can be removed during polishing than from enamel.[10] Polishing of exposed cementum and dentin is contraindicated.
  - Abrasion of the dentin may result in dentin hypersensitivity.[11]

D. Care of Restorations and Implants

- Use of coarse abrasives may create deep, irregular scratches in restorative materials. **Figure 1** shows a scanning electron photomicrograph of the damaged surface of a composite restoration polished with a rubber cup and coarse prophylaxis paste.
- Select a cleaning agent or a polishing agent recommended by the manufacturer of the restorative materials.[12-14]

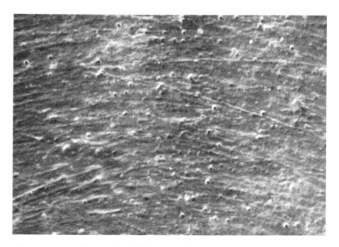

Figure 1 Scanning Electron Photomicrograph of a Composite Restoration Polished with Coarse Prophylaxis Paste

E. Heat Production

- Steady pressure with a rapidly revolving rubber cup or bristle brush and a minimum of wet abrasive agent can create sufficient heat to cause pain and discomfort for the patient.
- The pulp chamber in the teeth of children is large and may be more susceptible to heat.
- The rules for the use of cleaning or polishing agents include[8]:
  - Use light pressure (20 psi) at a slow, steady speed (2500–3000 rpm) of the rubber cup.
  - Use a moist cleaning or polishing agent; never use a dry powder due to the heat created.
  - Use a light patting motion and polish the tooth surface for 2–5 seconds.

IV. Effect on Gingiva

- Trauma to the gingival tissue can result, especially when the prophylaxis angle is operated at a high speed with heavy pressure and the rubber cup is applied for an extended period of time adjacent to gingival tissues.
- It may be best to delay stain removal after nonsurgical periodontal treatment (NSPT) to allow for healing of the sulcular tissue. If selective polishing is required, it can be done at the re-evaluation appointment following initial NSPT therapy.

Indications for Stain Removal

I. Removal of Extrinsic Stains

A. Patient Instruction

- Extrinsic stains often attach to the salivary pellicle and plaque biofilm layer of the tooth, so educating the patient on thorough dental biofilm removal is essential.[15]
- Patients who use tobacco should be counseled about cessation to reduce this cause of external stain. Tobacco cessation is described in Chapter 32.
- Components of the diet may also be a source for external stains, such as drinking tea, coffee, or red wine, so educate the patient about possible adjustments in intake to reduce stain.

B. Scaling and Root Debridement

- In addition to the use of cleaning or polishing agents during polishing procedures, stains can also be removed during scaling and root instrumentation.

- Example: Black line stain has been compared to calculus because it may be elevated from the tooth surface and may need to be removed by instrumentation.[16] (See Chapter 17.)

II. To Prepare the Teeth for Caries-Preventive Procedures

A. Placement of Pit and Fissure Sealant

- Follow manufacturer's directions. Sealants vary in their requirements.
- Avoid commercial oral prophylaxis pastes containing **glycerin**, oils, flavoring substances, or other agents. Glycerin and oils can prevent an optimum acid-etch and interfere with the adherence of the sealant to the tooth surface, causing the sealant to fail.
  - **Air-powder polishing** is one method of choice for preparing tooth surfaces for sealants; however, care must be taken to manage aerosols.[17,18] (See Chapter 35.)
  - An alternative is the use of a plain, fine pumice mixed with water when precleaning is necessary.
- If pumice is used, the tooth surface(s) needs to be rinsed thoroughly to remove the particles.

III. To Contribute to Patient Motivation

- Smooth, polished tooth surfaces may be easier to achieve once the patient has a biofilm and debris-free mouth and may contribute to patient motivation.

Clinical Application of Stain Removal

The decision to polish teeth is based on the individual patient's needs.

I. Summary of Contraindications for Polishing

The following list suggests some of the specific instances in which polishing either can be performed with a cleaning agent or is contraindicated.

A. No Visible Stain Extrinsic Stain

- If no stain is present, polishing with an abrasive polishing agent is not indicated.

B. Patients with Respiratory Problems

- Care must be taken to minimize the aerosols from the air–water syringe when rinsing in general,[5] but specifically for conditions at higher risk for infectious disease such as asthma, emphysema, cystic fibrosis, lung cancer, or patients requiring oxygen.
- This caution also applies to the use of air-powder polishers and spatter from prophylaxis polishing pastes.[5]

C. Tooth Sensitivity

- Abrasive agents can expose dentinal tubules in areas of thin cementum or dentin.
- The polishing of dentin and cementum is contraindicated.

D. Restorations

- Restorations and titanium implants may be scratched by abrasive prophylaxis polishing pastes.
- Tooth-colored restorations need to be polished with a cleaning agent, polishing paste specifically formulated for use on esthetic restorations, or the paste recommended by the manufacturer of the restorative material.[12-14]

II. Suggestions for Clinic Procedure

A. Provide Initial Education

- Daily dental biofilm removal to assist in dental stain control.
- Educate the patient that drinking coffee, tea, or red wine; tobacco; and/or marijuana is responsible for most dental stains.
- Provide patients with information about the types of dentifrices that are safe for stain control and those contraindicated due to excessive abrasiveness or chemical harshness.
- Initiate tobacco cessation when stain is primarily from tobacco use. (See Chapter 32.)

B. Remove Stain by Scaling

- Whenever possible, stains can be removed during scaling and root debridement.

C. Stain Removal Techniques

- Moist cleaning agent or low-abrasive prophylaxis paste.

- Slow-speed handpiece.
- Use the lightest pressure necessary for stain removal.
- Minimal heat production.
- Soft rubber cup at 90° to tooth surface with intermittent light applications.

Cleaning and Polishing Agents

There are two distinct types of agents used for "polishing" teeth: one is a cleaning agent, and the other is a polishing agent.

I. Cleaning Agents

- Unlike polishing agents, cleaning agents are round, flat, nonabrasive particles and do not scratch surface material but produce a higher luster than polishing agents.
  - Feldspar, sodium–aluminum silicate cleaning agent is a powder and can be mixed with water to make a paste for cleaning.

II. Polishing Agents

- Traditionally, abrasive agents have been applied with polishing instruments to remove extrinsic dental stains and leave the enamel surface smooth and shiny.
- Polishing agents act by producing scratches in the surface of the tooth or restoration created by the friction between the abrasive particle and the softer tooth or restorative surface.
- The cleaning and polishing process progresses from coarse abrasion to fine abrasion until the scratches are smaller than the wavelength of visible light, which is 0.05 μm.[8]
- When scratches of this size are created, the surface appears smooth and shiny—the smaller the scratches, the shinier the surface.
- For esthetic restorative surfaces, follow manufacturer instructions to choose the correct polishing agent.[12–14]

III. Factors Affecting Abrasive Action with Polishing Agents

During polishing, sharp edges of abrasive particles are moved along the surface of a material, abrading it by producing microscopic scratches or grooves. The rate of abrasion, or speed with which structural material is removed from the surface being polished, is governed by hardness and shape of the abrasive particles, as well as by the manner in which they are applied.

175

A. Characteristics of Abrasive Particles

- Shape: Irregularly shaped particles with sharp edges produce deeper grooves and thus abrade faster than do rounded particles with dull edges.
- Hardness: Particles must be harder than the surface to be abraded; harder particles abrade faster.
  - Many of the abrasives used in prophylaxis polishing pastes are 10 times harder than the tooth structure to which they are applied.[8]
  - **Table** 1 provides a comparison of the Mohs hardness value of dental tissues compared to agents commonly used in prophylaxis polishing pastes and substances used in cleaning agents.

Table 1 **Mohs Hardness Value of Dental Tissues Compared to Commonly Used Polishing Abrasive Particles**

	MOHS Hardness Value
Dental Tissues	
Enamel	5
Dentin	3.0–4.0
Cementum	2.5–3.0
Abrasive Agents in Polishing Pastes	
Zirconium silicate	7.5–8.0
Pumice	6.0–7.0
Silicone carbine	9.5
Boron	9.3
Aluminum oxide	9
Garnet	8.0–9.0
Emery	7.0–9.0
Zirconium oxide	7
Perlite	5.5
Calcium carbonate	3
Aluminum silicates	2
Sodium	0.5
Potassium	0.4

The Mohs hardness value of enamel, cementum, and dentin compared to the Mohs hardness value of abrasive materials commonly used in prophylaxis polishing pastes. The Mohs hardness value is indicative of a material's resistance to scratching. Diamonds have a maximum Mohs value of 10; talc has a minimum of Mohs hardness of 1.

- Body strength: Particles that fracture into smaller sharp-edged particles during use are more abrasive than those that wear down during use and become dull.
- Particle size (grit)
  - The larger the particles, the more abrasive they are and the less polishing ability they have.
  - Smaller (finer) abrasive particles achieve a glossier finish.
  - Abrasive and polishing agents are graded from coarse to fine based on the size of the holes in a standard sieve through which the particles will pass.[15]

B. Principles for Application of Abrasives

- Quantity applied: The more particles applied per unit of time, the faster the rate of abrasion.
  - Particles are suspended in water or other liquid to reduce heat produced by friction.
  - Frictional heat produced is proportional to the rate of abrasion; therefore, the use of *dry agents* is *contraindicated* for polishing natural teeth because of the potential danger of thermal injury to the dental pulp.
- Speed of application: The greater the speed of application, the faster the rate of abrasion.
  - With increased speed of application, pressure must be reduced.
  - Rapid abrasion also increases frictional heat.
- Pressure of application: The heavier the pressure applied, the faster the rate of abrasion.
  - Heavy pressure *is* contraindicated because it increases frictional heat.

IV. Abrasive Agents

The abrasives listed here are examples of commonly used agents. Some are available in several grades, and the specific use varies with the grade.

- For example, while a superfine grade might be used for polishing enamel surfaces and metallic restorations, a coarser grade would be used only for laboratory purposes.
- Abrasives for use daily in a dentifrice are a finer grade than those used for professional polishing.

A. Silex (Silicon Dioxide)

- XXX Silex: fairly abrasive.
- Superfine Silex: can be used for heavy stain removal from enamel.

B. Pumice

- Powdered pumice is of volcanic origin and consists chiefly of complex silicates of aluminum, potassium, and sodium.
- Pumice is the primary ingredient in commercially prepared prophylaxis pastes. The specifications for particle size are as follows:
  - Pumice flour or superfine pumice: least abrasive and can be used on enamel, dental amalgams, and acrylic resins.[8]
  - Fine pumice: mildly abrasive.
  - Coarse pumice: not for use on natural teeth.

C. Calcium Carbonate (Whiting, Calcite, Chalk)

- Less abrasive than pumice.[8]
- Various grades are used for different polishing techniques.

D. Tin Oxide (Putty Powder, Stannic Oxide)

- Polishing agent for teeth and metallic restorations.

E. Emery (Corundum)

Not used directly on the enamel.

- Aluminum oxide (alumina): the pure form of emery. Used for composite restorations and margins of porcelain restorations.
- Levigated alumina: consists of extremely fine particles of aluminum oxide, which may be used for polishing metals but are destructive to tooth surfaces.

F. Rouge (Jeweler's Rouge)

- Iron oxide is a fine red powder sometimes impregnated on paper discs.
- It is useful for polishing gold and precious metal alloys in the laboratory.

G. Diamond Particles

- Constituent of diamond polishing paste for porcelain surfaces.

V. Cleaning Ingredients

- Particles for cleaning agents differ from abrasive agents in shape and hardness.
- Particles used for cleaning agents include feldspar, alkali, and aluminum silicate.

A. Clinical Applications

Numerous commercial preparations for dental prophylactic cleaning and polishing preparations are available. Clinicians need more than one type available to meet the requirements of individual restorative materials.

B. Packaging

- Commercial preparations are in the form of pastes or powders.
- Some are available in measured amounts contained in individual plastic containers for one-time use to prevent cross contamination.
- Selection of a preparation is based on qualities of abrasiveness, consistency, and/or flavor for patient preference.

C. Enhanced Prophylaxis Polishing Pastes

Additives are included in prophylaxis polishing pastes to provide a specific function, such as enhancing the mineral surface of enamel, diminishing dentin hypersensitivity, or tooth whitening.

- Fluoride prophylaxis pastes
  - Application of fluoride by use of fluoride-containing prophylaxis polishing pastes cannot be considered a substitute for a professionally applied topical fluoride treatment.
  - Enamel surface: The greatest benefit of fluoride as a prophylaxis polishing paste additive occurs when the fluoride ions in the prophylaxis paste are released into the saliva.
    - The fluoride ions that become mixed in the saliva may become incorporated into the hydroxyapatite structure of the tooth, thus aiding in the remineralization of the tooth and improving enamel hardness.[19]
  - Clinical application: Use only an amount sufficient to accomplish stain removal to prevent excessive fluoride intake in a child. The paste may contain 4000–20,000 ppm fluoride ion.[20]
- Amorphous calcium phosphate and other forms of calcium and phosphate
  - Amorphous calcium phosphate and other formulations of calcium and phosphate, as additives to prophylaxis polishing pastes, have been shown to hydrolyze the tooth mineral to form apatite.[21]
  - When prophylaxis polishing pastes containing calcium and phosphate become mixed with saliva, the mineral ions may become incorporated into the hydroxyapatite structure

of the tooth, thus aiding in remineralization the enamel.[21-23]

- Fluoride, calcium, and phosphate
  - Fluoride, calcium, and phosphate prophylaxis pastes have the potential to have all three minerals incorporated into the hydroxyapatite structure of the tooth, thus aiding in remineralization to improve enamel hardness.
- Dentin hypersensitivity
  - The purpose of prophylaxis polishing pastes containing arginine, calcium, and bicarbonate/carbonate is to minimize dentin hypersensitivity.[22,23] Mixing these ingredients produces arginine bicarbonate and calcium carbonate. When applied with a rubber cup, these adjunctive ingredients can aid in temporarily occluding the dentinal tubules.

Procedures for Stain Removal (Coronal Polishing)

I. Patient Preparation for Stain Removal

A. Instruction and Clinical Procedures

- Review medical history to determine premedication requirements.
- Review intraoral charting and radiographs to locate all restorations.
- Provide education and hands-on practice with biofilm control techniques.
- Complete scaling, root debridement, and overhang removal.
- After scaling and other periodontal treatment, an evaluation is made to determine the need for **coronal polishing** for stain removal, polishing restorations, and dental prostheses.
- Inform the patient that polishing is a cosmetic procedure, not a therapeutic one.
- Explain the difference between cleaning and polishing agents.
- Check all restorations to ensure that the correct polishing agent has been selected.

B. Explain the Procedure

- Describe the noise, vibration, and grit of the polishing paste.
- Explain the frequent use of rinsing and evacuation with the saliva ejector.

C. Provide Protection for Patient

- Safety glasses worn for scaling should be kept in place to prevent eye injury or infection from the prophylaxis paste.
- Fluid-resistant bib over patient to keep moisture from skin and clothing.

D. Patient Position

- The patient is positioned for maximum visibility.

E. Patient Breathing

- Encourage the patient to breathe only through the nose.
- Less fogging of mouth mirror.
- Enhanced patient comfort.

II. Environmental Preparation

Environmental factors are described in Chapter 7.

A. Procedures to Lessen Aerosols Created

- Flush water through the tubing for 2 minutes at the beginning of each work period and for 30 seconds after each appointment.
- Request the patient rinse with an antimicrobial mouthrinse to reduce the numbers of oral microorganisms before starting instrumentation.[24]
- Use high-velocity evacuation to minimize droplet spatter and aerosols.[24]

B. Protective Barriers

- Protective eyewear and bib are necessary for the patient.
- The clinician should wear the appropriate personal protective equipment (PPE) per current OSHA and CDC guidelines.[24] (See Chapter 6.)

The Power-Driven Instruments

I. Handpiece

- A handpiece is used to hold rotary instruments.
- The three basic designs are straight, contra-angle, and right-angle.
- Instruments have been classified according to their rotational speeds, designated by revolutions per minute (rpm) as high speed and low (or slow) speed.
- Handpiece must be maintained and sterilized according to manufacturer's directions.

Table 2 Comparison of Disposable Prophylaxis Angles and Stainless-Steel Prophylaxis Angles

	Disposable Prophylaxis Angle	Disposable Angle with Abrasive-Impregnated Rubber Cup	Stainless Steel Prophylaxis Angle
Maintenance and care	One-time use, discard	One-time use, discard	Requires maintenance, sterilization
Attachments	Supplied with rubber cup from the manufacturer	Supplied with rubber cup from the manufacturer that is impregnated with one type of abrasive	Accepts variety of attachments: cups, brushes, and cone-shaped rubber points
Screw-in or snap-on rubber cups	Usually screw-in type cup		Will accept screw-in or snap-on cups and brushes
Advantages	Requires no maintenance or sterilization	Requires no additional prophylaxis paste	Can be used hundreds of times if maintained properly
Disadvantages	Not packaged with other attachments Creates refuse that is not biodegradable	Must have water and/or saliva as lubricant Creates refuse that is not biodegradable	Requires time to clean and maintain

A. Slow or Low Speed

- Low-speed handpieces are used for cleaning or polishing the teeth with a prophylaxis angle and rubber cup.
- *Speed*: Typical range is up to 5000 rpm for low-speed handpieces manufactured for dental hygienists. Other low-speed handpieces may have a higher range of rpms; air-driven.

II. Types of Prophylaxis Angles

- Types of prophylaxis angles are described in **Table 2**.
- Contra- or right-angle attachments to the handpiece for which polishing devices (rubber cup, bristle brush) are available. Contra-angle prophylaxis angles may have a longer shank and a wider angle between the rubber cup and shank to allow for greater reach when polishing posterior teeth and surfaces.
- Stainless steel with hard chrome, carbon, steel, or brass bearings.
- **Figure 2** shows examples of one-time use disposable contra-angle and right-angle prophylaxis angles and a stainless-steel prophylaxis angle.
- Stainless steel prophylaxis angles are sealed to prevent contamination, but there tends to be some leakage, so they need to be sterilized after each use following the manufacturer's instructions for maintenance.[25]
- Unless disposable, only instruments that can be sterilized should be used.

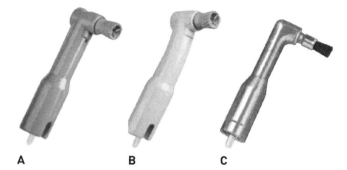

A   B   C

Figure 2 Prophylaxis Angles. **A:** Disposable right-angled prophylaxis angle with rubber cup attached. **B:** Disposable contra-angled prophylaxis angle with an attached rubber cup impregnated with a polishing agent (abrasive particles). **C:** Sterilizable stainless steel prophylaxis angle holding a cleaning or polishing brush on a mandrel.

III. Prophylaxis Angle Attachments

A. Rubber Polishing Cups

- Types: **Figure 3** shows several types of rubber polishing cups from which to choose. The internal designs and sizes have the same purpose, which is to aid in holding the prophylaxis polishing paste in the rubber cup while polishing. The ideal rubber cup design retains the prophylaxis polishing paste in the cup and releases the paste at a steady rate.
  - Slip-on (snap-on): with ribbed cup to aid in holding polishing agent.

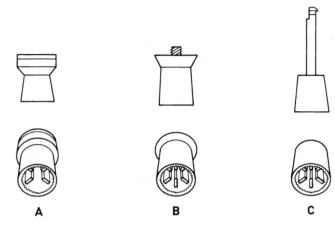

Figure 3 Rubber Cup Attachments. **A:** Slip-on or snap-on for button-ended prophylaxis angle. **B:** Threaded for direct insertion in right-angle. **C:** Mandrel stem for latch-type prophylaxis angle.

- Threaded (screw type): with plain ribbed cup or flange (webbed) type.
  - Mandrel mounted.
- Materials
  - Natural rubber: more resilient; adapts readily to fit the contours of the teeth.
  - Synthetic (non-latex): stiffer than natural rubber.
- Use: removal of stains from the tooth surfaces and polishing restorations.

B. Bristle Brushes

- Types
  - For prophylaxis angle: slip-on or screw type.
  - For handpiece: mandrel mounted.
- Materials: synthetic.
- Use:
  - Stain removal from deep pits and fissures and enamel surfaces away from the gingival margin.
  - A brush is contraindicated for use on exposed cementum or dentin.

C. Rubber Polishing Points

- **Figure** 4 shows an example of a rubber point that screws into a prophylaxis angle.
- Material
  - Natural rubber: flexible so that tip adapts to a variety of surfaces.
- Use
  - Stain removal and biofilm from proximal surfaces, embrasures, and around orthodontic bands and brackets.

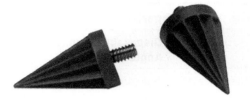

Figure 4 Flexible Rubber Point Has Screw Connection for a Prophylaxis Angle. Made with ribs or grooves to carry cleaning or polishing agent to difficult-to-reach areas.

IV. Uses for Attachments

A. Handpiece with Straight Mandrel

- Dixon bristle brush (type C, soft) for polishing removable dentures.
- Rubber cup on mandrel for polishing facial surfaces of anterior teeth.

Use of the Prophylaxis Angle

I. Effects on Tissues: Clinical Considerations

- Can cause discomfort for the patient if care and consideration for the oral tissues are not exercised to prevent unnecessary trauma.
- Tactile sensitivity of the clinician while using a thick, bulky handpiece is diminished and unnecessary pressure may be applied inadvertently.
- The greater the speed of application of a polishing agent, the faster the rate of abrasion. Therefore, the handpiece is applied at a low rpm.
- Trauma to the gingival tissue can result from too high a speed, extended application of the rubber cup, or use of an abrasive polishing agent.

II. Prophylaxis Angle Procedure

- Apply the polishing agent only where it is needed. See section *Contraindications*.

A. Instrument Grasp

- Modified pen grasp. (See Chapter 37.)

B. Finger Rest

- Establish a fulcrum firmly on tooth structure or use an exterior rest.
- Use a wide rest area when practical to aid in the balance of the large instrument. For example,

place pad of rest finger across the occlusal surfaces of premolars while polishing the molars.

- Avoid use of mobile teeth as finger rests.

C. Speed of Handpiece

- Use low speed to minimize frictional heat.
- Adjust rpm as necessary.

D. Use of Rheostat

- Apply steady pressure with foot to produce an even, low speed.

E. Rubber Cup: Stroke and Procedure

- Observe where stain removal is needed to prevent unnecessary rubber cup application.
- Fill rubber cup with polishing agent and distribute agent over tooth surfaces to be polished before activating the power.
- Establish finger rest and bring rubber cup almost in contact with tooth surface before activating power source.
- Using slowest rpm, apply revolving cup at a 90° angle lightly to tooth surfaces for 2 to 5 seconds. Use a light pressure so that the edges of the rubber cup flare slightly. The rubber cup needs to flare slightly underneath the gingival margin and onto the proximal surfaces.
- Move cup to adjacent area on tooth surface; use a patting or brushing motion.
- Replenish supply of polishing agent frequently.
- Turn handpiece to adapt rubber cup to fit each surface of the tooth, including proximal surfaces and gingival surfaces of fixed partial dentures.
- Start with the distal surface of the most posterior tooth of a quadrant and move forward toward the anterior; polish only the teeth that require stain removal. For each tooth, work from the gingival third toward the incisal third of the tooth.
- When two polishing agents of different abrasiveness are to be applied, use a separate rubber cup for each.
- Rubber cups, polishing points, and polishing brushes cannot be sterilized and are used only for one patient and then discarded.

F. Rubber Polishing Points

- Rubber polishing points can be used around orthodontic bands and brackets, on fixed bridges, and in wide interproximal spaces or embrasures.
- Rubber points are loaded with the cleaning or polishing agent in the grooves around the sides. The rubber points will need to be replenished frequently with paste after use on every one to two teeth.

G. Bristle Brush

- Bristle brushes are used selectively and limited to occlusal surfaces.
- Lacerations of the gingiva and grooves and scratches in the tooth surface, particularly the roots and restorations, can result when the brush is not used with caution.
- Soak stiff brush in hot water to soften bristles.
- Distribute mild abrasive polishing agent over occlusal surfaces of teeth to be polished.
- Place fingers of nondominant hand in a position to retract and protect cheek and tongue from the revolving brush.
- Establish a firm finger rest and bring brush almost in contact with the tooth before activating power source.
- Use slowest rpm as the revolving brush is applied lightly to the occlusal surfaces only. Avoid contact of the bristles with the soft tissues.
- Use a short stroke in a brushing motion; follow the inclined planes of the cusps.
- Move from tooth to tooth to prevent generation of excessive frictional heat. Avoid overuse of the brush. Replenish supply of polishing agent frequently.

H. Irrigation

- Irrigate teeth and interdental areas thoroughly several times with water from the syringe to remove abrasive particles. Care must be taken to minimize creation of aerosols.
- The rotary movement of the rubber cup or bristle brush can force the abrasive into the gingival sulci and irritate soft tissues.

Air-Powder Polishing

- Principles of selective stain removal are applied to the use of the air-powder polishing system (**Figure** 5). After biofilm control instruction, instrumentation, and periodontal debridement are completed, follow with an evaluation of need for stain removal.

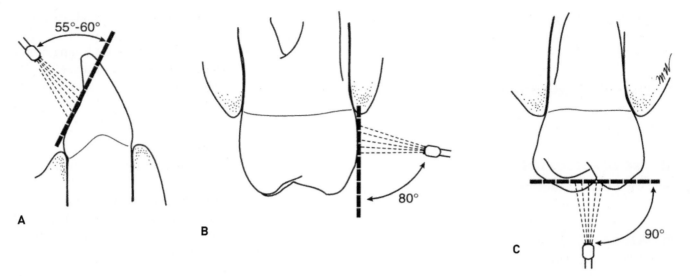

Figure 5 Air-Powder Polishing. Direct the aerosolized spray for **(A)** the anterior teeth at a 60° angle. **B:** The posterior teeth facial and lingual or palatal at an 80° angle. **C:** The occlusal surfaces at a 90° angle to the occlusal plane.

I. Principles of Application

- Air-powder systems manufactured by several companies are efficient and effective methods for mechanical removal of stain and biofilm.[26]
- Air-powder polishing systems use air, water, and specially formulated powders to deliver a controlled spray that propels the particles to the tooth surface.
    - Only powders approved by each air-powder polishing manufacturer are used in each brand of air-powder polishing unit.[26] The use of an unapproved powder in an air-powder polishing unit could void the warranty on the unit.
- The handpiece nozzle is moved in a constant circular motion, with the nozzle tip 4–5 mm away from the enamel surface.
- The spray is angled away from the gingival margin.
- The periphery of the spray may be near the gingival margin, but the center is directed at an angle less than 90° away from the margin.
- Complete directions for care of equipment and preparation for use of the device are provided by the individual manufacturer.

II. Specially Formulated Powders for Use in Air-Powder Polishing

Several manufacturers make and sell air-powder polishing powders.

- The abrasiveness of one brand of powder may differ from another brand, even though it is the same type of powder.[27]

A. Sodium Bicarbonate

- Sodium bicarbonate was the original powder used in air-powder polishing.[26]
- It is specially formulated with small amounts of calcium phosphate and silica to keep it free flowing.
- The Mohs hardness number for sodium bicarbonate is 3 and the particles average 74 µm in size.[27]
- The *only* type of sodium bicarbonate that can be used in air-powder polishing units is the type specially formulated for air-powder polishing.
- Sodium bicarbonate air-powder is available with flavorings.

B. Aluminum Trihydroxide

- Aluminum trihydroxide was the first air-powder developed as an alternative to sodium bicarbonate.
- Aluminum trihydroxide has a Mohs hardness value of 4 and the particles range in size from 80 to 325 µm.[27]

C. Glycine

- Glycine is an amino acid. For use in powders, glycine crystals are grown using a solvent of water and sodium salt.

- Glycine particles for use in air polishing have a Mohs hardness number of >4 and are 20–25 μm in size.[28]
- Glycine has been shown to be safe and effective for subgingival biofilm removal.[26,29]

D. Erythritol

- Erythritol is a nontoxic, chemically neutral, highly water-soluble polyol that is used as an artificial sweetener and food additive.
- Erythritol particles for use in air polishing have a Mohs hardness number of <2 and are 14 μm in size.[28]
- Erythritol has been shown to be safe and effective for subgingival biofilm removal.[28]

E. Calcium Carbonate

- Calcium carbonate is a naturally occurring substance that can be found in rocks.
- It is a main ingredient in antacids and is also used as filler for pharmaceutical drugs.
- Calcium carbonate has a Mohs number of 3 and particles are 45 μm in size.[26]

F. Calcium Sodium Phosphosilicate (Novamin)

- Calcium sodium phosphosilicate (Novamin) is a bioactive glass and has a Mohs hardness number of 6, making it the hardest air-polishing particle used in air-powder polishing powders.[27] The particles vary from 25 to 120 μm in size. This powder should not be used on any tooth structure or restorative material.[27]

III. Uses and Advantages of Air-Powder Polishing

- Requires less time, is ergonomically favorable to the clinician, and generates no heat.[26,29]
- Some air-polishing powders are less abrasive than traditional prophylaxis pastes, which makes the air-powder polisher ideal for stain and biofilm removal. However, some are much more abrasive and should only be used on surfaces that they will not damage.[27]
- Removal of heavy, tenacious tobacco stain and chlorhexidine-induced staining.
- Stain and biofilm removal from orthodontically banded and bracketed teeth and dental implants.[26,30]

- Before sealant placement or other bonding procedures.[26]
- Root detoxification for periodontally diseased roots by the periodontist during open periodontal surgery.[31]

IV. Technique

- A preprocedural antimicrobial rinse like 0.12% chlorhexidine is recommended to reduce the bacterial load and dispersion in this AGP.[24,26]
- Use of a high-volume evacuation (HVE) can reduce bacterial contamination up to 94.8%.[32]
- Increasing the water:powder ratio and adjusting the patient's position may also reduce the aerosols created.[32]

A. For Anterior Teeth

- Place the handpiece nozzle at a 60° angle to the facial and lingual surfaces of anterior teeth (**Figure 5A**).[26]

B. For Posterior Teeth

- Place the handpiece nozzle at an 80° angle to the facial and lingual surfaces (**Figure 5B**).[26]

C. For Occlusal Surfaces

- Place the handpiece nozzle at a 90° angle to the occlusal plane (**Figure 5C**).[26]

D. Incorrect Angulation

- Incorrect angulation of the handpiece can result in excessive aerosol production.
- The handpiece nozzle is never directed into the gingival sulcus or into a periodontal pocket with little bony support remaining, as this could result in facial emphysema (also known as a subcutaneous emphysema).[33]
- Facial emphysemas exhibit symptoms such as sudden soft tissue swelling with crepitus. If detected early, patients with facial emphysemas require observation and improve in 2–3 days.[33] There can be rare life-threatening complications so referral to a medical provider may be necessary.
- The closer the nozzle is held to the enamel, the more spray will deflect back into the direction of the clinician.
- When a clinician directs the handpiece at a 90° angle toward a facial, buccal, and some lingual

surfaces, the result is an immediate reflux of the aerosolized spray back onto the clinician.

- Changing the angle to the proper angulations of 60° and 80° will result in a change in the angle of the reflection, thus reducing the amount of reflux of aerosolized spray.

V. Recommendations and Precautions

A. Aerosol Production

- Air polishing is an AGP and therefore requires additional precautions to manage the aerosols and for PPE used by the clinician.[24,34] Suggestions for minimizing contamination and the effects of the aerosols include the following:
  - Patient uses a preprocedural antibacterial mouthrinse, particularly chlorhexidine.[35]
  - High-volume evacuation must be used to minimize aerosol dissemination.[24,36]
- See Chapter 6 for more information.

B. Protective Patient and Clinician Procedures

- Use protective eyewear, appropriate face mask, face shield, protective gown, and hair cover.
- Lubricate patient's lips to prevent the drying effect of the sodium bicarbonate using a nonpetroleum lip lubricant.
- Do not direct the spray toward the gingiva or other soft tissues, which can create patient discomfort and undue tissue trauma.
- Avoid directing the spray into periodontal pockets with bone loss or into extraction sites as a facial emphysema can be induced.

VI. Risk Patients: Air-Powder Polishing Contraindicated

The information from the patient's medical history is used and appropriate applications made. Antibiotic premedication is indicated for all the same patients who are at risk for any dental hygiene procedure. (See Chapter 11.)

A. Contraindications

- Physician-directed sodium-restricted diet (only for sodium bicarbonate powder).
- Respiratory disease or other condition that limits swallowing or breathing, such as chronic obstructive pulmonary disease.

- Patients with end-stage renal disease, Addison's disease, or Cushing's disease.
- Communicable infection that can contaminate the aerosols produced.
- Immunocompromised patients.
- Patients taking potassium, antidiuretics, or steroid therapy.
- Patients who have open oral wounds, such as tooth sockets, from oral surgery procedures.

B. Other Contraindications

- Root surfaces: Avoid routine polishing of cementum and dentin.
  - There is some evidence they can be removed readily during air-powder polishing if a sodium bicarbonate powder is used.[37]
  - However, research indicates that glycine[37] and erythritol[28,29] powders are safe for use subgingivally.
- Soft, spongy gingiva: The air-powder can irritate the free gingival tissue, especially if not used with the recommended technique.
  - Instruct the patient in daily biofilm removal.
  - Following scaling and periodontal debridement, postpone the stain removal until soft tissue has healed.
- Restorative materials: The use of air-powder polishing on composite resins, cements, and other nonmetallic materials can cause removal or pitting if an incorrect air polishing powder is used.[17,27] Manufacturer's recommendations for the use of a particular air polishing powder should be followed.[27]
  - **Table 3** provides a guide as to which restorative materials can be safely treated with the air-powder polishing powders containing sodium bicarbonate, aluminum trihydroxide, glycine, and erthyritol.[27,38]
  - Significant damage to margins of dental castings has been shown with incorrect usage of powder.

Polishing Proximal Surfaces

- Take care in the use of floss, tape, and finishing strips.
- Understanding the anatomy of the interdental papillae and relationship to the contact areas and proximal surfaces of the teeth is prerequisite to the prevention of tissue damage.

Table 3 Recommendations for Use of Air Polishing on Restorative Materials

Restorative Material	Polishing Powder Containing			
	Sodium Bicarbonate	Aluminum Trihydroxide	Glycine	Erythritol
Amalgam	Yes	No	Yes	Yes
Gold	Yes[a]	No	Yes	Yes
Porcelain	Yes[a]	No	Yes	Yes
Hybrid composite	No	No	Yes	Yes
Microfilled composite	No	No	Yes	Yes
Glass ionomer	No	No	Yes	Yes
Compomer	No	No	Yes	Yes
Luting agents	No	No	Yes	Yes

[a]Only if margin is avoided.

- Polish accessible proximal surfaces as much as possible during the use of the rubber cup in the prophylaxis angle.
- This can be followed by the use of dental tape with a polishing agent when indicated.

I. Dental Tape and Floss

A. Uses During Cleaning and Polishing

- Techniques for tape and floss application are described in Chapter 27.
- The same principles apply whether the patient or the clinician is using the floss.
- Finger rests are used to prevent snapping through contact areas.
- Stain removal with dental tape: Polishing agent is applied to the tooth, and the tape is moved gently back and forth and up and down curved over the area where stain was observed.
- Cleaning gingival surface of a fixed partial denture: A floss threader is used to position the floss or tape over the gingival surface. The agent is applied under the pontic, and the floss or tape is moved back and forth with contact on the bridge surface. Floss threaders are described and illustrated in Chapter 30.
- Flossing: Particles of abrasive agent can be removed by rinsing and by using a clean piece of floss applied in the usual manner.
- Rinsing and irrigation: Irrigate with air-water syringe to remove abrasive agent being careful to minimize aerosols.

The Porte Polisher

- Design
  - The porte polisher is a manual instrument designed especially for extrinsic stain removal or application of treatment agents such as for hypersensitive areas.
  - It is constructed to hold a wood point at a contra-angle. The wood points may be cone or wedge-shaped and made of various kinds of wood, preferably orangewood.[39] **Figure 6** illustrates a typical porte polisher.

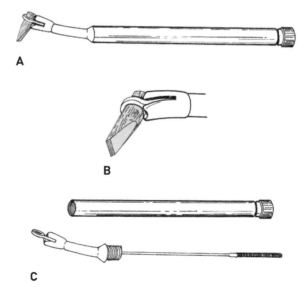

Figure 6 Porte Polisher. **A:** Assembled instrument shows position of wood point ready for instrumentation. **B:** Working end shows wedge-shaped wood point inserted. **C:** Disassembled, ready for autoclave.

- Grasp: The instrument is held in a modified pen grasp or palm grasp.
- Application: The wood point is applied to the tooth surface using firm; carefully directed; massaging, circular, or linear strokes to accommodate the anatomy of each tooth.
  - A firm finger rest and a moderate amount of pressure of the wood point provide protection for the gingival margin and efficiency in technique.
- Advantages
  - The porte polisher is useful for instrumentation of difficult-to-access surfaces of the teeth, especially malpositioned teeth.
  - No heat generation, no noise compared with powered handpieces, and minimal production of aerosols.
  - The porte polisher is portable and therefore is useful in any location, for example, for a bedbound patient.
- Disadvantages
  - It is time consuming and requires force.

Documentation

Documentation for a patient receiving tooth stain removal as part of the dental hygiene care plan for a maintenance appointment would include a minimum of the following:

- Review patient medical history with questions to determine health problems, recent medical examinations and treatments, and changes in medications.
- Current clinical examination findings: intraoral, extraoral, periodontal, and dental.
- With dental charting: identification of dental materials used in restorations that can influence choice of polishing agents. Identification would require use of radiographs and the intraoral dental charting.
- Dental hygiene examination for state of patient's personal daily self-care, calculus and biofilm deposits, sources for dental stains, products used for oral care, and dietary factors influencing the dentition and all oral tissues: questions answered about best choices for various products.
- A sample progress note may be reviewed in Box 1.

Factors to Teach the Patient

- How stains form.
- The importance of biofilm and calculus removal at maintenance appointments.
- The meaning of selective polishing and contraindications for polishing.
- Stains and biofilm removed by polishing can return promptly if biofilm is not removed faithfully on a schedule of two or three times each day.
- The options for stain removal that are appropriate for the patient.

Box 1 Example Documentation: Selection of Polishing Agent for a Patient with Esthetic Restorations

- **S**—A 36-year-old male patient presents for regular maintenance appointment. He comments on how pleased he is that his new implant crown and other esthetic restorations are not distinguishable from the color of his natural teeth. Updated medical history, medications, no changes.
- **O**—Blood pressure (115/75); extra-intraoral examinations: no findings; comprehensive periodontal examination: localized 3–4 mm, with bleeding on probing in 4 mm pockets in molar areas; supragingival calculus mand ant.; minimal biofilm with isolated areas of yellowish staining.
- **A**—Confirmed the material used for the various restorations and found that the patient has porcelain crowns on teeth numbers #2, 14, and anterior microhybrid composite restorations in teeth numbers #6, 7, 8, 10, and 11. Patient has an implant and porcelain crown on #9. Note: Microhybrid composite restorations and implant crown match the patient's natural teeth to the extent that it is difficult to identify the restorations.
- **P**—Gave patient new toothbrush with tongue cleaner on back and demonstrated the tongue cleaner. Reviewed oral-self care for areas areas of residual biofilm. Completed debridement. Avoided use of air polishing with sodium bicarbonate and prophy paste. Selected a cleaning agent to remove biofilm and isolated areas of yellowish staining.

Next regular appointment 4 months.
Signed: _____, RDH
Date: _____

References

1. American Dental Hygienists' Association. American Dental Hygienists' Association Position Paper on the Oral Prophylaxis. Published 1998. https://www.adha.org/resources-docs/7115_Prophylaxis_Postion_Paper.pdf. Accessed August 29, 2021.

2. Academy of Periodontology. Glossary of periodontal terms. https://members.perio.org/libraries/glossary. Accessed August 29, 2021.

3. Lanza A, Ruggiero A, Sbordone L. Tribology and dentistry: a commentary. *Lubricants*. 2019;7(6):52.

4. Tomás I, Diz P, Tobías A, Scully C, Donos N. Periodontal health status and bacteraemia from daily oral activities: systematic review/meta-analysis. *J Clin Periodontol*. 2012;39(3):213-228.

5. Innes N, Johnson IG, Al-Yaseen W, et al. A systematic review of droplet and aerosol generation in dentistry. *J Dent*. 2021;105:103556.

6. Centers for Disease Control and Prevention. Healthcare workers. Published February 11, 2020. https://www.cdc.gov/coronavirus/2019-ncov/hcp/infection-control-recommendations.html. Accessed September 11, 2021.

7. Ekmekcioglu H, Unur M. Eye-related trauma and infection in dentistry. *J Istanb Univ Fac Dent*. 2017;51(3):55-63.

8. Sawai MA, Bhardwaj A, Jafri Z, Sultan N, Daing A. Tooth polishing: the current status. *J Indian Soc Periodontol*. 2015;19(4):375-380.

9. Farooq I, Bugshan A. The role of salivary contents and modern technologies in the remineralization of dental enamel: a narrative review. *F1000Res*. 2020;9:171.

10. Pence SD, Chambers DA, van IG, Wolf RC, Pfeiffer DC. Repetitive coronal polishing yields minimal enamel loss. *J Dent Hyg*. 2011;85(4):10.

11. Liu X-X, Tenenbaum HC, Wilder RS, Quock R, Hewlett ER, Ren Y-F. Pathogenesis, diagnosis and management of dentin hypersensitivity: an evidence-based overview for dental practitioners. *BMC Oral Health*. 2020;20:220.

12. Can Say E, Yurdagüven H, Malkondu Ö, Ünlü N, Soyman M, Kazazoğlu E. The effect of prophylactic polishing pastes on surface roughness of indirect restorative materials. *Sci World J*. 2014;2014:e962764.

13. Yap AUJ, Wu SS, Chelvan S, Tan ESF. Effect of hygiene maintenance procedures on surface roughness of composite restoratives. *Oper Dent*. 2005;30(1):99-104.

14. Neme A, Frazier K, Roeder L, Debner T. Effect of prophylactic polishing protocols on the surface roughness of esthetic restorative materials. *Oper Dent*. 27(1):50-58.

15. Prathap S, Rajesh H, Boloor VA, Rao AS. Extrinsic stains and management: a new insight. *J Acad Indus Res*. 2013;1(8):435-442.

16. Żyła T, Kawala B, Antoszewska-Smith J, Kawala M. Black stain and dental caries: a review of the literature. *BioMed Res Int*. 2015;2015:e469392.

17. Cvikl B, Moritz A, Bekes K. Pit and fissure sealants—a comprehensive review. *Dent J*. 2018;6(2):18.

18. Botti R, Bossù M, Zallocco N, Vestri A, Polimeni A. Effectiveness of plaque indicators and air polishing for the sealing of pits and fissures. *Eur J Paediatr Dent*. 2010;11(1):15-18.

19. Mellberg JR, Nicholson CR, Ripa LW, Barenie J. Fluoride deposition in human enamel in vivo from professionally applied fluoride prophylaxis paste. *J Dent Res*. 1976;55(6):976-979.

20. Centers for Disease Control and Prevention (CDC). Recommendations for using fluoride to prevent and control dental caries in the United States. *MMWR Recomm Rep*. 2001;50(RR-14):1-42.

21. Zhao J, Liu Y, Sun W-B, Zhang H. Amorphous calcium phosphate and its application in dentistry. *Chem Cent J*. 2011;5:40.

22. Milleman JL, Milleman KR, Clark CE, Mongiello KA, Simonton TC, Proskin HM. NUPRO sensodyne prophylaxis paste with NovaMin for the treatment of dentin hypersensitivity: a 4-week clinical study. *Am J Dent*. 2012;25(5):262-268.

23. Khijmatgar S, Reddy U, John S, Badavannavar AN, Souza TD. Is there evidence for Novamin application in remineralization?: a systematic review. *J Oral Biol Craniofac Res*. 2020;10(2):87-92.

24. Centers for Disease Control and Prevention (CDC). Interim infection prevention and control guidance for dental settings during the coronavirus disease 2019 (COVID-19) pandemic. Published February 11, 2020. https://www.cdc.gov/coronavirus/2019-ncov/hcp/dental-settings.html. Accessed August 28, 2021.

25. Herd S, Chin J, Palenik CJ, Ofner S. The in vivo contamination of air-driven low-speed handpieces with prophylaxis angles. *J Am Dent Assoc*. 2007;138(10):1360-1365.

26. Dhande SR, Muglikar S, Hegde R, Ghodke P. Air-powder polishing: an update. *Recent Dev Med Med Res*. 2021;14(22):152-167.

27. Barnes CM, Covey D, Watanabe H, Simetich B, Schulte JR, Chen H. An in vitro comparison of the effects of various air polishing powders on enamel and selected esthetic restorative materials. *J Clin Dent*. 2014;25(4):76-87.

28. Kröger JC, Haribyan M, Nergiz I, Schmage P. Air polishing with erythritol powder – In vitro effects on dentin loss. *J Indian Soc Periodontol*. 2020;24(5):433-440.

29. Sultan DA, Hill RG, Gillam DG. Air-polishing in subgingival root debridement: a critical literature review. *J Dent Oral Bio*. 2017;2(10):1065.

30. Tuchscheerer V, Eickholz P, Dannewitz B, Ratka C, Zuhr O, Petsos H. In vitro surgical and non-surgical air-polishing efficacy for implant surface decontamination in three different defect configurations. *Clin Oral Invest*. 2021;25(4):1743-1754.

31. Schmidlin PR, Fujioka-Kobayashi M, Mueller H-D, Sculean A, Lussi A, Miron RJ. Effects of air polishing and an amino acid buffered hypochlorite solution to dentin surfaces and periodontal ligament cell survival, attachment, and spreading. *Clin Oral Invest*. 2017;21(5):1589-1598.

32. Khursheed DA. Managing periodontics patients during the SARS-CoV-2 pandemic. *J Int Oral Health*. 2020;12(8):85-89.

33. Alonso V, García-Caballero L, Couto I, Diniz M, Diz P, Limeres J. Subcutaneous emphysema related to air-powder tooth polishing: a report of three cases. *Aust Dent J*. 2017;62(4):510-515.

34. Centers for Disease Control and Prevention (CDC) HICPAC. Core infection prevention and control practices for safe healthcare delivery in all settings—recommendations of the HICPAC. Published September 10, 2021. https://www.cdc.gov/hicpac/recommendations/core-practices.html. Accessed September 17, 2021.

35. Koletsi D, Belibasakis GN, Eliades T. Interventions to reduce aerosolized microbes in dental practice: a systematic review with network meta-analysis of randomized controlled trials. *J Dent Res*. 2020;99(11):1228-1238.

36. Kumbargere Nagraj S, Eachempati P, Paisi M, Nasser M, Sivaramakrishnan G, Verbeek JH. Interventions to reduce contaminated aerosols produced during dental procedures for preventing infectious diseases. *Cochrane Database Syst Rev*. 2020;10:CD013686.

37. Bühler J, Schmidli F, Weiger R, Walter C. Analysis of the effects of air polishing powders containing sodium bicarbonate and glycine on human teeth. *Clin Oral Invest.* 2015;19(4):877-885.

38. Janiszewska-Olszowska J, Drozdzik A, Tandecka K, Grocholewicz K. Effect of air-polishing on surface roughness of composite dental restorative material—comparison of three different air-polishing powders. *BMC Oral Health.* 2020;20(1):30.

39. Tungare S, Paranjpe AG. Teeth polishing. In: *StatPearls.* StatPearls Publishing; 2021. http://www.ncbi.nlm.nih.gov/books/NBK513328/. Accessed September 22, 2021.

Tooth Bleaching

Heather Hessheimer, RDH, MS

CHAPTER OUTLINE

OVERVIEW OF TOOTH BLEACHING
- **I.** Bleaching versus Whitening
- **II.** Vital Tooth Bleaching versus Nonvital Tooth Bleaching
- **III.** History

VITAL TOOTH BLEACHING
- **I.** Mechanism of Bleaching Vital Teeth
- **II.** Tooth Color Change with Vital Tooth Bleaching
- **III.** Materials Used for Vital Tooth Bleaching
- **IV.** Vital Tooth Bleaching Safety
- **V.** Factors Associated with Efficacy
- **VI.** Reversible Side Effects of Vital Bleaching: Sensitivity
- **VII.** Irreversible Tooth Damage
- **VIII.** Modes of Vital Tooth Bleaching

NONVITAL TOOTH BLEACHING
- **I.** Procedure for Bleaching Nonvital Teeth
- **II.** Factors Associated with Efficacy

DENTAL HYGIENE PROCESS OF CARE
- **I.** Patient Assessment
- **II.** Dental Hygiene Diagnosis
- **III.** Dental Hygiene Care Plan
- **IV.** Implementation
- **V.** Evaluation and Planning for Maintenance

DOCUMENTATION

FACTORS TO TEACH THE PATIENT

REFERENCES

LEARNING OBJECTIVES

After studying this chapter, the student will be able to:

1. Discuss the mechanism, safety, and efficacy of tooth bleaching agents.
2. Identify specific tooth conditions and staining responses to tooth bleaching.
3. Differentiate reversible and irreversible side effects associated with the tooth bleaching process.
4. Assess appropriate interventions for tooth bleaching side effects.

Overview of Tooth Bleaching

Patients of all ages have concerns about the appearance of their teeth and expect their dental hygienists to guide them in their **esthetic** choices with evidence-based information. Because there are many causes of tooth discoloration, a review of Chapter 17 is recommended.

- Tooth **bleaching** may result in significantly whiter teeth and contribute to an increase in patient's self-confidence.
- A whiter smile may motivate the patient to maintain improved oral health, which is a significant benefit.

I. Bleaching versus Whitening

The terms "bleaching" and "**whitening**" have been used interchangeably, but are not the same:

- Tooth whitening refers to any process to lighten the tooth color.[1]
- Bleaching involves free radicals and the breakdown of chromagens.[1]

II. Vital Tooth Bleaching versus Nonvital Tooth Bleaching

- Teeth can be stained **intrinsically** and **extrinsically**.
- External tooth bleaching is used for both vital and nonvital teeth.
  - Agents for bleaching are applied to the external surfaces of the teeth.
  - Bleaching agents break down chemical bonds into larger pigmented organic molecules, called chromogens, making them refract light and appear lighter.[1]
- **Color** change can extend into the dentin to produce a whitened tooth.
- Nonvital teeth become intrinsically stained by blood breakdown products or agents from root canal therapy.[1]
- Nonvital tooth bleaching is a procedure performed by a dentist after root canal therapy using a rubber dam or other type of isolation.[2]
  - The bleaching agents are introduced into the pulp chamber.
  - The color of a single tooth is lightened to help it blend with the adjacent teeth.

III. History

A. Nonvital Tooth Bleaching History

- Bleaching of discolored, nonvital teeth was first described as early as 1864.[3]
- In 1961, the *walking bleach method* was introduced. The *walking bleach method* sealed a mixture of sodium perborate and water into the pulp chamber and retained it there between the patient's visits.[3]
- By 1963, the *walking bleach method* was modified to use water and 30% to 35% hydrogen peroxide instead of the sodium perborate and water. Result: improved lighter color of nonvital teeth.[3]

B. Vital Tooth Bleaching History

- In the 1960s, tooth lightening was observed after orthodontics used an antiseptic containing carbamide peroxide to promote tissue healing due to gingivitis.[3]
- In the 1980s, lighter tooth color was noted after advising patients to use carbamide peroxide in customized trays for antiseptic purposes following periodontal surgery.
- In 1989, the use of carbamide peroxide for the primary purpose of tooth bleaching was introduced.[3,4]
  - A custom tray was used to maintain the bleaching gel on the tooth surface for an extended time.
  - The procedure was known as nightguard vital bleaching (NGVB) and is a dentist-monitored process.
- No significant, long-term oral or systemic health risks have been associated with professional at-home tooth bleaching materials containing 10% carbamide peroxide or 3.5% hydrogen peroxide when professionally supervised.[5,6]

Vital Tooth Bleaching

The bleaching process is a subject of ongoing research and current theories about the mechanism of action involve a chemical change within the tooth structure.

I. Mechanism of Bleaching Vital Teeth

- Bleaching products penetrate enamel and dentin reaching the pulp within 5–15 minutes.[7-10]
- Bleaching products break down chromogens into smaller, less pigmented constituents that are locked in the enamel matrix and dentinal tubules.[1,9]
- The chemical reactions from bleaching products change the optical qualities of the tooth color.[11]

II. Tooth Color Change with Vital Tooth Bleaching

- The color of the teeth is influenced by thickness of enamel and underlying color of dentin.
- Color of both dentin and enamel are changed; primarily the dentin color is changed.
- Dentin color is either yellow or gray and can be seen through the enamel due to its **translucency**.
- Darker teeth take more time to lighten.
- Each tooth reaches a maximum color change. Additional bleaching product or contact time will not necessarily result in a lighter color.[1,5]
- Bleaching products cause teeth to become dehydrated during and after product administration. A lighter shade can result temporarily.[12]

- Color will stabilize approximately 2 weeks after bleaching.[10]

III. Materials Used for Vital Tooth Bleaching

- Both hydrogen peroxide and carbamide peroxide are used to lighten vital teeth.
- Hydrogen peroxide has a short working time because it begins to break down in 30–60 minutes[10]; carbamide peroxide has an extended working time.
- The chemicals are used alone or in combination.
- Bleaching materials need an appropriate viscosity to flow over the tooth surface, but not so excessive as to spread onto gingival and other oral tissues.

A. Hydrogen Peroxide

- Used directly or produced through a chemical reaction when carbamide peroxide breaks down (see **Figure** **1**).[11]
- Has a lower pH than carbamide peroxide, which may result in susceptibility to demineralization or erosion when used for longer treatment times than recommended.[1]
  - Takes less time per day, but more days, to change tooth color effectively.[6]
  - Higher concentrations of hydrogen peroxide may result in greater sensitivity and more color relapse after termination of bleaching.[13]

B. Carbamide Peroxide

- Active agent in many bleaching systems in a 10% concentration.
- Breaks down into hydrogen peroxide and urea. As shown in the flowchart (Figure 1), urea may

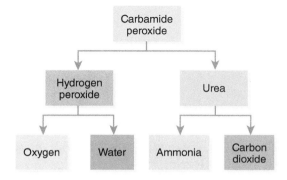

Figure **1** Hydrogen Peroxide and Carbamide Peroxide Product Breakdown. Flowchart to show breakdown of bleaching products. Hydrogen peroxide breaks down into oxygen and water; carbamide peroxide breaks down into hydrogen peroxide and urea, which further break down as shown.

further break down into ammonia with high pH to facilitate bleaching.
- Has slow release: 50% of peroxide released in 2 hours and remainder of peroxide in 6 hours, resulting in less sensitivity.[10]
  - At neutral pH, 10% solution safe and has similar efficacy as more concentrated solutions with less sensitivity.[5] A 10% solution has not been shown to affect the hardness of dental enamel.[14]

C. Desensitizers

- Materials to reduce the sensitivity side effect of bleaching may be added to bleaching systems.
- Materials can be:
  - Incorporated into the bleaching gel.
  - Applied to teeth before bleaching.
  - Given for use in trays before, during, and after treatment.
- Material used:
  - **Potassium nitrate**: creates a calming effect on pulp by affecting the transmission of nerve impulses.[15,16]
  - Sodium fluoride: aids in remineralization and reducing sensitivity.[16]
  - Calcium phosphate and **amorphous calcium phosphate**: aid in reducing sensitivity and remineralization.[17]

D. Other Ingredients

- Carbopol: a water-soluble resin used as a thickening agent
  - Prolongs the release of hydrogen peroxide from carbamide peroxide.
  - Promotes quicker results.
- Glycerin: a gel to thicken and control the flow of bleaching agent to prevent overextending onto gingival tissues.
- Sodium hydroxide: a cleaning agent.
- **Surfactants**: help to lift and remove extrinsic stains.
- Flavoring: aids in patient satisfaction and compliance.

IV. Vital Tooth Bleaching Safety

A. Tooth Structure

- Both hydrogen peroxide 3.5% and carbamide peroxide 10% are considered safe to lighten the color of teeth when professionally monitored.[10]
- Carbamide peroxide 10% will cause fewer changes in the enamel matrix.[14]

- Research is inconsistent in regard to pulpal necrosis from the heat produced during laser-activated treatment.[18,19]

B. Soft Tissue

- Hydrogen peroxide is caustic and may cause burning and bleaching of the gingiva and any exposed oral tissue.[3]
- Hydrogen peroxide 10% concentration or higher has greater incidence of gingival irritation.[6]
- Ill-fitting or overfilled trays may cause product spillage onto soft tissues, resulting in tissue burning.[6]

C. Restorative Materials

- Restorative material color will not be lightened by bleaching.
- Complications with current restorations may include[1]:
  - Increased surface roughness.
  - Change in surface color.
  - Increased microleakage.
- After bleaching, new restorative procedures need to be delayed for 2 weeks to allow for color stabilization.[10,20]
- Bonding needs to be delayed for 2 weeks due to significantly reduced bonding strength associated with recently bleached tooth surface.[10,20]
- Bleaching chemicals containing hydrogen peroxide may:
  - Cause porosity in restorative materials due to the lower pH, resulting in surface changes in surface texture and hardness.[21]
  - Increase mercury release from amalgam restorations, giving off a green hue.[21]
  - Increase solubility of some dental cements.[20]

D. Systemic Factors

- The use of tooth-bleaching products containing hydrogen peroxide or carbamide peroxide has not been shown to increase the risk of oral cancer in the general population, including those persons who abuse alcohol and/or are heavy cigarette smokers.[22]
- The effects of accidental ingestion of hydrogen peroxide or carbamide peroxide depend on the amount and concentration ingested.[3]
  - Effects of small amounts may include sore throat, nausea, vomiting, abdominal distention, and ulcerations of the oral mucosa, esophagus, and stomach.

Box 1 Medications Associated with Potential Photosensitivity and Hyperpigmentation

- Acne medications
- Antiarrhythmic drugs
- Antibiotics
- Anticancer drugs
- Antidepressants
- Antihistamines
- Antiparasitics
- Antipsychotics
- Antiseizure medications
- Arthritis medications
- Birth control medications
- Coal tar
- Diuretics
- Hypoglycemics
- Nonsteroidal anti-inflammatory drugs
- Phenothiazines[23]
- Retinoids[23]
- Steroids
- Sulfur-containing drugs
- Targeted anticancer therapies (BRAF, EGFR, VEGFR, MEK, and Bcr-Abl tyrosine kinase inhibitors)
- Tranquilizers[23]

  - Large amounts can be fatal, so it is essential to keep it out of the reach of children.
- Medications that may be associated with photosensitivity and hyperpigmentation when light-activated bleaching agents are used are listed in **Box 1.**

E. Cautions and Contraindications Associated with Vital Tooth Bleaching

- Treatment considerations may include:
  - Subjective determination when tooth shade is acceptable.
  - Patients with unrealistic personal expectations.
  - Poor patient compliance with treatment results in suboptimal outcomes.
  - Patients with tooth conditions that do not respond favorably to vital tooth bleaching (see **Table 1**).
- Children and adolescents
  - The American Academy of Pediatric Dentistry (AAPD) discourages full-arch cosmetic bleaching for patients with a mixed dentition, but encourages judicious use of vital and nonvital bleaching due to the negative

Table 1 Decision Making for Tooth Bleaching

Tooth Condition	Response to Tooth Bleaching	Special Considerations
Yellow color	Normally excellent	Resistant yellow may be tetracycline stain
Enamel white spots	Do not bleach well or may get lighter during bleaching	■ Eventually background color lightens resulting in less noticeable white spots ■ Goes through splotchy stage before background color whitens ■ Microabrasion may lessen white spots if less than one-third through enamel
Brown fluorosis stains	Respond 80% of the time	Microabrasion techniques done after bleaching and color stabilization may improve final result
Nicotine stains	Require longer treatment	May take 2–3 mo of nightly application
Tetracycline stains	Multicolored band may not respond well. ■ Gray most difficult ■ Dark grays only get lighter ■ Dark cervical has poorest prognosis	Requires 3-6 mo of daily bleaching
Minocycline stains	Will respond; will take longer than yellow stain	■ Type of tetracycline stain ■ Gives gray hue
Root exposure	Does not respond to bleaching	Better treated with periodontal coverage
Dentinogenesis imperfecta and amelogenesis imperfecta	No significant improvement with bleaching	Inherited conditions resulting in defective dentin and enamel, respectively
Microcracks	Become whiter than rest of tooth	Bright light or magnification required during assessment to view; may appear streaky during bleaching process
Anterior lingual amalgams	Become more visible after bleaching	Replacement with very light composite restoration before bleaching
Dental caries	Not to be bleached	■ Decay removal ■ Temporary restoration followed by bleaching and final restoration after color stabilization. Carbamide peroxide may increase sensitivity
Dark canines	Require longer bleaching	Isolated canine treatment until color match
Attrition	Incisal edges do not respond	Composite restorations added to incisal edges after bleaching
Aging	Excellent	More youthful appearance; root surfaces exposure likely
Translucent teeth	Bleaching will increase translucency at incisal	Translucent areas will appear darker after bleaching due to contrast

self-image that may arise from a discolored tooth or teeth.[24]

- Current AAPD recommendations for children and adolescent use include[24]:
  - Delaying treatment until after permanent teeth have erupted.
  - Use of a custom-fabricated tray to limit amount of bleaching gel.
  - Close supervision.
- Tooth bleaching is contraindicated in the following patients:
  - Pregnant and lactating women.

Light-activated bleaching is contraindicated for patients who are:

- Light sensitive.
- Taking a photosensitive medication.
- Receiving photochemotherapeutic drugs or treatments such as psoralen and ultraviolet radiation.

Exposure to ultraviolet radiation produced by some lights must be avoided for those at increased risk for or with a history of skin cancer, including melanoma.

- Use of photosensitive medications (see Box   1).
- Laser light/power bleaching contraindicated for some patients as described in **Box   2**.

V. Factors Associated with Efficacy

- Some tooth conditions will not respond to tooth bleaching; other tooth conditions will respond slowly (Table   1).[10]
- The initial color of the teeth and type of stain present will affect the final color change.[10]
- Specific indications for bleaching and methods of treatments are listed in **Table   2**.
- Attrition: occlusal wear through enamel exposes the darker underlying dentin.
- Concentration of bleaching agent.
- Ability of agent to reach the stain molecules.
- Duration of contact of the active bleaching agent: the longer the duration, the greater the degree of bleaching.
- Number of times the agent is applied to obtain desired results: darker teeth tend to require more treatment applications.
- Temperature of agent: heat will result in faster oxygen release, but speed of color change may not be altered.

A. Intrinsic

- Tetracycline and minocycline staining
  - Tetracycline particles incorporate into dentin calcium during mineralization of unerupted teeth. Result: discolored dentin resistant to bleaching.[10]
  - Minocycline, a derivative of tetracycline, can discolor erupted teeth.[10]

Table   2 Indications for Tooth Bleaching and Methods of Treatment

Indication	Method to Treat
Discolored, endodontically treated tooth	Internal bleaching; in-office or walking
Single or multiple discolored teeth	External bleaching: in-office one to three visits or custom trays worn 2–6 weeks
Surface staining	Dental prophylaxis and brushing with whitening dentifrice
Isolated brown or white discoloration, shallow depth in enamel	Microabrasion followed by neutral sodium fluoride applications
White discoloration on yellowish teeth	Microabrasion followed by custom tray bleaching

- Tetracycline and minocycline staining severity varies. A comparison of before and after bleaching of brown tetracycline staining is shown in **Figure   2**.
  - *First-category staining*: light-yellow to light-gray responds to bleaching.
  - *Second-category staining*: darker and more extensive yellow-gray responds to extended bleaching time.
  - *Third-category staining*: intense dark gray-blue banding stains. Severe third-category staining may require porcelain veneers for satisfactory esthetic result.
  - Some tetracycline stains will require 1–12 months to achieve a satisfactory result.
- Fluorosis
  - Fluorosis results from ingesting excessive fluoride during tooth development resulting in white or brown spots on teeth.
  - Bleaching does not change white spots, but lightens the background color, making the contrast less noticeable.[10]
  - White spots go through a splotchy stage during bleaching but will return to baseline.
  - Amorphous calcium phosphate may be effective in lessening the white spots if lesion is less than one-third through enamel.[25]
  - Brown discoloration responsive to bleach 80% of the time.[10]
  - Resin infiltration or **microabrasion** may be recommended to decrease additional brown discoloration.[10,26]

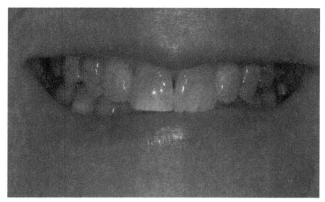

A

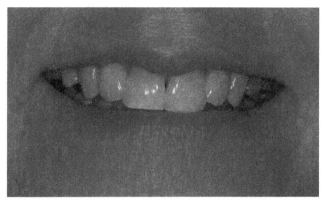

B

Figure 2 Before and After Bleaching of Moderate Tetracycline-Stained Teeth. **A:** Patient before treating. **B:** Patient after being treated with 10% carbamide peroxide for 4 months. Some tetracycline-stained teeth will require up to 12 months to achieve improved results. Those with severe gray stain or banded staining may require porcelain veneers to achieve an acceptable cosmetic result.

Images courtesy of Dr. Van B. Haywood, DMD, Professor, Dental College of Georgia, Augusta University.

- Tobacco
  - Tobacco stains: require 1–3 months of nightly treatment due to the tenacity of the stain.

B. Extrinsic

- Interactions with bleaching agents.
  - Staining agents may compromise treatment.[1]
  - Advise patient to avoid:
    - Coffee and tea.
    - Dark sodas or soft drinks.
    - Red wine.
    - Soy sauce.
    - Tobacco.
- Chromogenic bacteria.
- Biofilm accumulation.
- Topical medications.

C. Longevity of Results

- Relapse of shade occurs almost immediately as newly bleached, dehydrated teeth rehydrate.
- As months and years pass, teeth may discolor and darken again, especially if stain-inducing activities continue.
- To maintain shade, periodic bleaching procedures are performed or repeated.

VI. Reversible Side Effects of Vital Bleaching: Sensitivity

The most common side effects of bleaching are tooth tingling and sensitivity. An aching sensation can occur because of the insult of peroxide on nerves: a reversible pulpitis.[10]

- Mild-to-moderate tooth sensitivity is reported in as many as 75% of patients.[3,20]
- Primarily occurs in the first 2 weeks of treatment and may last days to months after cessation of bleaching.
- Side effects resolve completely as teeth become accustomed to bleaching.
- Not correlated with increased wear time.
  - Lower concentrations have been used for up to 12 months (i.e., in bleaching tetracycline stain) and do not exhibit greater sensitivity.[10]
  - Higher concentrations of hydrogen peroxide may result in greater sensitivity.
- Patients with prior history of tooth sensitivity may be more at risk to develop sensitivity during bleaching.[3,10]
- Vulnerable tooth surfaces include:
  - Exposed root surfaces and dentin appear to increase risk of developing sensitivity and need to be protected from bleaching material.
  - Teeth with unrestored abfraction lesions tend to have more sensitivity.
- Addition of desensitizing materials decreases sensitivity.
- Treatments to reduce tooth sensitivity are listed in **Table 3**.

VII. Irreversible Tooth Damage

A. Root Resorption

- Can occur after bleaching, particularly after intracoronal, nonvital tooth bleaching when heat is applied during the technique.[3,27]
- Internal and external resorption may become apparent several years after bleaching.[3]

Table 3 Desensitization Procedures for Bleaching

Pretreatment	■ Brush on or use the bleaching tray with a desensitizing toothpaste containing potassium nitrate, without sodium lauryl sulfate, which removes the smear layer from dentin, beginning 2 weeks before bleaching. ■ Use toothpaste with prescription strength sodium fluoride. ■ Use toothpaste that includes calcium carbonate.
During treatment	■ Continue to use desensitizing toothpaste, which includes sodium fluoride or potassium nitrate, daily between treatments. Amorphous calcium phosphate may be used as well. ■ Increase time intervals between treatments. ■ Reduce exposure time of bleaching materials. ■ Limit the amount in the tray to prevent tissue contact.
Postbleaching	■ Sensitivity diminishes with time. ■ Continue daily use of desensitizing dentifrice and amorphous calcium phosphate. ■ Have professional fluoride varnish application. ■ Avoid foods and beverages with temperature extremes or that contain acidic elements.

- Occurs usually in cervical third of the tooth.[3]
- Cause may be related to a history of trauma.[3]
- May lead to tooth loss.[3]
- Bleaching agents should not be placed on exposed cementum to avoid complications.

B. Tooth Fracture
- May be related to removal of tooth structure or reduction of the microhardness of dentin and enamel.[28]
- More common with nonvital tooth bleaching.[29]
- May lead to tooth loss.

C. Demineralization
- Demineralization with slight surface pitting can result from a hydrogen peroxide concentration above 15%.[30]

- Patient with over-the-counter (OTC) product may not seek or follow professional advice and attempt to get the teeth whiter by using the product more often than recommended.
- Remineralization should be initiated early and fluoridated carbamide peroxide gels may be a good choice to aid remineralization.[31]
- Remineralization protocols are described in Chapter 25.

D. Erosion
- Products containing acidic pH may result in tooth erosion over time.
- The higher the percentage of hydrogen peroxide, the lower the pH.
- More common with OTC bleaching products.

VIII. Modes of Vital Tooth Bleaching
- A comparison of the advantages and disadvantages of professionally applied and professionally dispensed/professionally monitored systems and the OTC systems is listed in **Table 4**.
- The different methods of tooth bleaching can achieve similar, effective results, although the mode of delivery, length of treatment, and ease of treatment vary.

A. Professionally Applied
- Professionally applied bleaching may be performed with high concentrations of 30% to 40% hydrogen peroxide or 35% to 44% carbamide peroxide.
- Bleaching gels are administered by a dental professional and are not for at-home use.
- Some systems use activation or enhancement with a light or heat source (**Figure 3**).
  - Local anesthesia should not be used in order to monitor heat-provoked sensitivity.
  - Heat applied or produced by the use of light may cause an adverse effect such as necrosis of the pulp of the tooth.[32]
  - Additional issues associated with the use of a light-activated bleaching are listed in Box 2.
- Laser-safe/ultraviolet light protection of eyes for anyone in the treatment room is required.
- Gingival sensitivity or irritation may occur.[10]
  - Rubber dam or an equivalent technique, such as a liquid light-cured resin dam, should be used to isolate the caustic agents from contact with soft tissues.

Table 4 Comparisons of Modes of Tooth Bleaching Systems

Methods	Advantages	Disadvantages
Professionally applied utilizing laser/ultraviolet light system procedure	■ Performed as part of comprehensive care ■ Treatment may be combined with trays and professional grade home bleaching materials ■ Professional product selection ■ Patient education. ■ Follow-up, evaluation of effectiveness ■ Sensitivity treatment ■ Compliance guaranteed ■ Quickest result	■ Higher cost ■ Higher risk for sensitivity
Professionally dispensed, includes professional grade product and trays	■ Performed as part of comprehensive care ■ Appropriate patient selection ■ Professional product selection ■ Patient education ■ Follow-up, evaluation of effectiveness ■ Sensitivity treatment; patient can also use less often if sensitive ■ Choice of comfortable time and place for application ■ Potential for best result	■ Cost ■ Longer time to whiten than professionally applied ■ Patient compliance
Over-the-counter	■ Lowest cost ■ Easier access to purchase ■ Immediate start ■ Choice of comfortable time and place for application ■ Short exposure time	■ No comprehensive exam ■ Slowest and least effective results ■ Noncustomized delivery ■ Compliance issues ■ Bulky fit for patient ■ Results and tissue response not monitored ■ Limited effects due to short exposure time ■ Unsupervised

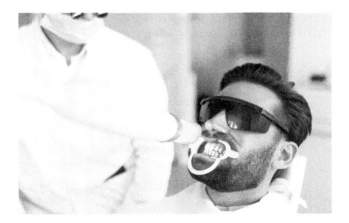

Figure 3 Laser Tooth Whitening Treatment
© Aywan88/E+/Getty Images

- Take care to assure the liquid light-cured resin dam is in the interproximal spaces to protect gingival tissue.
- Improvements in paint-on rubber dams, cheek, lip retractors, and lower concentrations

of peroxide have made in-office bleaching safer for the patient.

- Treatment may take one to six applications for optimal results.
- Time for each application varies between different products; ranges from 30- to 60-minute treatment.
- Laser/power bleaching treatment plan may also involve use of **bleaching trays** for home use.

B. Professionally Dispensed/ Professionally Monitored

- Also called bleaching trays, external bleaching, at-home bleaching.
- Study model preparation
  - An impression of the teeth is taken to prepare the cast for fabrication of the tray.
  - Inspect impression to ensure all anatomy is present without bubbles or voids.
  - Dental stone is poured into the impression with little delay to avoid distortion.

- Place impression on vibration plate while slowly pouring stone mixture in impression to avoid bubbles on the cast surface.
- After entire arch is filled with stone mixture, let solidify for 1 hour. Remove cast from impression and inspect for voids.
- An ideal cast is trimmed into a horseshoe shape with the central incisors perpendicular to the base to allow proper suction during tray formation.
- With a moderate grasp, place the back of cast on model trimmer pushing lightly.
- Hold the cast with the occlusal plane parallel to wheel until vestibule is removed.
- Light-cured block-out resin can be placed on the surfaces of teeth to be bleached. A 1-mm border with no block-out should be maintained to allow proper fit of bleaching tray to the tooth.
- Tray preparation
  - Thin, vacuum-formed custom trays are made for each dental arch to be bleached.
  - Place prepared cast on base of vacuum former and place sheet of thin tray material in holder. Raise to heating element and heat tray material until it sags 1 inch.
  - Lower material to the vacuum base and allow machine to suction material around cast for 1 minute.
  - Carefully remove from base since material may be hot. Cool completely before removing cast from material.
  - Trays should be trimmed with small, sharp scissors in a smooth motion to produce uniform edges.
  - As shown in **Figure 4**, trays are either scalloped at gingival margin or unscalloped and trimmed 1–2 mm from deepest portion of gingival margin, taking care to cut around the incisive papilla and frena.
  - Unscalloped trays seal better and result in less gingival irritation.[10]
  - Trays are fitted to the patient and adjusted to ensure bleaching material will not come into contact with soft tissues.
- Digital impressions
  - An intraoral scanner is inserted into the oral cavity and moved over the surface of the teeth to create a digital image.
  - The image is displayed on a computer screen and used for fabrication of bleaching trays.
- Patient instruction
  - Instructions and bleaching materials for use in the trays at home should be provided.

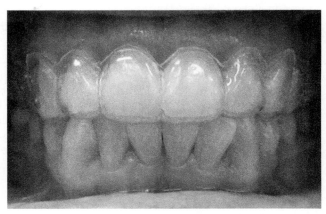

A

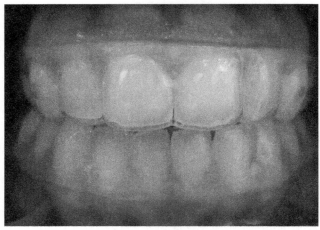

B

Figure 4 Scalloped and Unscalloped Bleaching Tray Designs. Either scalloped or unscalloped trays may be used. **A:** Scalloped trays aim to protect the gingiva and exposed root surfaces. **B:** Unscalloped trays are more comfortable and take less preparation time. Patients need to be warned to avoid overfilling trays.

  - Patient should practice placing correct amount of bleaching gel to demonstrate understanding.
  - Once or twice daily application for 1–2 weeks is usually recommended if lack of sensitivity and other side effects permit. Maximum color change obtained with consistent compliance (see **Figure 5**).
  - The enamel may become more porous during treatment[13]; therefore, patient should be advised to avoid staining agents.
- Patient retains the trays after completion of bleaching to reuse for touch-ups as needed.
- Professionally dispensed bleaching products are commonly recommended after professionally applied bleaching procedures to maintain and promote results.

C. OTC Products

- OTC products may use generic bleaching trays (**Figure 6**).
- When asked about use of the self-directed product, a dental hygienist should stress the need for

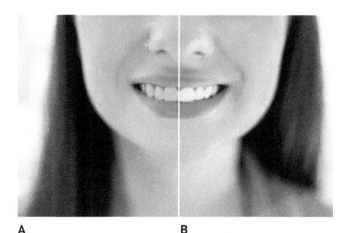

A　　　　　　　　**B**

Figure 5 Professionally Monitored At-Home Bleaching Tray Treatment. **A:** Before treatment. **B:** After treatment.

© SimonSkafar/E+/Getty Images

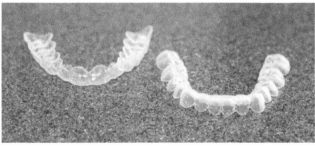

A

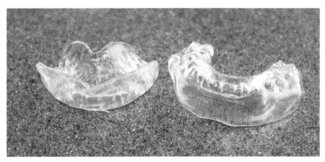

B

Figure 6 Comparison of Professional and OTC Bleaching Trays. **A:** Scalloped professionally dispensed bleaching trays. Professionally dispensed trays are fitted to the patient using impressions, casts, and flexible plastic for custom fit. **B:** Over-the-counter (OTC) bleaching trays made by patient at home and are bulkier.

Photo courtesy Heather Hessheimer, RDH, MS.

professional examination and supervision; the products can cause harm if misused, may irritate tissues, or cause systemic illness if ingested.

- May be recommended to help maintain results of professionally applied and professionally dispensed methods of bleaching.
- The dental professional must be informed of patient's proposed use of OTC products to discuss risks and possible interaction with any proposed dental treatment.
- An oral evaluation is recommended before use of the at-home or OTC products, as well as appropriate dental and periodontal treatment including calculus, stain, and biofilm removal.
- Delivered with various packaging, viscosities, and flavors (**Box 3**).

Box 3 Over-the-Counter Bleaching Preparations

Strips
- Hydrogen peroxide is delivered on polyethylene film strips.
- Strips are placed on the teeth up to two times per day for 30 minutes for about 2 weeks.

Prefabricated Trays
- Thin-membrane tray loaded with bleaching agent is adapted to maxillary or mandibular arch.
- Usually worn 30–60 minutes daily for 5–10 days.

Paint-on
- Carbamide peroxide is incorporated into a thick gel that is painted on the teeth selected to be bleached.
- An advantage to this method is that individual teeth may be bleached.

Dentifrice
- Some have more abrasive materials to remove extrinsic stains.
- Owing to short exposure time, the bleaching agent in the dentifrice has little effect on staining.
- Some contain hydrogen peroxide; others contain agents that may deter further attachment of stains to the teeth.

Mouthrinse
- Contain a variety of active ingredients to bleach teeth, remove stains, or prevent stain retention.
- Content of alcohol is avoided in selection of mouthrinse.

Nonvital Tooth Bleaching

Also called *walking bleach method* and *internal bleaching*, nonvital tooth bleaching involves the bleaching of a single, endodontically treated tooth that is discolored.

- Alternative to more invasive correction, such as a post and core with crown.
- Performed by a dentist.
- Requirements for procedure:
  - Healthy periodontium.
  - Successfully obturated root canal filling.
  - Root canal filling is sealed off with a restorative material before treatment to prevent bleaching agent from reaching periapical tissue.

I. Procedure for Bleaching Nonvital Teeth

- Hydrogen peroxide and/or sodium perborate is placed in the pulp chamber, sealed, and left for 3–7 days, as outlined in **Box 4**.
- Hydrogen peroxide and sodium perborate may be synergistic and very effective in bleaching the tooth.
- The process is repeated until a satisfactory result is obtained.
- Once a satisfactory result is obtained, the pulp chamber is sealed with glass ionomer cement.
- Appoint patient 2 weeks later to place permanent, bonded, composite-resin restoration in access cavity to allow dissipation of residual oxygen that would interfere with efficacy of bonding agent.
- If unsuccessful after repeated attempts, techniques for vital tooth bleaching or an alternative restorative procedure, such as a post and core with crown, can be attempted.

II. Factors Associated with Efficacy

- Results usually last longer than external tooth bleaching.
- There is no universal standard for what is considered acceptable esthetics.
  - Personal background, culture, and patient's image of esthetics are factors.
  - The dentist initially may not identify a patient's esthetic issues in the same way that the patient identifies them.
- Careful communication and agreement about the course of treatment and the expected result of treatment before the start of bleaching by the patient is essential.

Box 4 Procedure for Nonvital Tooth Bleaching

Periodontally healthy, endodontically treated tooth:
1. Photograph of the tooth to be bleached with shade guide.
2. Provide dental hygiene services to remove extrinsic stain and calculus.
3. Probe circumferentially to determine the outline of the cementoenamel junction.
4. Rubber dam isolation is applied to prevent contamination of root canal therapy.
5. Prepare access cavity. Remove all endodontic obturation material, sealer, cement, and necessary restorative material without removing more dentin than necessary.
6. Remove 2–3 mm of obturation material from the root canal to level below the crest of the gingival margin.
7. Irrigate access cavity with copious amount of water and dry well without desiccating.
8. Root canal therapy is sealed off, commonly with glass ionomer cement or other filling material.
9. Medicament is placed in pulp chamber.
10. Pulp chamber is sealed with a temporary restoration.
11. Patient returns in 3–7 days for evaluation.

Aforementioned procedure is repeated several times until desired result is obtained. To finalize procedure:
1. Rubber dam isolation.
2. Temporary restoration on medicament is removed.
3. Pulp chamber is irrigated thoroughly with water.
4. Coronal restoration is placed; generally a composite material.
5. Photograph tooth with corresponding shade guide for records.

Dental Hygiene Process of Care

I. Patient Assessment

- Review of medical history; identify any contraindications for bleaching.
- Complete dental assessment, including the following:
  - Complete extraoral and intraoral examination with oral cancer screening.
  - Updated radiographs.

- Comprehensive dental exam.
  - The presence of cavitated dental caries is a contraindication for bleaching. A lesion is prepared and restored with a temporary restoration to be replaced with permanent matching restoration upon completion of bleaching.
  - To identify abscesses or nonvital teeth, which would require endodontic therapy before bleaching.
- Comprehensive periodontal examination including areas of recession. Cementum needs to be protected from bleaching material to avoid potential internal and/or external resorption.
- Determine initial tooth shade either manually with a shade guide (**Figure 7**) or electronically

with a spectrophotometer (**Figure 8**). **Box 5** provides tips for manually selecting a tooth shade.
- Obtain photographic record of tooth shade without lipstick or strong clothing colors that may interfere with accurate assessment. Use the canine

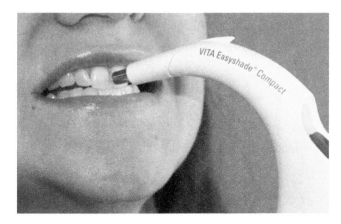

Figure 8 Digital Photographic Record of Tooth Shade. Electronic digital shade guides provide objective records.

Photo courtesy Heather Hessheimer, RDH, MS.

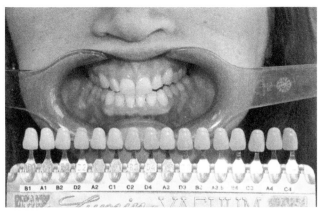

A

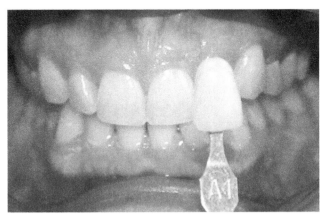

B

Figure 7 Manual Selection of Tooth Shade. Patient's shade taken, recorded, and photographed in natural light or color-corrected lighting after extrinsic stain removal before bleaching. **A:** Several manufacturers provide color ranges with as many as 29 shades.
B: Patient's shade and photograph are recorded at each visit while in bleaching treatment.

Photo courtesy Heather Hessheimer, RDH, MS.

Box 5 Tips for Manually Selecting Tooth Shade

Three concepts should be considered when determining tooth shade: hue, chroma, and value. *Hue* refers to the color of a tooth. Some teeth are more yellow while others are more red or gray. *Chroma* refers to the saturation, or intensity of the color. *Value* is the lightness or brightness of the color. When selecting tooth shade, it is best to start with selecting the proper *value*.

1. Arrange shade guide on the *value* scale with incisal edges oriented for maxilla.
2. Limit extra light sources in the room. Have patient face natural lighting if possible.
3. Remove any distracting colors from view, such as wiping off lipstick or covering brightly colored clothing.
4. Rest eyes by looking at light-gray color prior to shade matching.
5. Hold shade guide close to patient's teeth so shadow of the upper lip will be similar and select the *value* that best represents their tooth brightness. When debating between two shades, select the lighter of the two.
6. Next select the chroma that best correlates in that *value* range.
7. Finally, confirm the *hue* of the selected shade is appropriate for the tooth being matched.

for base color. Color will be gray or yellow. Confirm with patient.

- Identify those factors that would lead to a guarded prognosis for bleaching, such as:
  - Unrealistic expectations of the patient.
  - History of sensitive teeth.
  - Extremely dark gingival third of tooth visible during a smile.
  - Extensive white spots that are very visible.
  - Temporomandibular joint dysfunction or bruxism that would make wearing bleaching trays uncomfortable and potentially aggravate condition.
  - Inability to tolerate the taste of the product.
- Identify contraindications for at-home bleaching, including the following:
  - Unwillingness or inability to comply with at-home treatment routines.
  - Excessive existing restorations not requiring replacement.
  - Pregnancy or lactation.

II. Dental Hygiene Diagnosis

Distortions in body image can include obsessive teeth whitening so it is important to identify when the request for whitening becomes excessive and make appropriate referral.

III. Dental Hygiene Care Plan

- Plan dental hygiene therapy and preventive procedures.
- Choose appropriate bleaching method.
  - Discussion of procedure, risks, and realistic results.
  - Plan with patient for anticipated needs after bleaching, such as replacement of existing tooth-colored restorations that will not match after bleaching.
- List procedure and risks.
- Encourage questions.
- Obtain informed consent and patient's signature.

IV. Implementation

- Education to aid the patient in optimal biofilm removal as it may also help reduce sensitivity.
- Dental hygiene therapy: debridement of all soft and hard deposits along with extrinsic stains.
- Pretreatment desensitization when indicated. Recommended procedures for pretreatment,

during treatment, and post-bleaching are listed in Table 3.

- Premedication with anti-inflammatory pain medication when indicated for sensitivity.
- Preparation of trays: impression and construction.
- Provide patient education and instructions for use with an emphasis on the following:
  - Tooth sensitivity treatment and sensitivity prevention.
  - Effective daily biofilm removal before bleaching material use to prevent additional extrinsic stain accumulation.
  - Avoid or minimize foods and beverages that stain teeth such as coffee, red wine, and use of tobacco to maximize results.
  - Use of nonabrasive whitening dentifrice.
  - Avoidance of overfilling tray to protect soft tissue and exposed cementum.
  - Removal of excess bleaching material after use.
  - Avoidance of swallowing bleaching material due to irritation of materials to mucosa.

V. Evaluation and Planning for Maintenance

- Monitor appointments as needed to assess patient compliance, results, and sensitivity.
- At continuing care appointments, compare tooth color with tooth color guide. Take follow-up photos as appropriate for records.
- Tooth color from bleaching relapses with time.
- Plan for repeat of bleaching process at appropriate intervals.

Documentation

Documentation in the patient's permanent record when planning tooth bleaching includes a minimum of the following:

- Current oral conditions.
- Consent to treat related to tooth bleaching.
- Services provided including necessary records for tooth shade.
- Impressions and preparation of the trays.
- Demonstration of tray filling, positioning, timing, and cleaning.
- Instructions given to patient.
- Planned follow-up care and appointments.
- Patient problems or complaints expressed.
- An example documentation is shown in **Box** **6**.

- **S**–Patient states she is unhappy with the color of teeth. Patient states she has sensitive teeth.
- **O**–Tooth shade: C-1; appears to have only yellow stain. Patient's medical and dental histories present no contraindications for tooth bleaching. Radiographs and dental examination reveal absence of cavitated caries.
- **A**–Patient presents with a deficit in wholesome body image as evidenced by her statement she is self-conscious of tooth color.
- **P**–Consent for treatment signed and copy given to patient. Completed prophylaxis with all extrinsic stain removed. Intraoral photographs obtained to document tooth color. Impressions and preparation of bleaching trays. Dispensed three syringes of carbamide peroxide 10%. Patient instructed to brush with potassium nitrate product for 2 weeks before beginning bleaching process; after beginning bleaching use of carbamide peroxide 10% every other day.

Patient demonstrated dispensing correct amount of bleaching gel into tray. Patient states tray provides comfortable fit; understanding of sensitivity treatment; and willingness to return for follow-up appointment. Next steps: Patient scheduled for follow-up appointment 2 weeks after bleaching process initiated.

Signed: _____, RDH

Date: _____

Factors to Teach the Patient

- Why a complete oral cancer screening and dental examination, including radiographs and periodontal evaluation, is performed before any form of bleaching is initiated.
- During bleaching, teeth and gingival tissues may become sensitive for a period of time.
- If sensitivity is experienced, use a desensitizing product, discontinue bleaching, or delay next treatment.
- Regardless of method, color relapse occurs in a relatively short period of time.
- Excessive use of bleaching products may be harmful. Follow manufacturer's directions.
- Existing tooth-colored restorations will not change color, and therefore may not match and may need to be replaced after bleaching.

References

1. Carey CM. Tooth whitening: what we now know. *J Evid-Based Dent Pract*. 2014;14 Suppl:70-76.
2. Coelho AS, Garrido L, Mota M, et al. Non-vital tooth bleaching techniques: a systematic review. *Coatings*. 2020;10(1):61.
3. Dahl JE, Pallesen U. Tooth bleaching—a critical review of the biological aspects. *Crit Rev Oral Biol Med*. 2003; 14(4):292-304.
4. Haywood VB. History, safety, and effectiveness of current bleaching techniques and applications of the nightguard vital bleaching technique. *Quintessence Int*. 1992;23(7):471-488.
5. de Geus JL, Wambier LM, Boing TF, Loguercio AD, Reis A. At-home bleaching with 10% vs more concentrated carbamide peroxide gels: a systematic review and meta-analysis. *Oper Dent*. 2018;43(4):E210-E222.
6. American Dental Association. Whitening. Oral Health Topics. Published October 30, 2020. https://www.ada.org/en/member-center/oral-health-topics/whitening. Accessed November 4, 2021.
7. Bharti R, Wadhwani K. Spectrophotometric evaluation of peroxide penetration into the pulp chamber from whitening strips and gel: an in vitro study. *J Conserv Dent JCD*. 2013;16(2):131-134.
8. Llena C, Martínez-Galdón O, Forner L, Gimeno-Mallench L, Rodríguez-Lozano FJ, Gambini J. Hydrogen peroxide diffusion through enamel and dentin. *Materials*. 2018;11(9):1694.
9. Ubaldini ALM, Baesso ML, Medina Neto A, Sato F, Bento AC, Pascotto RC. Hydrogen peroxide diffusion dynamics in dental tissues. *J Dent Res*. 2013;92(7):661-665.
10. Haywood VB, Sword RJ. Tray bleaching status and insights. *J Esthet Restor Dent*. 2021;33(1):27-38.
11. Pereira Sanchez N, Aleksic A, Dramicanin M, Paravina RD. Whitening-dependent changes of fluorescence of extracted human teeth. *J Esthet Restor Dent*. 2017;29(5):352-355.
12. Hatırlı H, Karaarslan EŞ, Yaşa B, Kılıç E, Yaylacı A. Clinical effects of dehydration on tooth color: how much and how long? *J Esthet Restor Dent*. 2021;33(2):364-370.
13. Mokhlis GR, Matis BA, Cochran MA, Eckert GJ. A clinical evaluation of carbamide peroxide and hydrogen peroxide whitening agents during daytime use. *J Am Dent Assoc*. 2000;131(9):1269-1277.
14. Zanolla J, Marques A, da Costa DC, de Souza AS, Coutinho M. Influence of tooth bleaching on dental enamel microhardness: a systematic review and meta-analysis. *Aust Dent J*. 2017;62(3):276-282.

15. Martini EC, Favoreto MW, Rezende M, de Geus JL, Loguercio AD, Reis A. Topical application of a desensitizing agent containing potassium nitrate before dental bleaching: a systematic review and meta-analysis. *Clin Oral Investig.* 2021;25(7):4311-4327.

16. Wang Y, Gao J, Jiang T, Liang S, Zhou Y, Matis BA. Evaluation of the efficacy of potassium nitrate and sodium fluoride as desensitizing agents during tooth bleaching treatment—a systematic review and meta-analysis. *J Dent.* 2015;43(8):913-923.

17. Oldoini G, Bruno A, Genovesi AM, Parisi L. Effects of amorphous calcium phosphate administration on dental sensitivity during in-office and at-home interventions. *Dent J.* 2018;6(4):E52.

18. Sari T, Celik G, Usumez A. Temperature rise in pulp and gel during laser-activated bleaching: in vitro. *Lasers Med Sci.* 2015;30(2):577-582.

19. De Moor RJG, Verheyen J, Verheyen P, et al. Laser teeth bleaching: evaluation of eventual side effects on enamel and the pulp and the efficiency in vitro and in vivo. *Sci World J.* 2015;2015:835405.

20. Tredwin CJ, Naik S, Lewis NJ, Scully C. Hydrogen peroxide tooth-whitening (bleaching) products: review of adverse effects and safety issues. *Br Dent J.* 2006;200(7):371-376.

21. Attin T, Hannig C, Wiegand A, Attin R. Effect of bleaching on restorative materials and restorations—a systematic review. *Dent Mater Off Publ Acad Dent Mater.* 2004;20(9):852-861.

22. Munro IC, Williams GM, Heymann HO, Kroes R. Tooth whitening products and the risk of oral cancer. *Food Chem Toxicol Int J Publ Br Ind Biol Res Assoc.* 2006;44(3):301-315.

23. Lugović-Mihić L, Duvančić T, Ferček I, Vuković P, Japundžić I, Ćesić D. Drug-induced photosensitivity - a continuing diagnostic challenge. *Acta Clin Croat.* 2017;56(2):277-283.

24. American Academy of Pediatric Dentistry. Policy on the use of dental bleaching for child and adolescent patients. *Pediatr Dent.* 2018;40(6):92-94.

25. Abdullah Z, John J. Minimally invasive treatment of white spot lesions—a systematic review. *Oral Health Prev Dent.* 2016;14(3):197-205.

26. Gugnani N, Pandit IK, Gupta M, Gugnani S, Soni S, Goyal V. Comparative evaluation of esthetic changes in nonpitted fluorosis stains when treated with resin infiltration, in-office bleaching, and combination therapies. *J Esthet Restor Dent.* 2017;29(5):317-324.

27. Sulieman M. An overview of bleaching techniques: 2. Night guard vital bleaching and non-vital bleaching. *Dent Update.* 2005;32(1):39-40, 42-44, 46.

28. Elfallah HM, Bertassoni LE, Charadram N, Rathsam C, Swain MV. Effect of tooth bleaching agents on protein content and mechanical properties of dental enamel. *Acta Biomater.* 2015;20:120-128.

29. Kazemipoor M, Azad S, Farahat F. Concurrent effects of bleaching materials and the size of root canal preparation on cervical dentin microhardness. *Iran Endod J.* 2017;12(3):298-302.

30. Grazioli G, Valente LL, Isolan CP, Pinheiro HA, Duarte CG, Münchow EA. Bleaching and enamel surface interactions resulting from the use of highly-concentrated bleaching gels. *Arch Oral Biol.* 2018;87:157-162.

31. Bollineni S, Janga RK, Venugopal L, Reddy IR, Babu PR, Kumar SS. Role of fluoridated carbamide peroxide whitening gel in the remineralization of demineralized enamel: an in vitro study. *J Int Soc Prev Community Dent.* 2014;4(2):117-121.

32. Benetti F, Lemos CAA, de Oliveira Gallinari M, et al. Influence of different types of light on the response of the pulp tissue in dental bleaching: a systematic review. *Clin Oral Investig.* 2018;22(4):1825-1837.

Sealants

Jill C. Moore, EdD, MHA, BSDH, RDH

CHAPTER OUTLINE

LEARNING OBJECTIVES

After studying this chapter, the student will be able to:

1. Describe the development and purposes of dental sealant materials.
2. Explain the types of sealant materials and list the criteria of an ideal dental sealant material.
3. List indications and contraindications for placement of dental sealants.
4. Describe the clinical procedures for placement and maintenance of a dental sealant.
5. Explain the factors that affect sealant penetration.
6. Identify factors to document a dental sealant placement in the patient record.

Introduction

A pit and fissure **sealant** is an organic **polymer** (resin) that flows into the pit or fissure of a posterior tooth and bonds by mechanical retention to the tooth.

- Placement of dental sealants is an evidence-based preventive recommendation that can significantly reduce the incidence of dental caries.[1]
- As part of a complete preventive program, pit and fissure sealants are indicated for selected patients.
- Topically applied fluorides protect smooth tooth surfaces more than occlusal surfaces; dental sealants reduce the incidence of occlusal dental caries.
- The incidence of new pit and fissure caries can be lowered by 86% if the sealant is retained at 1 year, 78.6% at 2 years, and 58.6% at 4 years.[2]
- Sealant application is a part of a complete prevention program, not an isolated procedure.
- As an isolated procedure, the patient (and parent) may misunderstand the specific role of sealants in prevention.
- Other surfaces and other teeth still need other methods of preventive protection.

I. Development of Sealants

Sealants were developed by Dr. Michael Buonocore and a group of dental scientists at the Eastman Dental Center in Rochester, New York.[3]

- Early research focused on the need to prepare the enamel surface so a dental material would adhere.
- They demonstrated that, by using an **acid-etchant** process, the enamel could be altered to increase retention.
- The research proved to be a major breakthrough, particularly in esthetic and preventive dentistry.[3,4]

II. Purposes of the Sealant

- Provides a physical barrier to "seal off" the pit or fissure.
- Prevents oral bacteria and their nutrients from collecting within the pit or fissure to create the acid environment necessary for the initiation of dental caries.
- Fills the pit or fissure as deep as possible and provide tight smooth margins at the junction with the enamel surface.[5,6]
- Provides continued protection in the depth of the micropore even when the sealant material is worn or cracked away on the surface around the pit or fissure, and new sealant material can be added for repair and to reseal the enamel/sealant junction.[5]

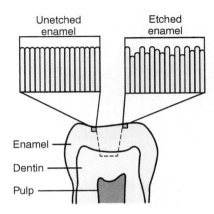

Figure 1 Dental Sealant Adhesion.

III. Purposes of the Acid Etch

- To produce irregularities or **micropores** in the enamel.
- To allow the liquid resin to penetrate into the micropores and create a bond or mechanical locking.
- **Figure 1** demonstrates the microscopic change of the enamel before and after acid etch is placed.

Sealant Materials

The variety of available sealant materials provides options for both the patient and clinician. The clinician decides which material will be most beneficial depending on:

- An assessment of patient needs and caries risk.
- Sealant placement environment.
- Available supplies.

I. Criteria for the Ideal Sealant[3]

- Achieve prolonged **bonding** to the enamel.
- Be biocompatible with oral tissues.
- Offer a simple application procedure.
- Be a free-flowing, low-**viscosity** material capable of entering narrow fissures.
- Have low solubility in the oral environment.

II. Classification of Sealant Materials

- A majority of sealants in clinical use are made of **Bis-GMA** (bisphenol A–glycidyl methylacrylate).[5] The techniques of application vary slightly among available products; follow manufacturer's directions.
- There is no difference in the preventive effect of resin-based or glass-ionomer cement. Resin-based

application will generate aerosols and glass-ionomer cement can be placed without generating aerosols.[7] Follow updated Centers for Disease Control and Prevention guidance specific to aerosol generating procedures (AGPs). See Chapter 6 for more on AGPs.

A. Classification by the Method of Polymerization

- Self-cured or **autopolymerized**
  - Preparation: material supplied in two parts. When the two are mixed, they quickly polymerize (harden).
  - Advantage: no **curing** light required.
  - Disadvantages: mixing required; working time limited because **polymerization** begins when the material is mixed.
- Visible light-cured or **photopolymerized**
  - Preparation: material hardens when exposed to a special curing light.
  - Advantages: no mixing required; increased working time due to control over start of polymerization.
  - Disadvantages: extra costs and disinfection time required for curing light, protective shields, and/or glasses.

B. Classification by Filler Content

- Filled
  - Purpose of filler: to increase **bond strength** and resistance to abrasion and wear.
  - Fillers: glass and quartz particles give hardness and strength to resist occlusal forces.
  - Effect: viscosity of the sealant is increased. Flow into the depth of a fissure varies.
- Unfilled
  - Clear, does not contain particles.
  - Less resistant to abrasion and wear.
  - May not require occlusal adjustment after placement, so provides an advantage for school and community health programs where sealants are placed.
- Fluoride releasing
- Purpose: to enhance caries resistance.
- Action: remineralization of **incipient caries** at the base of the pit or fissure.

C. Classification by Color

- Available: clear, tinted, and opaque.
- Purpose: quick identification for evaluation during maintenance assessment.

- Effect: clear, tinted, or opaque sealants do not differ in retention.

Indications for Sealant Placement

Individual patient benefit will depend on the following:

- Health, diet, and lifestyle.
- Age of tooth and past caries experience.
- Tooth anatomy.

I. Patients at Risk for Dental Caries (Any Age)

The following risk factors will lead to an increased risk of dental caries:

- Xerostomia: from medications or other reasons.
- Patient undergoing orthodontic treatment.
- Incipient pit and fissure caries (limited to the enamel) with no radiographic evidence of caries on an adjacent proximal surface.
- Low socioeconomic status.
- Diet high in sugars.
- Inadequate daily oral health care.

II. Selection of Teeth

- Newly erupted: place sealant as soon as the tooth is fully erupted.[8]
- Occlusal contour: when pit or fissure is deep and irregular, as illustrated in **Figure 2**.

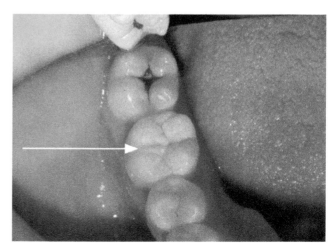

Figure 2 Molar Tooth with Pits and Fissures. Tooth #30 with deep fissures is selected for placing a dental sealant. Note the amalgam filling on tooth #31, which is evidence of previous dental caries experience.

Photograph courtesy of Jill Moore, EdD, MHA, BSDH, RDH, School Oral Health Consultant, Michigan Department of Health and Human Services.

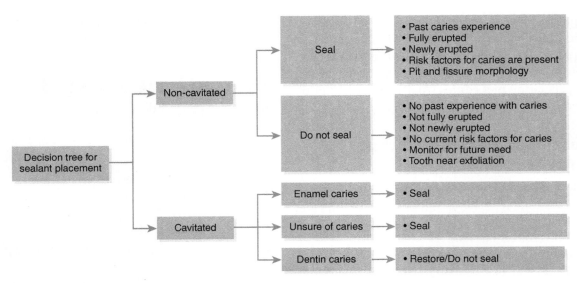

Figure 3 Decision Tree for Sealant Placement. Flowchart to assist in decision making for placement of sealants.

Developed by Jill C. Moore, EdD, MHA, BSDH, RDH.

- Caries history: other teeth restored or have carious lesions.
- **Figure 3** is a flowchart to assist in decision making.

III. Contraindications for Sealant Placement

- Radiographic evidence of adjacent proximal dental caries.
- Pit and fissures are well coalesced and self-cleansing; low caries risk.
- Tooth not completely erupted.
- Primary tooth near exfoliation.

Penetration of Sealant

Penetration of sealant material to the depth of the fissure depends on the following:

- Configuration of the pit or fissure.
- Presence of deposits and debris within the pit or fissure.
- Properties of the sealant itself.

I. Pit and Fissure Anatomy

The shape and depth of pits and fissures vary considerably even within one tooth. (**Figure 4A**) Anatomic differences include:

- Wide V-shaped (**Figure 4B**) or narrow V-shaped fissures.
- Long narrow pits and grooves reach, or nearly reach, the dentinoenamel junction (**Figure 4C**).

- Long constricted fissures with a bulbous terminal portion (**Figure 4D**) that may take a wavy course, which may not lead directly from the outer surface to the dentinoenamel junction.

II. Contents of a Pit or Fissure

A pit or fissure may contain the following:

- Dental biofilm, pellicle, debris.
- Rarely but possibly intact remnants of tooth development.

III. Effect of Cleaning

- Cleaning the tooth prior to acid etching can increase sealant retention.
- Use of an air polisher or laser prior to acid etching is not well supported by the literature, mainly because of added cost.[9]
- Cleaning the tooth with a toothbrush and water is ideal because the narrow, long fissures are difficult to clean completely.[10]
- Removal of pumice used for cleaning and thorough washing are necessary for retention of the sealant.
- Cleaning the tooth with pumice prior to dental sealant placement is avoided; if used, complete removal of pumice is necessary.
- Retained cleaning material can block the sealant from filling the fissure and can also get mixed with the sealant.

IV. Amount of Penetration

- Wide V-shaped and shallow fissures are more apt to be filled by sealants (Figure 4B).

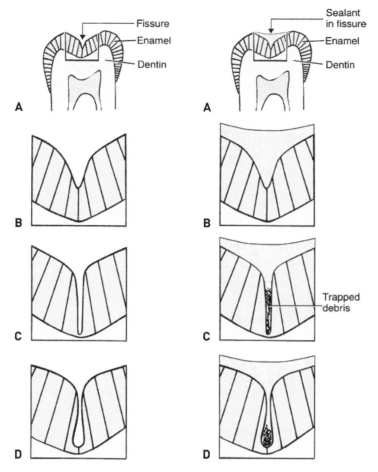

Figure 4 Occlusal Fissures. Drawings made from microscopic slides show variations in the shape and depth of fissures both before and after sealant placement. **A:** Tooth with section enlarged for (B–D). **B:** Wide V-shaped fissure shows full sealant penetration. **C:** Long narrow groove that nearly reaches the dentinoenamel junction. **D:** Long constricted form with a bulbous terminal portion.

- Although ideally the sealant penetrates to the bottom of a pit or fissure, such penetration is frequently impossible.
- Microscopic examination of pits and fissures after sealant application has shown the sealant material often does not penetrate to the bottom because residual debris, cleaning agents, and trapped air prevent passage of the material (Figure 4C–D).
- The bacteria in incipient dental caries at the base of a well-sealed pit or fissure have no access to nutrients required for survival.

Clinical Procedures

To achieve high dental sealant retention rates:

- Treat each quadrant separately while placing sealants on all eligible teeth.

- Use the four-handed method with an assistant:
  - To ensure moisture control.
  - To work efficiently and save time.
- Follow manufacturer's directions for each product.
- Success of treatment (retention) depends on the precision in each step of the application.
- Retention of sealant depends on maintaining a dry field during etching and sealant placement.
- Step-by-step clinical procedures and equipment/supplies needed for the placement of a dental sealant are illustrated in **Table 1**. Additional details for each step are provided in Sections I through IX.

I. Patient Preparation

- Explain the procedure and steps to be performed.
- Provide patient with ultraviolet (UV)-protective safety eyewear for protection from:

Table 1 Steps for Placement of a Photopolymerized Dental Sealant

Step	Illustration	Description	Equipment and Supplies
Step 1	 Courtesy of Jill Moore, RDH, BSDH, MHA, EdD, School Oral Health Consultant, Michigan Department of Health and Human Services.	Patient preparation ■ Seat patient comfortably. ■ Provide patient education materials and answer questions. ■ Provide ultraviolet (UV)-protective eyewear for protection from chemicals and curing light.	■ Patient education materials ■ Safety glasses for patient
Step 2	 Courtesy of Susan J. Jenkins, RDH, MS, CAGS, Forsyth School of Dental Hygiene, MCPHS University.	Tooth preparation ■ Clean the tooth with a toothbrush. ■ Ensure the tooth is free from debris, external stain, and calculus prior to sealant placement.	■ Toothbrush ■ Examination instruments (mirror and explorer)
Step 3	 Courtesy of Jill Moore, RDH, BSDH, MHA, EdD, School Oral Health Consultant, Michigan Department of Health and Human Services. Courtesy of Jill Moore, RDH, BSDH, MHA, EdD, School Oral Health Consultant, Michigan Department of Health and Human Services.	Tooth isolation ■ Maintain a working field that is not contaminated by saliva during all steps of sealant placement. ■ Options include: • Rubber dam (not shown) • Cotton rolls on the mandibular arch (top left) • Triangular bibulous pad to cover the parotid duct for the maxillary arch (lower left) • Commercial isolation system with light and high speed suction (**Figure 5A**) • Note: Take care to moisten all cotton prior to removal to avoid sticking to dry mucosa.	■ Rubber dam set up (optional) ■ Cotton rolls and holders (**Figure 5B**) ■ Bibulous pads (lower left)
Step 4	 Courtesy of Susan J. Jenkins, RDH, MS, CAGS, Forsyth School of Dental Hygiene, MCPHS University. Courtesy of Jill Moore, RDH, BSDH, MHA, EdD, School Oral Health Consultant, Michigan Department of Health and Human Services.	Acid etch ■ Dry entire area for 20–30 sec with air/water syringe. ■ Maintain a dry field. Use a commercial etchant applicator (shown), brush, or cotton pellet to dispense etchant material. ■ Place the acid etch only within the grooves and fissures where the sealant will be placed (shown at lower left). ■ Note: Follow manufacturer's directions for application time; usually between 15 and 60 sec.	■ Air/water syringe ■ Acid-etch material and applicator, brush, or cotton pellet

Step	Illustration	Description	Equipment and Supplies
Step 5	Courtesy of Jill Moore, RDH, BSDH, MHA, EdD, School Oral Health Consultant, Michigan Department of Health and Human Services.	Rinse and air dry tooth ■ Place the high-velocity evacuation system over the tooth. ■ Rinse the tooth with the air/water syringe. ■ Spray water until the surface is free of etch (30–60 sec). ■ Spray air with an air/water syringe until dry. ■ Re-isolate if necessary.	■ High-velocity evacuation system ■ Air/water syringe
Step 6	Courtesy of Jill Moore, RDH, BSDH, MHA, EdD, School Oral Health Consultant, Michigan Department of Health and Human Services.	Evaluate for complete etching ■ A completely etched tooth will have a chalky-white appearance when dry. ■ If the surface does not appear chalky, repeat the acid-etch step.	■ Air/water syringe ■ Mouth mirror for retraction and indirect vision
Step 7	Courtesy of Susan J. Jenkins, RDH, MS, CAGS, Forsyth School of Dental Hygiene, MCPHS University.	Place sealant material ■ Continue to maintain a dry field. ■ Use external fulcrum (fingers resting lightly on patient's chin or cheek). ■ Place the wet sealant material in the prepared pits and fissures. ■ Adjust flow so sealant material is deposited only within the grooves, pits, and fissures.	■ Sealant material and applicator ■ Slow-speed saliva ejector to help maintain dry field
Step 8	Courtesy of Susan J. Jenkins, RDH, MS, CAGS, Forsyth School of Dental Hygiene, MCPHS University.	Cure sealant If using light-polymerized sealant material: ■ Ensure clinician and patient have UV-protective eye protection. ■ Cover entire tooth with light and cure for 20–30 sec in accordance with manufacturer's instructions. If using self-curing sealant material: ■ Maintain dry field and allow drying time as indicated in manufacturer's instructions.	■ UV-protective goggles/glasses for patient and clinicians ■ Curing light ■ Saliva ejector to help maintain dry field
Step 9	Courtesy of Jill Moore, RDH, BSDH, MHA, EdD, School Oral Health Consultant, Michigan Department of Health and Human Services.	Final/cured sealant ■ Gently check for voids in the sealant material with explorer. ■ Additional material can be added if the surface is not contaminated or wet.	■ Mirror and explorer ■ Saliva ejector to help maintain dry field ■ Additional sealant material, if needed, to fill voids

(continues)

Step	Illustration	Description	Equipment and Supplies
Step 10	 Courtesy of Susan J. Jenkins, RDH, MS, CAGS, Forsyth School of Dental Hygiene, MCPHS University	Check occlusion ■ Use articulating paper to locate high spots and adjust as needed. ■ Unfilled sealant material will wear down via normal attrition. ■ Filled sealant material will require occlusal adjustment.	■ Articulating paper ■ Holder
Step 11	 Courtesy of National Institute of Dental and Craniofacial Research. https://www .nidcr.nih.gov/sites/default/files/2017-11 /seal-out-tooth-decay-parents.pdf.	Follow-up ■ Provide patient education materials for the patient to take home. ■ Answer patient's questions. ■ Re-evaluate sealants at each subsequent maintenance appointment.	■ Excellent patient education materials are available for free from the National Institute of Dental and Craniofacial Research website (www .nidcr.nih.gov /orderpublications/).

Photographs in Steps 2, 4A, 7, 8, and 10 courtesy of Susan J. Jenkins, RDH, PhD, Forsyth School of Dental Hygiene, MCPHS University. Photograph in Step 11 courtesy of National Institute of Dental and Craniofacial Research. https://www.nidcr.nih.gov/sites/default/files/2017-11/seal-out-tooth-decay-parents.pdf. Additional photographs courtesy of Jill Moore, EdD, MHA, BSDH, RDH, School Oral Health Consultant, Michigan Department of Health and Human Services.

- Chemicals used during etching and sealant placement.
- The UV light from the curing lamp.

II. Tooth Preparation

A. Purposes

- Remove deposits and debris.
- Permit maximum contact of the etch and the sealant with the enamel surface.
- Encourage sealant penetration into the pit or fissure.

B. Methods

- Examine the tooth surfaces: remove calculus and stain.
- For a patient with no stain or calculus, apply toothbrush filaments straight into occlusal pits and fissures.
- Suction the pits and fissures with a high-velocity evacuator.
- Gently use the explorer tip to remove debris and bacteria from the pit or fissure and suction again to remove loosened material.
- Evaluate the need for additional cleaning; brushing may be sufficient.

III. Tooth Isolation

A. Purposes of Isolation

- Maintaining a dry tooth is the single most important factor in sealant retention.
- Keep the tooth clean and dry for optimal action and bonding of the sealant.
- Eliminate possible contamination by saliva and moisture from the breath.
- Keep the materials from contacting the oral tissues, being swallowed accidentally, or being unpleasant to the patient because of their flavor.

B. Rubber Dam Isolation

- Rubber dam application is the method of choice for complete isolation. This method is especially helpful when more than one tooth in the same quadrant is to be sealed.
- Rubber dam is essential when profuse saliva flow and overactive tongue and oral muscles make retraction and consistent maintenance of a dry, clean field impossible.
- When a quadrant has a rubber dam and anesthesia for restoration of other teeth, teeth indicated for sealant can be treated at the same time.

- Use local anesthesia when application of the clamp cannot be tolerated by the patient.
- Rubber dam may not be possible when a tooth needed to hold the clamp is not fully erupted.

C. Cotton-Roll Isolation

- Patient position: tilt the head to allow saliva to pool on the opposite side of the mouth.
- Position cotton-roll holder. **Figure 5A** shows the placement of two types of cotton-roll holders.
- Place a saliva ejector.
- Apply triangular saliva absorber (**bibulous pad**) over the opening of the parotid duct in the cheek.
- Take care to prevent saliva contamination from entering the area to be etched.

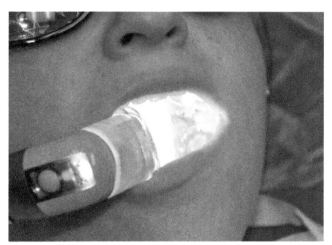

A

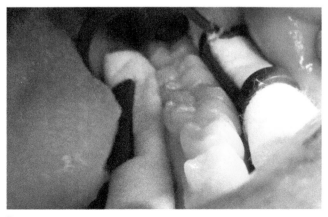

B

Figure 5 Tooth Isolation. **A:** Demonstrates a commercial isolation system which has an internal light and high evacuation suction. This system will allow for two-handed sealant placement. **B:** Illustrates a disposable plastic cotton roll holder used to isolate teeth in a mandibular quadrant.

Photographs courtesy of Jill Moore, EdD, MHA, BSDH, RDH, School Oral Health Consultant, Michigan Department of Health and Human Services.

D. Additional Isolation Options

- Commercially available isolation systems (**Figure 5B**) that can be attached to the dental unit offer intraoral quadrant isolation, illumination, and suction.

IV. Acid Etch

A. Dry the Tooth

- Purposes
  - Prepare the tooth for acid etch.
  - Eliminate moisture and contamination.
- Use clean, dry air
  - Clear water from the air/water syringe by releasing the spray into a sink.
  - Test for absence of moisture by blowing on a mouth mirror or other dry surface.
- Air dry the tooth for at least 10 seconds.

B. Apply Etchant

- Action
  - Creates micropores to increase the surface area and provide retention for the sealant.
  - Removes contamination from the enamel surface.
  - Provides antibacterial action.
- Etchant solution forms
  - Phosphoric acid: 15% to 50%, depends on the product and manufacturer.
  - Liquid: low viscosity allows good flow into the pit or fissure but may be difficult to control.
  - Gel: tinted gel with thick consistency allows increased visibility and control but may be difficult to rinse off the tooth surface.
  - Semi-gel: tinted, with enough viscosity to allow good visibility, control, and rinsing ease.
- Etchant timing varies from 15 to 60 seconds. Follow manufacturer's instructions for each product.
- Etchant delivery
  - Liquid etch: use a small brush, sponge, or cotton pellet; continuously pat rather than rub, when applying to keep the surface moist.
  - Gel and semi-gel: use a syringe, brush, or manufacturer-supplied single-use cannula.

V. Rinse and Air Dry Tooth

- Rinse thoroughly; apply continuous suction to prevent saliva from reaching the etched surface.
- Dry for 15–20 seconds and maintain a dry field through isolation.

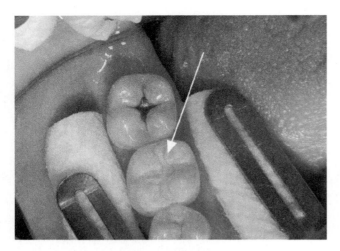

Figure 6 Placement of Dental Sealant Material. Appropriate placement of a dental sealant will completely fill pits and fissures, but not compromise occlusion by overfilling to a high, flat surface.

Photograph courtesy of Jill Moore, EdD, MHA, BSDH, RDH, School Oral Health Consultant, Michigan Department of Health and Human Services.

VI. Evaluate for Complete Etching

- Dry and examine the etched surface.
- Repeat etching process if the surface does not appear chalky white.

VII. Place Sealant Material

Follow manufacturer's instructions included in the sealant material package. General instructions include:

- Avoid overmanipulation of sealant materials to prevent producing air bubbles.
- Use the disposable implement supplied in the sealant material package for application.
- Flow minimal amount into all pits and fissures; do not overfill to a high, flat surface.
- **Figure 6** illustrates a correctly filled dental sealant surface.

VIII. Cure Sealant

- If using a light-cured sealant material:
  - Leave the liquid sealant material in place for 10 seconds to allow for optimum penetration.
  - Use UV-blocking eye protection for both the clinician and patient.
  - Apply the curing light for 20–30 seconds in accordance with the manufacturer's instructions. Cover the entire tooth surface with the light to ensure complete polymerization.

- If using an autopolymerized sealant material, consult the manufacturer's instructions for curing time.

IX. Evaluate Cured Sealant

- Check for voids gently with explorer: additional sealant material can be added if the surface is not contaminated or wet.

X. Check Occlusion

- Use **articulating paper** to locate high spots; adjust as required.
- Occlusal wear: unfilled sealants wear down via normal attrition to the correct height; **filled sealants** require occlusal adjustment.

XI. Follow-Up

- Educate the patient.
- Administer fluoride treatment.
- Re-evaluate at each subsequent appointment.

Maintenance

Dental sealants need to be in place to prevent caries, and should be checked for the following[11]:

- Retention.
- Need for replacement when sealant is missing or partially retained.

I. Retention

- At each continuing care appointment, or at least every 6 months, each sealant needs to be examined for retention and to identify deficiencies that may have developed.
- Properly placed dental sealants can be retained for many years.[1,2]

II. Factors Affecting Retention

- During placement: precision of technique with exclusion of moisture and contamination.
- Patient self-care: advise patient to avoid biting or chewing on hard surfaces such as a pencil or ice cubes.
- Dental hygiene care: avoid using an air-powder polisher on intact sealants during maintenance appointments.[12]

III. Replacement

- Consult the manufacturer's instructions.
- Tooth preparation: same as for original application.
- Removal of firmly attached sections of retained sealant is not usually necessary.
- Re-etching of the tooth surface prior to replacement of a dental sealant is always essential.

School-Based Dental Sealant Programs

- Healthy People 2030 Objectives call for an increase in children and adolescents who have received dental sealants.
- Many states in the United States are not meeting national goals for delivering dental sealants to low-income children.[13]
- Delivery of dental sealants in school-based settings is a proven strategy[13,14] that can:
  - Effectively increase the percentage of children in communities who receive dental sealants.
  - Reduce the risk for decay for high-risk children.
- Many such school-based programs provide additional preventive services such as screening, prophylaxis, topical fluoride application, and oral health education.[11]
- Programs that provide sealants are an effective adjunct to preventive care provided in traditional dental care settings.[1,2]
- **Figure 7** shows a portable dental unit set up in a classroom in a public school The tent is incorporated to assist in controlling aerosols and spatter in a public setting.

Documentation

Documentation in the record of a patient receiving a sealant contains a minimum of the following:

- Reason for selection of certain teeth for sealants; informed consent of patient, parent, or other caregiver.
- Type of sealant used, preparation of tooth, manner of isolation, patient cooperation during administration; postinsertion instructions given.
- Sample documentation for placement of dental sealants may be reviewed in **Box 1**.

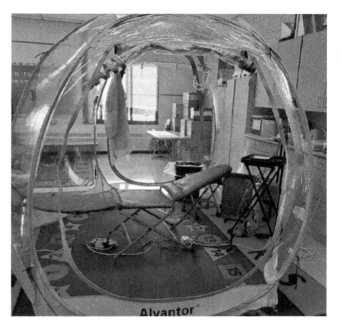

Figure 7 Delivery of Dental Sealants in a School-Based Program Using Portable Dental Equipment Set Up in the School Library.

Photograph courtesy of Jill Moore, EdD, MHA, BSDH, RDH , School Oral Health Consultant, Michigan Department of Health and Human Services.

Box 1 Example Documentation: Placement of Dental Sealants

- **S**—A 12-year-old male patient presents for dental sealant placement.
- **O**—Occlusal contour and previous history of dental caries in primary dentition indicate need for sealant placement for second molars; X-rays indicate no dental caries on proximal surfaces of second molars. Tooth #30 partially erupted with operculum.
- **A**—Need to wait until #30 is completely erupted to place sealant.
- **P**—Reviewed sealant education materials with mother and patient. Mother provided consent for placement of the recommended sealants. Sealants placed on #3-O, 14-O, 14-L, 19-O, 19-B pit using right-side, then left-side isolation. Autopolymerized opaque sealant material used with 15% acid etch, applied as per manufacturer's directions. Patient tolerated treatment well, no gagging, minimal saliva, easy isolation.

Next steps: Schedule in 1 month to re-examine for sealant placement on #30 and retention check on 3, 14, and 19.

Signed: _____, RDH

Date: _____

Factors to Teach the Patient

- Sealants are part of a total preventive program. They are not substitutes for other preventive measures. Limitations of dietary sucrose, refined carbohydrate intake, use of fluorides, and dental biofilm control are major factors along with sealants for prevention of dental caries.
- What a sealant is and why such a meticulous application procedure is required.
- What can be expected from a sealant; how long it may last and how it prevents dental caries.
- Need for examination of the sealant at frequent, scheduled maintenance appointments, and need for replacement when missing or chipped.
- Avoid biting hard items such as a pencil, hard candy, or ice cubes to increase sealant retention.

References

1. Ahovuo-Saloranta A, Forss H, Walsh T, et al. Sealants for preventing dental decay in the permanent teeth. *Cochrane Database Syst Rev.* 2013;(3):CD001830.
2. Beauchamp J, Caufiel PW, Crall JJ, et al. Evidence-based clinical recommendations for the use of pit-and-fissure sealants: a report of the American Dental Association Council on Scientific Affairs. *J Am Dent Assoc.* 2008;139(3):257-268.
3. Handleman SL, Shey Z. Michael Buonocore and the Eastman Dental Center: a historic perspective on sealants. *J Dent Res.* 1996;75(1):529-534.
4. Cueto EI, Buonocore MG. Sealing of pits and fissures with an adhesive resin: its use in caries prevention. *J Am Dent Assoc.* 1967;75(1):121-128.
5. Wright JT, Tampi MP, Graham L, et al. Sealants for preventing and arresting pit-and-fissure occlusal caries in primary and permanent molars. *J Am Dent Assoc.* 2016;147(8):631-645.
6. Wright JT, Crall JJ, Fontana M, et al. Evidence-based clinical practice guideline for the use of pit-and-fissure sealants. A report of the American Dental Association and the American Academy of Pediatric Dentistry. *J Am Dent Assoc.* 2016;147(8):672-682.
7. Eden E, Frencken J, Gao S, Horst JA, Innes N. Managing dental caries against the backdrop of COVID-19: approaches to reduce aerosol generation. *Br Dent J.* 2020;229(7):411-416.
8. Jaafar N, Ragab H, Abedrahman A, Osman E. Performance of fissure sealants on fully erupted permanent molars with

incipient carious lesions: a glass-ionomer-based versus a resin-based sealant. *J Dent Res Dent Clin Dent Prospects.* 2020;14(1):61-67.
9. Bagherian A, Sarraf Shirazi A. Preparation before acid etching in fissure sealant therapy: yes or no?: a systemic review and meta-analysis. *J Am Dent Assoc.* 2016;147(12):943-951.
10. Deery C. Brushing as good as handpiece prophylaxis before placing sealants. *Evid Based Dent.* 2010;11:79-80.
11. Sreedevi A, Brizuela M, Mohamed S. Pit and fissure sealants. *StatPearls*; 2021. https://www.ncbi.nlm.nih.gov/books/NBK448116/. Accessed October 3, 2022.
12. Pelka MA, Altmaier K, Petschelt A, Lohbauer U. The effect of air-polishing abrasives on wear of direct restoration materials and sealants. *J Am Dent Assoc.* 2010;141(1):63-70.
13. PEW Center on the States. *States Stalled on Dental Sealant Programs: A 50-State Report.* Washington, DC: The PEW Charitable Trusts; 2015. http://www.pewtrusts.org/~/media/assets/2015/04/dental_sealantreport_final.pdf. Accessed September 9, 2021.
14. Children's Dental Health Project. *Dental Sealants: Proven to Prevent Decay.* Washington, DC: Children's Dental Health Project; 2014:21. https://www.cdhp.org/resources/314-dental-sealants-proven-to-prevent-tooth-decay. Accessed September 9, 2021.

Sutures and Dressings

Susan J. Jenkins, RDH, PhD

CHAPTER OUTLINE

LEARNING OBJECTIVES

After studying this chapter, the student will be able to:

1. State the functions and purposes of sutures and periodontal dressings.
2. Describe the differences between absorbable and nonabsorbable sutures.
3. Describe the procedure for suture removal.
4. Describe the procedure for periodontal dressing placement and periodontal dressing removal.
5. Explain approaches for managing biofilm with the periodontal dressing in place and upon removal.

Many periodontal surgical procedures require sutures and dressings. The dental hygienist will often participate in the patient's oral self-care instruction at initial placement and during postoperative care.

Sutures

I. The Ideal Suture Material

- A **suture** is a strand of material used to control bleeding, stabilize the wound edges in the proper position, protect the wound, and aid in patient comfort.[1]
  - Sutures are necessary in many oral surgical procedures when a surgical wound must be closed, a flap positioned, or tissue grafted.
- Historically, a wide range of suture materials has been used, including silk, cotton, linen, and animal tendons and intestines.
- The ideal suture material is nonallergenic, easy to handle, and sterile; has adequate **tensile strength**; does not interfere with healing; causes minimal inflammatory reaction; and has some capacity to stretch to allow for wound edema.[1,2]
  - Ultimately, the ideal suture does not exist and each surgeon must select the best suture material based on the surgical procedure to be performed and patient and wound characteristics.[2]

II. Functions of Sutures

- Close periodontal wounds and secure grafts in position.
- Assist in maintaining **hemostasis**.
- Reduce posttreatment discomfort.
- Promote primary intention healing.
- Prevent underlying bone exposure.
- Protect a healing surgical wound from foreign debris and trauma.

III. Characteristics of Suture Materials

A. Biologic Characteristics

The biologic characteristics of suture materials include the following[1]:

- Sterility.
- Reabsorption ability.
- Tolerability: creates minimal inflammatory reaction in the tissue.

B. Physical Characteristics

Physical characteristics of suture materials include the following[1]:

- Tensile strength.
- Flexibility: ability to twist and tie knot without breaking.
- Plasticity: ability to maintain new shape.
- Elasticity: ability of material to stretch and return to original shape.
- Maneuverability: easy to handle and able to create a small knot.
- Fluency: passes through tissue with minimal trauma.
- Length and diameter: various lengths and diameters are available.

IV. Classification of Suture Materials

A. Type of Material Used

- Two types of suture materials are used[1]:
  - Natural: classified into animal origin (i.e., catgut and silk) and vegetal origin (i.e., cotton and linen).
  - Synthetic: developed to reduce tissue reactions and unpredictable rates of absorption commonly found in natural sutures.

B. Absorption Properties

- Absorbable sutures
  - Natural absorbable sutures: digested by body enzymes.
    - Plain gut: monofilamentous, derived from purified collagen of sheep or cattle and lasts about 8 days before beginning to degrade.[1]
    - Chromic gut: contain chromatic salts to delay enzyme resorption for 18 days.[1]
- Synthetic resorbable sutures: broken down by **hydrolysis**, a process in which water slowly penetrates the suture filaments to cause a breakdown of the suture's polymer chain.
  - Example: polyglactin (Vicryl), poliglecaprone (Monocryl), and polydioxanone (PDS II).
- Nonabsorbable sutures: not digested by body enzymes or hydrolyzation; patient returns for removal usually after 1 week.
  - Natural nonabsorbable
    - Silk.
  - Synthetic nonabsorbable
    - Nylon (Ethilon).
    - Polyester (Ethibond).
    - Polypropylene (Prolene).

- ◦ Polytetrafluoroethylene (PTFE) (Gore-Tex).
- ◦ Coated sutures: Suture material coated with the antibacterial agents chlorhexidine may provide antibacterial efficacy and oral biofilm inhibition, reducing surgical site infections.[1,3,4]
- Although nonabsorbable silk sutures have been widely used, research is showing silk sutures increase inflammation at the suture site due to bacterial accumulation, increasing patient discomfort and increased healing time. All suture material attract bacteria.[5,6]
  - Of the nonabsorbable suture material, nylon sutures have demonstrated the lowest bacterial accumulation.
- Current trends are favoring adsorptive suture materials. Ultimately, suture choice is determined by the provider.

C. Number of Strands

- Monofilament suture: single strand of material; typical of gut, nylon, PTFE, and other synthetic sutures.[1]
- Multifilament suture: several strands twisted or braided together: typical of silk, nylon, polyglycolic acid, polyester, and other synthetic sutures.[1]

D. Diameter of Suture Material

- Numbers range from 1 to 10 and are associated with diameter.
- Thin sutures have the greatest number of zeros from 1-0 to 12-0.

V. Selection of Suture Materials

Choosing the appropriate suture material for a specific procedure is critical both for patient comfort and tissue health. Suture selection is based on the following[2]:

- Preference and experience of the surgeon.
- Characteristics of the tissue and the presence of saliva.
- Characteristics of the wound such as length and tissue type (mucosa vs. attached gingiva).
- Cosmetic implications.
  - Examples of suture types surgeons may use for specific procedures are listed in **Table 1.**

Needles

Many types of suturing needles are available. Their use and selection are primarily based on specific procedures, location for use, and clinician's preference.

Table 1 Selection of Suture Material

Suture Types	Specific Dental Procedures
Silk, nonabsorbable, braided	Periodontal flaps and closure
Nylon, monofilament	Periodontal flaps and closure
Polyester, braided	Periodontal flaps and closure
Gut, absorbable	Extraction socket, bone grafting, free-gingival grafting
Absorbable preferred: nonabsorbable used when pain and swelling may be anticipated	Implant flap closure

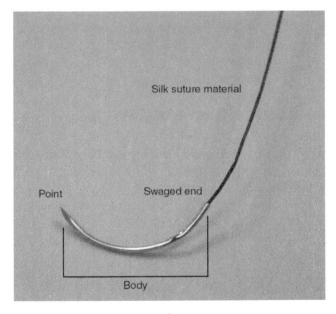

Figure 1 Suture Needle Components

Courtesy of Susan Jenkins, MCPHS University Forsyth School of Dental Hygiene.

I. Needle Components

- Swaged end (eyeless)
  - The **swaged** end allows the suture material and needle to act as one unit (**Figure 1**).
- Body
  - Shape/curvature
    - ◦ Straight.
    - ◦ Half-curved.
    - ◦ Curved 1/4, 3/8, 1/2, 5/8 (**Figure 2**).
  - Diameter
    - ◦ Gauge or size; finer for delicate surgeries.

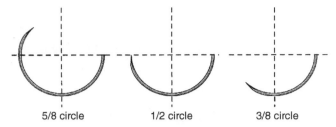

5/8 circle   1/2 circle   3/8 circle

Figure   **2** Suture Needles. A curved needle is manipulated with a needle holder. The 3/8 curve is most effective for closure of skin and mucous membranes and is a needle of choice in many dental and periodontal surgeries.

- The body is the strongest part of the needle that is grasped with the needleholder during the surgical procedure.
- The swaged end is the weakest part of the body.
- Point
  - Point of the needle extends from the extreme tip of the needle to the widest part of the body.
  - Each needle point is designed and manufactured to penetrate tissue with the highest degree of sharpness.

II. Needle Characteristics

- Material
  - Most needles are made of stainless steel formulated and sterilized for surgical use.
- Attachment
  - Majority of needles are permanently attached to suture material.
  - Eliminates need for threading and unnecessary handling.
- Cutting edge (**Figure**   **3**)
  - Reverse cut: the sharpest needle[3]; has two opposing cutting edges, with a third located on the outer convex curve of needle.
  - Conventional cut: consists of two opposing cutting edges and a third within the concave curvature of the needle.
- Requirements
  - Needle point: designed to meet the needs of specific surgical procedures.
    - Sharp enough to penetrate tissues with minimal resistance.
    - Rigid enough to resist bending, yet are flexible.
    - Sterile and corrosion resistant.
  - Surgical needles: intended to carry suture material through tissues with minimal trauma.

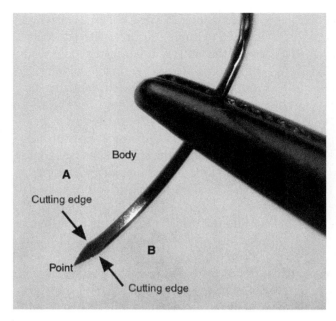

Figure   **3** Suture Needles. Shapes of Points. Triangle shows cross section of needle point. **A:** Conventional cutting with third cutting edge on the inside of the needle curvature. **B:** Reverse cutting with a third of cutting edge on the outer curvature of the needle, used for difficult-to-penetrate tissue, such as skin.

Courtesy of Susan Jenkins, MCPHS University Forsyth School of Dental Hygiene.

Knots

The book *Surgical Knots and Suturing Techniques*[7] describes a variety of surgical knots. Only a few are used in dentistry.

- Type of knot used will depend on the:
  - Specific procedure.
  - Location of the incision.
  - Amount of stress the wound will endure.
- Square knots are most frequently used in dentistry because they are the easiest and most reliable.

I. Knot Characteristics

- The knot is tied as small as possible.
- Completed knot needs to be firm to reduce slipping.
- Excessive tension should be avoided to prevent breakage or trauma to the tissue.

II. Knot Management

- The knot is tied on the facial aspect for easier access for removal.
- A 2- to 3-mm suture "tail" is left to assist in locating the suture for removal.

Suturing Procedures

- Many different patterns of suturing are used. Assisting and observing during the surgical procedure can be an educational experience for the dental hygienist.
- General types of sutures used in the oral cavity are described next.

I. Blanket (Continuous Lock)

- Each stitch is brought over a loop of the preceding one, thus forming a series of loops on one side of the incision and a series of stitches over the incision (**Figure 4A**).
- Uses: to approximate the gingival margins after **alveolectomy**.

II. Interrupted

- **Figure 4B** shows a series of interrupted sutures.

III. Continuous Uninterrupted

- A series of stitches tied at one or both ends.
- Examples of sutures that may be applied in a series are the sling or suspension and the blanket.

IV. Circumferential

- Suture that encircles a tooth for suspension and retention of a flap.

V. Interdental

- Flaps are on both the lingual and facial sides; interdental **ligation** joins the two by passing the suture through each interdental area (**Figure 4C**). Coverage for the interdental area can be accomplished by **coapting** the edges of the papillae.

VI. Sling or Suspension

- When a flap is only on one side, facial or lingual, the sutures are passed through the interdental papilla, around the tooth, and into the adjacent papilla (**Figure 4D**).
- The suture is adjusted so that the flap can be positioned for correct healing.

Procedure for Suture Removal

- Removal schedule: 7 days after the surgery and no longer than 14 days to prevent tissue infection and promote healing.

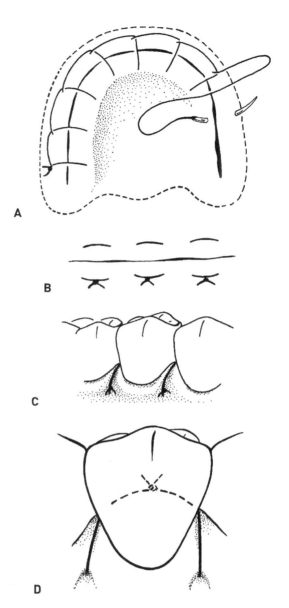

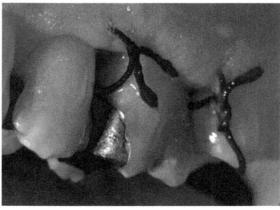

Figure 4 Types of Sutures. **A:** Blanket stitch. **B:** Interrupted, individual sutures. **C:** Interdental individual sutures. **D:** Sling or suspension suture tied on the lingual (dotted line) **E:** Interrupted silk sutures in place 1-week postsurgery.

Courtesy of Dr. Robert Lewando, Boston, MA.

I. Review Previous Documentation

- Medical history.
- Surgical procedures.
- Patient reactions to healing.
- Current surgery: number and type of sutures placed.

II. Sterile Clinic Tray Setup

- Sterile mouth mirror.
- Sterile cotton pliers.
- Sterile curved sharp scissors with pointed tip (suture scissors).
- Gauze.
- Topical anesthetic: type that can be applied safely on an abraded or incompletely healed area.
- Cotton pellets.
- Saliva ejector tip.

III. Preparation of Patient

- Patient history check
  - Patients with valvular heart disease require consultation with the cardiologist.[8]
    - Sutures are colonized by bacteria and should be removed as soon as possible once adequate wound healing has occurred.[1,2,9]
    - Suture removal can cause bacteremia.[5,6,10-12]
- Patient examination
  - Observe healing tissue around the suture(s) (**Figure 4E**).
  - Record any deviations in color, size, shape of the tissue, adaptation of a flap, or coaptation of an incision healing by first intention.
- Preparation of the sutured area
  - Sutures placed without a dressing may have debris lodged in them at the time of removal.
  - Irrigate and/or swab with a cotton tip applicator or cotton pellet.
  - 0.12% chlorhexidine mouthrinse or 3% peroxide can be used to dip the cotton tip applicator to aid in debris removal.
  - Follow with another rinse or wipe gently with a gauze sponge.
  - Place and adjust saliva ejector.

IV. Steps for Removal

- The suture removal procedure described here and illustrated in **Figure 5** is for a single interrupted suture.

- The same principles apply for the ends and each segment of a continuous suture, wherever suture material can pass through the soft tissue.
- Steps
  1. Review the surgeon's chart notes to determine the number of sutures placed and visually locate them prior to beginning suture removal.
  2. Use caution when removing a periodontal dressing to prevent tearing a suture that may have become embedded in the dressing, causing the patient significant discomfort.
  3. Once the sutures are exposed, carefully remove debris by irrigating with water and/or use antiseptic/antimicrobial like 0.12% chlorhexidine mouthrinse on a cotton tip applicator or cotton pellet.
  4. Gently grasp the ends of the suture above the knot with the cotton plier held in the nondominant hand. Gently draw the suture up several millimeters if possible and hold with slight tension (Figure 5A). A finger rest is needed for control.
  5. With the scissors in the dominant hand, insert one blade of the scissors just under the suture knot on one thread of the suture material (Figure 5B).
  6. Hold knot end up with the cotton plier and pull gently to allow suture to exit through the side opposite where it was cut (Figure 5C).
  7. Place each suture on a piece of gauze and proceed to remove the next suture.
  8. Count the total number of sutures removed to ensure they were all removed.
     - During healing, sutures can become loosened, misplaced, or occasionally covered by tissue.
     - A remaining suture can lead to infection and possible abscess.
  9. Irrigate with water or antiseptic. Apply gauze with slight pressure on any bleeding spots.
  10. Provide proper postsuture removal instructions both verbally and in writing.
  11. Observe all tissue and record observations, noting any adverse reactions or bleeding.

Periodontal Dressings

Historically, periodontal dressings were thought to prevent wound infection and enhance healing; however, current evidence does not support this.[13,14] The use of a periodontal dressing is based on the personal preference and judgment of the clinician.

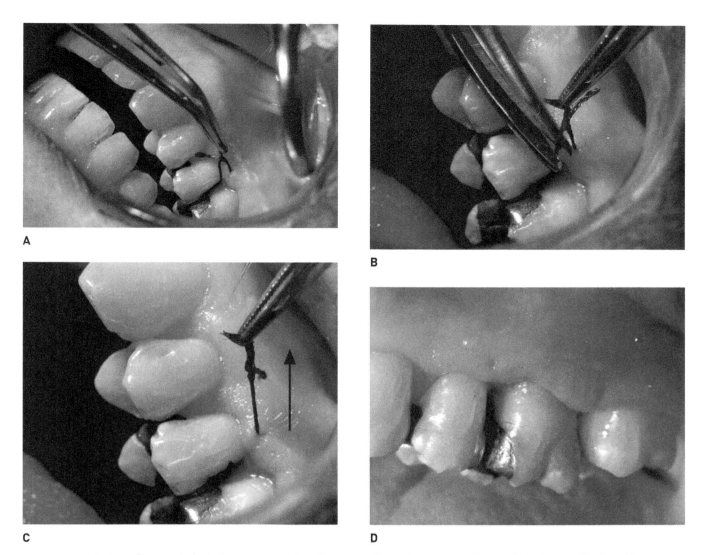

Figure 5 Suture Removal. **A:** Suture grasped by pliers near the entrance into tissue. **B:** Suture pulled gently up while scissor is inserted close to the tissue and cut. **C:** Suture is held up for vertical removal. **D:** Suture is pulled gently to bring it out on the side opposite from where it was cut. The object is to prevent the external part of the suture from passing through the tissue and introducing infectious material.

Courtesy of Dr. Robert Lewando, Boston, MA.

I. Purposes and Uses

- The purposes and uses of periodontal dressing include the following[10-15]:
  - Reduce pain following surgery.
  - Provide a physical barrier to external irritation and trauma, and may reduce bacterial colonization of the suture material.
  - Help prevent posttreatment bleeding by securing initial clot formation.
  - Support mobile teeth during healing.
  - Minimize tooth hypersensitivity.
  - Assist in shaping or molding newly formed tissue, in securing a flap, or in immobilizing a graft.

- Possible use after nonsurgical periodontal therapy has also been proposed to enhance periodontal outcomes, but more research is needed.[16]

II. Characteristics of Acceptable Dressing Material

An acceptable dressing material has the following characteristics:

- Preparation, placement, and removal will take place with minimal discomfort to the patient.
- Material adheres to itself, teeth, and adjacent tissues and maintains retention within interdental areas.

- Provides stability and flexibility to withstand distortion and displacement without fracturing.
- Is nontoxic and nonirritating to oral tissues.
- Possesses a smooth surface that will resist accumulation of dental biofilm.
- Will not traumatize tissue or stain teeth and restorative materials.
- Possesses an aesthetically acceptable appearance.

Types of Dressings

Traditionally, dressings were classified into two groups: those that contained **eugenol** and those that did not. With the development of new products, "noneugenol-containing" dressings have been reclassified into **chemical-cure** and **visible light-cure** (*VLC*) materials. They are available as ready-mix, paste–paste, or paste–gel preparations.

I. Zinc Oxide with Eugenol Dressing

- Example: Kirkland periodontal pack.

A. Advantages

- Consistency: firm and heavy—provides support for tissues and flaps.
- Slow setting: extended working time.
- Preparation and storage: can be prepared in quantity and stored (frozen) in work-size pieces.

B. Disadvantages

- Taste: sharp, unpleasant taste.
- Tissue reaction: irritating; hypersensitivity reactions can occur.
- Consistency: the dressing is rough, hard and brittle, breaks easily, and encourages dental biofilm retention.

II. Chemical-Cured Dressing

- Two examples of chemical-cured dressings are PerioCare and Coe-Pak.

A. Basic Ingredients

- Coe-Pak: most commonly used two-paste system.[15]
  - Base paste: zinc oxide with added oils and gums.
  - Catalyst paste: resins, fatty acids, and chlorothymol as an antibacterial agent.

- Coe-Pak is available in regular and fast set; hand mix or cartridge delivery.
- PerioCare: two-paste system.[15]
  - One paste contains metal oxides and oil.
  - The other paste contains a gel rosin and fatty acids.

B. Advantages

- Consistency: pliable, easy to place with light pressure.
- Smooth surface: comfortable to patient; resists biofilm and debris deposits.
- Taste: acceptable.
- Removal: easy, often comes off in one piece.

III. Visible Light-Cured (VLC) Dressing

- VLC dressing (Barricaid VLC) is available in a syringe for direct application.
- The same light-curing unit used for composite restorations and sealants is used.

A. Advantages

- Color: more like gingiva than other dressings and often preferred in anterior areas.
- Setting: cured in increments with a light-curing unit.
- Removal: easy, often comes off in one piece.

IV. Collagen Dressing

- Absorbable collagen dressings (e.g., CollaCote) used to promote wound healing.[15]
- Contributes to decreased inflammation and subsequent reduced discomfort.[17]
- Special use in periodontal surgery for a collagen patch dressing: for protection of graft sites of the palate during healing.
- Formed into a bullet shape to use for deep biopsy sites.[15]
- Available in individual unit sterile packages.
- Collagen dressing may be placed on clean moist or bleeding wounds.

V. Alternative Material for Periodontal Dressing

- *Curcumin (Tumeric) Gel*[18]
  - Anti-inflammatory and antioxidant properties reduce inflammation and discomfort and increase healing.
  - Reduces edema.
  - Topical application.

Clinical Application

I. Dressing Placement

- General procedure
  - For all types of dressing, follow the manufacturer's instructions. Each product has unique properties that require special handling.
- Retention
  - Mold the dressing by pressing at each interproximal site to cover interdental tissue (**Figure 6A**). Do not extend over the height of contour of each tooth.
  - **Border mold** to prevent displacement by the tongue, cheeks, lips, or frena (**Figure 6B-C**).
  - Check the occlusion and remove areas of contact.

II. Characteristics of a Well-Placed Dressing

- Dressings placed in keeping with biologic principles contribute to healing and are more comfortable for the patient.
- A satisfactory dressing (**Figure 6D-E**) has the following characteristics:
  - Is secure and rigid. A movable dressing is an irritant and can promote bleeding.
  - Has as little bulk as possible, yet is bulky enough to give strength.
  - Locks mechanically interdentally and cannot be displaced by action of tongue, cheek, or lips.
  - Covers the entire surgical wound without unnecessary overextension.
  - Fills interdental area and adequately covers the treated area to discourage retention of debris and dental biofilm.

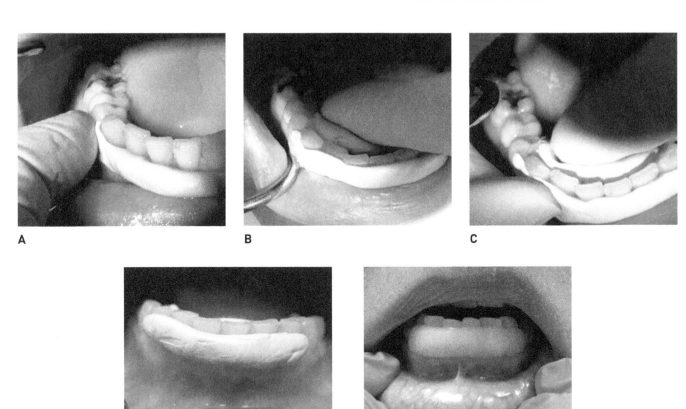

A   B   C

D   E

Figure 6 Periodontal Dressing. **A:** Gently pressing the facial periodontal dressing into the interproximal space. **B:** Gently pushing the lingual periodontal dressing into the interproximal space. **C:** Gently pressing the dressing from the buccal and lingual to help "lock" the dressing in place. **D:** Correct placement of the periodontal dressing. A dressing must cover the surgical wound without unnecessary overextension and fill interdental areas to lock the dressing between the teeth. It is molded in the vestibule and around frena to allow movement of the lips, cheeks, and tongue with no displacement of the dressing. **E:** Reso-Pac (Hager Worldwide), a hydrophilic, more esthetically pleasing periodontal dressing.

Courtesy of Susan Jenkins, MCPHS University Forsyth School of Dental Hygiene.

- Possesses a smooth surface to prevent irritation to cheeks and lips while resisting debris and biofilm retention.

III. Patient Dismissal and Instructions

- Patient is not dismissed until bleeding or oozing from under a dressing has stopped.
- Written instructions are necessary to reinforce those that are provided verbally. **Table 2** lists items to discuss with the patient before discharge.

Dressing Removal and Replacement

During healing, epithelium begins to cover a wound in 5–6 days and complete epithelial healing in 7–14 days.[19] The dressing may be left in place for 7 to 10 days, as determined by the surgeon.

Keep the following factors relative to dressings in mind:

- If the dressing becomes dislodged before the removal appointment, the healing tissue needs to be evaluated.

Table 2 Instructions for Posttreatment Care

Factor	Instructions to Patient	Purpose of Instruction
Information for the patient about the dressing	■ Dressing will protect the surgical wound. ■ Do not disturb the dressing. ■ Allow it to remain until the next appointment.	■ An informed patient is more likely to be more compliant.
Care during the first few hours	■ Do not eat anything that requires chewing. ■ Use only cool liquids. ■ Stay quiet and rest. ■ If a periodontal dressing was placed, it will not set for a few hours.	■ Do not touch or disturb the surgical area. ■ Dressing will become set or become hard.
Local anesthesia	■ Be careful not to bite lip, cheek, or tongue. ■ Avoid foods that require chewing, hot liquids, and spicy foods until anesthesia has worn off.	■ Prevent trauma to lips, cheeks, and tongue. ■ Rest and be quiet.
Discomfort after local anesthesia wears off	■ Fill any prescriptions provided by the dentist or periodontist and follow directions. ■ Do not take more than directed. ■ Avoid aspirin. ■ Call the dental office if pain persists.	■ Pain control. ■ Aspirin can interfere with blood-clotting mechanisms. ■ The patient will be more prepared to manage any postoperative discomfort when appropriately informed.
Ice pack or cold compress	■ Apply every 30 minutes for 15 minutes; or 15 minutes on, then 15 minutes off. ■ Use as directed only.	■ Prevent swelling from edema.
Bleeding	■ Slight bleeding within the first few hours is not unusual. ■ Blood clot must not be disturbed. ■ Do not suck on the area or use straws.	■ When bleeding seems persistent or excessive, please call the dental office immediately.
Dressing care and retention	■ Avoid disturbing the dressing with the tongue or trying to clean under it. ■ Small particles may chip off, which is not a problem unless sharp edges irritate the tongue or the dressing becomes loose. ■ Call the dentist if the entire dressing or a large portion falls off before the fifth day. ■ Rinse with a saline solution; rinse with chlorhexidine 0.12% morning and evening after brushing teeth.	■ Dressing is needed for wound protection. ■ Epithelium covers wound by fifth or sixth day in normal healing.

Factor	Instructions to Patient	Purpose of Instruction
Use of tobacco and tobacco products	■ Do not smoke; avoid all tobacco products. ■ A heavy smoker must make every effort to decrease quantity of tobacco used. The dental hygienist may suggest a nicotine patch to aid in preventing withdrawal symptoms and aid the patient in abstaining from tobacco use.	■ Heat and smoke irritate the gingiva and delay healing.
Rinsing	■ Do not rinse on the day of treatment. ■ Second day: Use saline solution made with 1/2 teaspoon (measured) in 1/2 cup of warm water every 2–3 hours. ■ Begin chlorhexidine 0.12% b.i.d. (twice a day).	■ Might disturb blood clot. ■ Saline cleanses and aids healing.
Toothbrushing and flossing	■ Continue to maintain optimal personal oral self-care in untreated areas. ■ Lightly brush occlusal surface over dressing material. ■ Use extra soft or soft brush dampened with warm water, and carefully clean film from dressing. ■ Clean the tongue.	■ Dental biofilm control essential to reduce the number of oral microorganisms. ■ Odor and taste control. ■ Oral sanitation.
Diet	■ Use highly nutritious foods for healing. ■ Follow the MyPlate guide. (See Chapter 33.) ■ Use soft-textured diet. ■ Avoid highly seasoned, spicy, hot, sticky, crunchy, and coarse foods.	■ Healing tissue requires a healthy diet and specific comfort foods. ■ Use soft foods to protect the dressing from breakage or displacement.
Mastication	■ Avoid foods that require excessive chewing such as hard, crunchy, or sticky foods. ■ Chew only on the untreated side. ■ Use ground meat or cut meat into small, bite-sized pieces.	■ To protect the dressing while it protects the surgical site.

- When the dressing remains intact for 4 or 5 days, replacement may not be necessary.
- When replacement is indicated, the dressing is replaced in its entirety rather than patched.
- Instruct the patient to proceed with daily biofilm removal and rinsing using an antimicrobial agent.
- Schedule follow-up appointment for the patient.

I. Patient Examination

- Question patient about and record posttreatment effects or discomfort. Record length of time the dressing remained in place.
- Examine the mucosa around the dressing and record its appearance.

II. Procedure for Removal

- Insert a smooth instrument such as a plastic instrument under the border of the dressing and gently apply lateral pressure.

- Watch for sutures lodged in the dressing. If present, cut before removing the dressing.
- Remove fragments of dressing gently with cotton pliers to avoid scratching the thin epithelial covering of the healing tissue.
- Observe tissue and record its appearance. Note any deviations from normal healing that is expected within the number of days.
- Use a scaler for removal of fragments adhering to tooth surfaces and near the gingival margin.
- Use an air–water syringe with a gentle stream of *warm* water. Warm diluted mouthrinse may soothe the healing area.

III. Dressing Replacement Procedure

- Topical anesthetic may be necessary to prevent patient discomfort.
- Use a soft dressing with minimal pressure during application.

IV. Patient Oral Self-Care Instruction

Biofilm control follow-up is essential after final dressing removal.

- Use an extra soft or soft toothbrush on the treated area, paying careful attention to biofilm removal at the gingival margin.
- Increase intensity of care on the treated area each day, with a return to normal oral self-care procedures by day 3 or 4.
- Rinse with 0.12% chlorhexidine gluconate twice daily during the healing period. Gently force liquid between the teeth when swishing.
- Recommend a dentifrice with sodium fluoride for caries prevention and a prescription fluoride may be indicated depending on the patient's caries risk.
- If the patient experiences postsurgical sensitivity, recommend a dentifrice containing a desensitizing agent. Suggestions for coping with sensitivity are found in Chapter 41.

V. Follow-Up

The return for observation of the surgical areas can be scheduled in 1–2 weeks, depending on the patient's progress and treatment planning.

Documentation

Detailed documentation is required at each patient visit. The appointment is dated and signed by the attending clinician.

- At the time of surgical treatment include in the patient's permanent record at least the following:
  - Vital signs.
  - Anesthesia: type, location, number and size of carpules, and patient response to anesthesia.
  - Sutures: type, location, and number placed.
  - Dressing: specific type and area placed.
  - Provide instructions to patient prior to dismissal.

- Date and signature by attending dentist or periodontist and surgical assistant.
- Dressing and suture removal
  - Tissue examination: tissue response.
  - Patient comments of posttreatment effects, discomfort.
  - Number of sutures removed: compare with number placed.
  - Patient instruction for continued care.
  - Date and signature by attending dental hygienist.
- Sample documentation may be reviewed in Box 1.

Box 1 Example Documentation: Sutures and Dressings

S—Patient presents for postsurgical dressing removal between teeth 11 and 15. Patient states no postsurgical problems.

O—Tissue bled slightly during dressing removal. Removed four sutures; confirmed four sutures were placed during surgery. Patient responded well.

A—Dr. examined area; no additional dressing needed; patient discharged with posttreatment instructions.

P—Patient instructed to call if any problems; patient to return for 2-week follow up appointment.

Signed: _____, RDH

Date: _____

Factors to Teach the Patient

- Provide the posttreatment instructions as outlined in Table 2.
- Care of the mouth during the period after treatment while wearing a periodontal dressing.
- Reasons for not using aspirin for pain relief.
- Inform and explain why tobacco use is detrimental and delays healing. Encourage cessation of use of all forms of tobacco.
- Discuss the importance of regular periodontal maintenance after treatment is complete.

References

1. Minozzi F, Bollero P, Unfer V, Dolci A, Galli M. The sutures in dentistry. *Eur Rev Med Pharmacol Sci.* 2009;13(3):217-226.
2. Selvi F, Cakarer S, Can T, et al. Effects of different suture materials on tissue healing. *J Istanb Univ Fac Dent.* 2016;50(1):35-42.
3. Burkhardt R, Lang NP. Influence of suturing on wound healing. *Periodontol 2000.* 2015;68(1):270-281.
4. Ahmed I, Boulton AJ, Rizvi S, et al. The use of triclosan-coated sutures to prevent surgical site infections: a systematic review and meta-analysis of the literature. *BMJ Open.* 2019;9(9):e029727.
5. Asher R, Chacartchi T, Tandlich M, Shapira L, Pollak D. Microbial accumulation on different suture materials

following oral surgery: a randomized controlled study. *Clin Oral Investig.* 2019;23:559-565.

6. Dimova C, Popovaka M, Evrosimovskka B, et al. Various suturing material and wound healing process after oral surgery procedure—a review. *J Hyg Eng Des.* 2020;95-100.

7. Giddings FD. *Book of Surgical Knots and Suturing Techniques.* 3rd ed. Fort Collins, CO: Giddings Studio Publishing; 2009.

8. Nishimura RA, Otto CM, Bonow RO, et al. 2017 AHA/ACC focused update of the 2014 AHA/ACC guideline for the management of patients with valvular heart disease: A report of the American College of Cardiology/American Heart Association Task Force on clinical practice guidelines. *J Am Coll Cardiol.* 2017;70(2):252-289.

9. Giglio JA, Rowland RW, Dalton HP, et al. Suture removal-induced bacteremia: a possible endocarditis risk. *J Am Dent Assoc.* 1992;123(1):65-70.

10. Banche G, Roana J, Mandras N, et al. Microbial adherence on various intraoral suture materials in patients undergoing dental surgery. *J Oral Maxillofac Surg.* 2007;65(8): 1503-1507.

11. Otten JE, Wiedmann-Al-Ahmad M, Jahnke H, Pelz K. Bacterial colonization on different suture materials: a potential risk for intraoral dentoalveolar surgery. *J Biomed Mater Res B Appl Biomater.* 2005;74(1):627-635.

12. King RC, Crawford JJ, Small EW. Bacteremia following intraoral suture removal. *Oral Surg Oral Med Oral Pathol.* 1988;65(1):23-27.

13. Soheilifar S, Bidgoli M, Faradmal J, Soheilifar S. Effect of periodontal dressing on wound healing and patient satisfaction following periodontal flap surgery. *J Dent.* 2015;12(2):151-156.

14. Dumville JC, Gray TA, Walter CJ, et al. Dressings for the prevention of surgical site infection. *Cochrane Database Syst Rev.* 2016;12:CD003091.

15. Kathariya R, Jain H, JadhavT. To pack or not to pack: the current status of periodontal dressings. *J Appl Biomater Funct Mater.* 2015;13(2):e73-e86.

16. Monje A, Kramp AR, Criado E, et al. Effect of periodontal dressing on non-surgical periodontal treatment outcomes: a systematic review. *Int J Dent Hyg.* 2016;14(3):161-167.

17. Vinay Kumar MB, Naraganan V, Jalaluddin M, et al. Assessment of clinical efficacy of different periodontal dressing materials on wound healing: a comparative study. *J Contemp Dent Pract.* 2019;20(8):896-900.

18. Meghana MVS, Deshmukh J, Devarathanamma MV, Asif K, Jyothi L, Sindhura H. Comparison of effect of curcumin gel and noneugenol periodontal dressing in tissue response, early wound healing, and pain assessment following periodontal flap surgery in chronic periodontitis patients. *J Indian Soc Periodontol.* 2020;24(1):54-59.

19. Hämmerle CH, Giannobile WV, Working Group 1 of the European Workshop on Periodontology. Biology of soft tissue wound healing and regeneration: consensus report of Group 1 of the 10th European Workshop on Periodontology. *J Clin Periodontol.* 2014;41(suppl 15):S1-S5.

Index